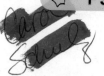

THE
HARRIET LANE
HANDBOOK
A Manual for
Pediatric House Officers

**FOURTEENTH
EDITION**

THE HARRIET LANE HANDBOOK

A Manual for Pediatric House Officers

**FOURTEENTH
EDITION**

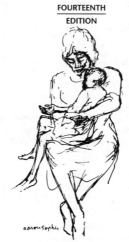

aaronsophy

*The Harriet Lane Service
Children's Medical and Surgical Center of
The Johns Hopkins Hospital*
editor
MICHAEL A. BARONE, M.D.

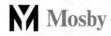

St. Louis Baltimore Boston Carlsbad Chicago Naples New York
Philadelphia Portland London Madrid Mexico City Singapore
Sydney Tokyo Toronto Wiesbaden

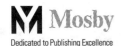

Mosby
Dedicated to Publishing Excellence

A Times Mirror Company

Publisher Anne S. Patterson
Editor Laura DeYoung
Senior Developmental Editor Sandra Clark Brown
Project Manager Dana Peick
Production Editor Jeffrey Patterson
Manufacturing Supervisor Karen Lewis
Book Designer Amy Buxton

FOURTEENTH EDITION

Printed in the United States of America
Composition by Black Dot
Printing/binding by Malloy

Mosby-Year Book, Inc.
11830 Westline Industrial Drive
St. Louis, MO 63146

ISBN 0-8151-4944-1
    97 98 99 00 / 9 8 7 6 5 4 3 2

This 14th edition of the Harriet Lane Handbook is dedicated to Frank Aram Oski, M.D. Throughout his career, Dr. Oski has strived to improve the lives of children with contributions in the areas of pediatric hematology, childhood nutrition, child advocacy, and medical education. Countless numbers of those who care for children (particularly parents) have benefitted from his work and will continue to do so for years to come. His ongoing commitment to his patients, students, and colleagues sets a lasting example for us all.

FOREWORD

The Harriet Lane Handbook was first published 43 years ago—before the Editor and contributors of the fourteenth edition were born. The daily life of the pediatric resident is no less hurried or complicated now then it was then. And now, as then, pediatric residents of the Harriet Lane Service of Johns Hopkins Hospital incorporate what they learn from their faculty and colleagues into the care of their patients. It is this information that Dr. Michael Barone, Chief Resident of the Harriet Lane Service for 1996, has helped each senior resident select and compile to make up the fourteenth edition. Each table, figure, and paragraph has been chosen because its content has been found useful, if not essential, in the evaluation and management of sick and/or healthy children. We hope this handbook will become your trusted partner in the care of your patients.

Julia A. McMillan, M.D.
Deputy Director, Department of Pediatrics,
Residency Program Director,
Johns Hopkins University School of Medicine,
Baltimore, Maryland

PREFACE

In 1950, Dr. Harrison Spencer, the Chief Resident in the Harriet Lane Home at the Johns Hopkins Hospital, spoke of developing a manual of essential information for residents in Pediatrics. Over the next few years the book began to take shape. During the chief residency of Dr. William Waring, the senior house officers would meet every Friday night after rounds to work on the manual's material. This continued throughout the chief residency of Dr. Henry Seidel, and in 1953 the first edition of the Harriet Lane Handbook was distributed to the residents. Still very active in the Department of Pediatrics today, Dr. Seidel, being the book's first editor, has humbly reminded me that "It was Harrison's idea." The first four editions of the book were distributed in the form of loose sheets to be placed in a small pocket binder. Through the efforts of Year-Book Medical publishers and then editor, Dr. Jerry Winkelstein, the Harriet Lane Handbook became widely available with the publication of the fifth edition. The rest is history.

The current revision process takes place every three years. Under the direction of the Chief Resident, the senior residents review, modify, and develop material for each chapter. Over the years, new chapters have been added when deemed necessary. The challenge, as always, is to include information most useful to the reader in a portable package. After many sessions of planning and close attention to letters from the readers, we bring you the fourteenth edition.

If the average reader uses the Handbook at all like we do, the Formulary will be turned to most often. Thanks to the efforts of the contributors listed below and Dr. Carlton K.K. Lee, this section has been completely revised and updated. One will note a slightly different three column format and the addition of the *therapeutic class* for each medication. These classifications should not be considered comprehensive but should be helpful for quickly determining uses of unfamiliar drugs. This Handbook also includes the first chapter on Adolescent Medicine with information on contraceptive methods and adolescent health supervision. Information regarding pediatric trauma care has been provided in the Burns chapter and the Genetics chapter has been completely revised with an emphasis on the diagnosis and early therapy of metabolic diseases. Thanks to the efforts of Ms. Jeanne Cox, M.S., R.D., the reader is provided with a comprehensive and user friendly Nutrition formulary and practical information about childhood nutrition assessment. The reader will also note a new color plate section in the Hematology chapter. The slides are courtesy of the Dr. William Zinkham. The important message here is that, even in this age of automated everything and sometimes prohibitive laboratory standards, it is still important to "look at the smear." Ms. Josie Pirro, R.N. has provided the Handbook with the unique and outstanding illustrations in the Procedures chapter. The artwork at the section headings is the work of the late Mr. Aaron Sopher, an artist whose timeless illustrations of the Harriet Lane Home were made some 25 years ago.

I am indebted to the 22 senior residents (20 in Pediatrics, 1 in Child Neurology, and 1 in Anesthesia/Critical Care) whose tremendous efforts throughout the year created this fourteenth edition, all the while continuing their strenuous clinical duties and teaching our interns. In addition, many faculty have provided valuable guidance and advice for the preparation of the chapters. The names of the main faculty advisors appear below. There were many others, however, either approached in the hallways or "curbsided", who provided equally valuable information. On behalf of the contributors, I thank them all. The contributors are as follows:

Resident	Chapter	Advisor
Dr. Edith Bernosky	Neonatology	Dr. Susan McCune
Dr. Kim C. Brownell	Adolescent Medicine	Dr. Alain Joffe
Dr. Kathleen J. Chen	Nephrology	Dr. Barbara Fivush
Dr. Christopher T. Clemens	Immunology	Dr. Howard Lederman
	Immunoprophylaxis	Dr. Mark Steinhoff
Dr. Michael T. Crocetti	Cardiology	Dr. W. Reid Thompson
	Radiology	Dr. Jane Benson
Dr. Elizabeth H. Cuervo	Formulary	Carlton K. K. Lee, Pharm.D.
	Drugs in Renal Failure	
	Special Drug Topics	
Dr. Robert A. Dudas	Trauma/Burns	Dr. Charles N. Paidas
		Dr. C. Jean Ogborn
Dr. Karen S. Galloway	Analgesia and Sedation	Dr. Myron Yaster
Dr. Donald L. Gilbert	Neurology	Dr. Thomas Crawford
Dr. Rebecca B. Gould	Formulary	Carlton K. K. Lee, Pharm.D.
	Special Drug Topics	
Dr. Michelle L. Hearns	Endocrinology	Dr. Leslie Plotnick
Dr. Xenia B. Hom	Fluids and Electrolytes	Dr. Fred J. Heldrich
		Dr. Mathuram Santosham
	Blood Chemistries/ Body Fluids	Dr. John S. Andrews
Dr. Nina S. Kadan-Lottick	Formulary	Carlton K.K. Lee, Pharm.D.
	Special Drug Topics	
Dr. Lucia H. Lee	Formulary	Carlton K.K. Lee, Pharm.D.
	Special Drug Topics	
Dr. Eric B. Levey	Development	Dr. Bruce Shapiro
	Pulmonology	Dr. Gerald Loughlin
Dr. Ellen M. Neuhaus	Emergency Management	Dr. Allen R. Walker
Dr. Denise M. O'Grady	Procedures	Dr. Mary Clyde Pierce
Dr. Beth D. Rockcress	Hematology	Dr. James Casella
Dr. Prantik Saha	Poisonings	Dr. Martin Pusic
Dr. Jennifer C. Shores	Cardiology	Dr. W. Reid Thompson
	Genetics	Dr. Ada Hamosh
Dr. Marion R. Sills	Infectious Diseases	Dr. Rodney Willoughby
	Microbiology	
Dr. Adam Y. Slote	Gastroenterology	Dr. Maria Oliva
Jeanne Cox, M.S., R.D.	Nutrition	Dr. Jose Saavedra

It should be no surprise to past users of the Harriet Lane Handbook that this edition could not be possible without the collective efforts of the previous editors. For this, we thank Drs. Harrison Spencer, Henry Seidel, Herbert Swick, William Friedman, Robert Haslam, Jerry Winkelstein (for editions 5 *and*

6), Dennis Headings, Kenneth Schuberth, Basil Zitelli, Jeffrey Biller, Andrew Yeager, Cynthia Cole, and Mary Greene. I especially thank Drs. Kevin Johnson and Peter Rowe for their work on previous editions and for the advice and support they gave me throughout my year as Chief Resident.

We are grateful to the rest of the 1995–1996 Harriet Lane house staff for their committment, enthusiasm, and for always striving for the highest standard.

Senior Assistant Residents
Laura Domenech
Jeanne Nunez

Assistant Residents
Susan A. Bardwell
Kirsten M. Brinkmann
R. Clark Brown
Michael D. Cabana
Susan J. Chaitovitz
Christine Chiello
Miriam R. Goodstein
Robert Iannone
Rebecca F. Jacobs
Christina S. Johns
M. Heather Johnson
Debra L. Kruse
Cynthia R. LaBella
Margaret A. Leary
David M. Loeb
John C. Lovejoy
Bradley S. Marino
Soheil Meshinchi
Beverly E. Naiman
Theresa T. Nguyen
James W. Rice
George K. Siberry
Katie L. Snead
Kristine A. Torjesen

Interns
Sook-Hee Ahn
Rosemary I. Ashman
John D. Barbe
Piers C. Barker
Steve Y. Cho
Maria T. Curet-Salim
Diane A. Ferran
Travis F. Ganunis
Laura I. Gerald
W. Christopher Golden
Mitchell A. Goldstein
Scott D. Krugman
Gaurav Kumar
Angela R. LaRosa
Robert C. Macauley, Jr.
M. Catherine Mailander
Munisha Mehra
Teri S. Metcalf
Vinod K. Misra
Colleen H. O'Brien
Marjorie S. Rosenthal
Martha Ann Brewer Sharkey
Hui-Hsing Wong

We thank all the nurses, Child Life specialists, pharmacists, members of Nutrition Support Service, social workers, and other staff for making a children's hospital a stimulating and promising place to work. Mr. Kenneth Judd deserves special credit for his energy and dedication to the Hopkins' house staff. We all know we could not get through the days without this extraordinary individual.

On a more personal note, I thank Dr. Julia McMillan for the tireless effort she gives to the pediatrics residents and for teaching me insight and leadership. It has been my pleasure to work with such a friend and colleague for the past five years, and it is safe to say that I could not have survived this year without her. I have also been very fortunate to work closely with Dr. George Dover. I thank him for his guidance and wish him the best as he begins his tenure as the Chairman of the Department of Pediatrics at Johns Hopkins.

I owe a great deal to Drs. Michael G. Burke and Frederick Heldrich. Together they have taught me not only a love for general pediatrics, but the balance necessary in the lives of every physician. They will always be role models for me.

A special thanks to Ms. Leslie Burke, Jeanne Butta, R.N., Kathy Miller and especially Ms. Monica Casella for all their support and for keeping me smiling throughout this year. In addition, thanks to Mr. Wayne Reisig, our departmental librarian, for saving me countless hours of time doing literature searches and running down references during manuscript preparation.

I have learned that the process of organizing such a unique manuscript has its surprises. I thank the staff at Mosby, especially Ms. Laura DeYoung, Sandra Clark Brown, Dana Peick, and Mr. Jeff Patterson for keeping me on track and for their countless days (and nights) of overtime.

I am forever grateful to my parents and the rest of my family for their unconditional support and for always tolerating the holidays apart. Finally, I thank my wonderful wife Deirdre and our daughters Emily Louise and Meredith Grace for all the sacrifices they have made while showing understanding and strength beyond what any husband and father could ask for. You are the best part of my life.

Michael A. Barone, M.D.
Chief Resident 1995–1996
Editor

CONTENTS

PART I

Pediatric Acute Care

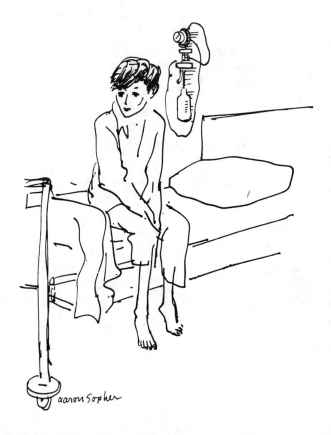

aaron Sopher

EMERGENCY MANAGEMENT

1

I. AIRWAY

A. Assessment

1. Establish open airway with head-tilt/chin-lift maneuver. If neck injury is suspected, jaw-thrust should be used.
2. Rule out foreign body, anatomic, or other obstruction.

B. Management

1. Equipment
   a. Oral airway
      1) Poorly tolerated in conscious patient.
      2) Size: With flange at teeth, tip reaches angle of jaw.
      3) Length ranges from 4–10 cm.
   b. Nasopharyngeal airway
      1) Relatively well tolerated in conscious patient. Rarely provokes vomiting, laryngospasm.
      2) Size: Length = tip of nose to angle of jaw.
      3) Diameter: 12–36 French.
2. Intubation: Sedation and paralysis recommended unless patient is unconscious or a newborn.
   a. Equipment
      1) Endotracheal tube (ETT): Size = (age + 16)/4 = internal diameter. Uncuffed ETT in patients less than 8 years old. Depth of insertion (at the teeth or lips) is approximately 3 × ETT size.
      2) Laryngoscope blade: Generally, a straight (Miller) blade is used in patients <6–10 years old; straight or curved (MacIntosh) blades in older patients (Table 1.1).
      3) Bag and mask attached to 100% oxygen.

TABLE 1.1.

Age	ETT size	Laryngoscope blade	Mask
Premie	2.5–3.0	0	0
Newborn	3.0–3.5	1	0
Infant	3.5–4.0	1	0–1
1 y	4.0–4.5	1.5	1
3 y	4.5–5.0	2	1–2
6 y	5.0–5.5	2	2
10 y	6.0–6.5	2	3
Adolescent	7.0–7.5	3	3
Adult	7.5–8.0	3	3

ETT, Endotrachial tube.

        4) ETT stylets: Not to extend beyond the distal end of the ETT.
        5) Suction: Large bore (Yankauer) suction catheter or 14–18 French suction catheter.
        6) Nasogastric (or orogastric) tube: Size from nose to angle of jaw to xyphoid process.
        7) Monitoring equipment for electrocardiogram (ECG), pulse oximetry, blood pressure.
    b. Procedure
        1) Preoxygenate with 100% O_2 via bag and mask.
        2) Administer intubation medications (Table 1.2).
        3) Have assistant apply cricoid pressure to prevent regurgitation (Sellick maneuver).
        4) With patient lying supine on a firm surface, head midline and slightly extended, open mouth with right thumb and index finger.
        5) Hold laryngoscope blade in left hand. Insert blade into right side of mouth, sweeping tongue to the left out of line of vision.
        6) Advance blade to epiglottis. With straight blade, lift laryngoscope straight up, directly lifting the epiglottis until cords are visible. With curved blade, the tip of blade rests in the vallecula (between the base of tongue and epiglottis). Lift straight up to elevate the epiglottis and visualize the cords.

7) While maintaining direct visualization, pass the ETT from the right corner of the mouth through the cords.

8) Verify ETT placement by listening for breath sounds under both axillae. Ensure that they are equal and are louder than those heard over the stomach. Confirm position by x-ray.

C. Rapid Sequence Intubation

Note: Titrate drug doses to achieve desired effect (see Table 1.2 and Fig. 1.1).

TABLE 1.2.

Drug	Dose (IV)	Comments
1. PREOXYGENATE	Bag-mask, 100%	
2. VAGOLYTIC		
Atropine	0.01–0.02 mg/kg (min 0.1 mg, max 1 mg)	Prevents bradycardia and reduces oral secretions.
3. ANESTHETIC		
Lidocaine (optional)	1–2 mg/kg	Blunts ICP spike, cough reflex, and cardiovascular effects of intubation. Beneficial in elevated ICP.
4. CRICOID PRESSURE		
5. SEDATIVE/HYPNOTIC		
Thiopental	2–6 mg/kg	May cause hypotension, myocardial depression. Decreases ICP. Use low dose in hypovolemia.
Ketamine	1–4 mg/kg	May ↑↑ICP, ↑ BP, ↑ HR, ↑ oral secretions. Causes bronchodilatation, emergence delirium.

(Continued.)

TABLE 1.2. (cont.)

Drug	Dose (IV)	Comments
Midazolam	0.05–0.1 mg/kg	May cause ↓ BP, ↓ HR, respiratory depression.
Fentanyl	1–5 mcg/kg	Fewest hemodynamic effects of all opioids. Chest wall rigidity with high dose or rapid administration, which can be reversed with naloxone.
6. PARALYTIC		
Succinylcholine	1–2 mg/kg	Onset 30–60 sec. Duration 3–10 min. Contraindicated in burns, massive trauma, neuromuscular disease, and eye injuries. Elevates ICP. Nonreversible.
Pancuronium	0.04–0.1 mg/kg	Onset 70–120 sec. Duration 45–90 min. Contraindicated in renal failure and tricyclic antidepressant use. May reverse in 45 min with neostigmine.
Vecuronium	0.1 mg/kg	Onset 70–120 sec. Duration 30–90 min. Minimal effect on BP or HR. May reverse in 30–45 min.

ICP, Intracranial pressure; *BP*, blood pressure; *HR*, heart rate.

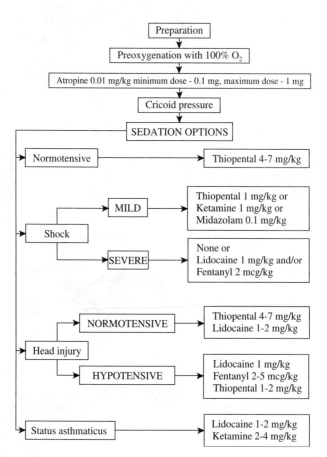

FIG. 1.1. Treatment algorithm for sedative choices for intubation. *(From Nichols D et al, editors:* Golden hour: the handbook of advanced pediatric life support, *ed 2, St Louis, 1996, Mosby.)*

II. BREATHING
A. Assessment
Once airway is established, evaluate air exchange. Examine for evidence of abnormal chest wall dynamics, such as tension pneumothorax or central problems such as apnea.
B. Management
Positive pressure ventilation (application of 100% oxygen is never contraindicated in resuscitation situations).
1. Mouth-to-mouth or nose-to-mouth breathing if in situation where no supplies are available. Provide two slow breaths (1–1.5 sec per breath) initially, then 20 breaths/min. One breath every fifth chest compression in cardiopulmonary resuscitation (CPR).
2. Bag-mask ventilation rate of 20 breaths/min. Assess chest expansion and breath sounds.
3. Endotracheal intubation (see p. 2).

III. CIRCULATION
A. Assessment
1. Assess pulse (central and peripheral) and capillary refill (assuming extremity is warm): <2 seconds is normal, 2–5 seconds is delayed, and >5 seconds is markedly delayed and suggests shock. Decreased mental status may be a sign of inadequate perfusion.
2. Blood pressure (BP) is one of the least sensitive measures of adequate circulation in children.

Hypotension = systolic BP <[70 + (2 × age in years)]

For normal values by age, refer to Chapter 7.
B. Management
1. Chest compressions (Table 1.3)

TABLE 1.3.

	Location	Depth (in)	Rate (per min)
Infants	1 finger breadth below intermammary line	0.5–1	100
Children	2 finger breadths above lower end of sternum	1–1.5	80

2. Fluid resuscitation
    a. Initial fluid should be lactated Ringers (LR) or normal saline. Bolus with 20 ml/kg over 5–15 min. Reassess. If no improvement, consider repeat bolus with 20 ml/kg of same fluid. Reassess. If replacement requires >40 ml/kg or if acute blood loss, consider 5% albumin, plasma, or blood at 10 ml/kg. See also Chapter 11 for deficit replacement.
    b. If cardiogenic etiology is suspected, fluid resuscitation may worsen clinical status.
3. Pharmacotherapy: See inside front cover for arrest drug guidelines.

Note: Consider early administration of antibiotics or corticosteroids if clinically indicated.

IV. ALLERGIC EMERGENCIES (Anaphylaxis)
A. Initial Management
1. Epinephrine (1:1000) 0.01 ml/kg subcutaneously (SC) (maximum 0.3 ml). Repeat Q15 min as needed.
2. Supply 100% oxygen. Establish airway if necessary. Place on cardiac monitor. Establish intravenous (IV) access.
3. H_1-receptor antihistamine: Diphenhydramine 1–2 mg/kg IM/IV/PO (max 50 mg).
4. Corticosteroids help prevent late phase of the allergic response. Methylprednisolone 2 mg/kg IV bolus, then Q6 hr.

B. Bronchospasm
1. Nebulized albuterol 0.05–0.15 mg/kg in 3 ml NS Q15min as needed.
2. Aminophylline 6 mg/kg IV bolus, then continuous infusion (see dosages in Formulary).

C. Hypotension
1. Place in Trendelenburg position.
2. Rapid administration of NS 20 ml/kg IV. Repeat bolus as necessary.
3. Epinephrine (1:10,000) 0.01 mg/kg (0.1 ml/kg) may be given IV over 2–5 min while an epinephrine or dopamine infusion is being prepared. (See Infusion Table on front cover for details on preparation and dosages.)

V. **RESPIRATORY EMERGENCIES**

The hallmark of upper airway obstruction is inspiratory stridor, whereas lower airway obstruction is characterized by cough, wheeze, and a prolonged expiratory phase.

A. **Asthma**

The mortality rate in children with asthma continues to rise in the United States.

1. **Assessment:** Heart rate (HR), respiratory rate (RR), O_2 saturation, peak expiratory flow rate, use of accessory muscles, pulsus paradoxus, dyspnea, alertness, color

2. **Initial management**
   a. Oxygen to keep saturations >93%–95%
   b. Inhaled beta-agonists: Nebulized albuterol 0.05–0.15 mg/kg/dose every 20 min for 3 doses
   c. If very poor air movement or if unable to cooperate with a nebulizer, give epinephrine (1:1000) 0.01 ml/kg SC (max 0.3 ml) Q15 min × 3 or terbutaline 0.01 mg/kg SC Q15 min × 3 doses.
   d. Start corticosteroids if no response after one nebulizer or if steroid dependent. Prednisone 1-2 mg/kg PO Q24 hr or methylprednisolone 2–8 mg/kg/24hr IV ÷ Q6 hr if severe.

3. **Further management if incomplete or poor response**
   a. Continue nebulization therapy Q20–30 min and space interval as tolerated.
   b. Alternative nebulized bronchodilators
      1) Ipratropium bromide 0.5 mg nebulized with albuterol (as above) OR
      2) Atropine sulfate 0.05 mg/kg in 2.5 ml NS (min 0.25 mg, max 1 mg) Q6–8 hr
   c. Aminophylline 6 mg/kg IV bolus, then continuous infusion (dosages in Formulary)

4. Intubation of acute asthmatics is dangerous and should be reserved for impending respiratory arrest.

B. **Upper Airway Obstruction**

Most commonly caused by foreign body aspiration or infection.

1. Epiglottitis: This is a true emergency requiring immediate intubation. Any manipulation, including aggressive physical exam, attempt to visualize the epiglottis, venipuncture, or IV placement may precipitate complete obstruction. If epiglottitis is suspected, definitive air-

way placement should precede all diagnostic procedures. A prototypic "epiglottitis protocol" may include the following:

a. Unobtrusively give O_2 (blow-by). Make patient NPO.
b. Have parent accompany child to allay anxiety.
c. Have physician accompany patient at all times.
d. Summon predetermined "epiglottitis team" (most senior pediatrician, anesthesiologist, and otolaryngologist in hospital).
e. Management options
   1) If unstable (unresponsive, cyanotic, bradycardic), emergent intubation.
   2) If stable with high suspicion, escort patient with team to operating room for endoscopy and intubation under general anesthesia.
   3) If stable with moderate or low suspicion, obtain lateral x-ray exam to confirm. Epiglottitis team must accompany patient at all times.
f. After airway is secured, draw cultures of blood and epiglottis surface. Begin antibiotics to cover H. influenzae (type B), S. pneumoniae, group A streptococci.

2. Croup
   a. Mild (no stridor at rest): Cool mist therapy, minimal disturbance, hydration, antipyresis
   b. Moderate to severe
      1) Mist tent or humidified oxygen mask near the child's face.
      2) Racemic epinephrine (2.25%) 0.05 ml/kg/dose in 3 ml NS, no more than Q1–2 hr; or, nebulized epinephrine 0.5 ml/kg of 1:1000 (1 mg/ml) in 3 ml NS. Hospitalize if more than 1 nebulization is required. Observe 4–6 hours if discharge is planned.
      3) Dexamethasone 0.6 mg/kg IM once. Oral steroids may be adequate.
      4) Nebulized steroids have been shown to be effective in mild to moderate croup where available. Budesonide 2 mg/4 ml NS via nebulization.
   c. If child fails to respond as expected to the above therapy, consider evaluation by otolaryngology or anesthesiology. Consider retropharyngeal abscess, bacterial tracheitis, subglottic stenosis, and epiglottitis.

3. Foreign body aspiration: Occurs most often in children <5 years old. Involves hot dogs, candy, peanuts, grapes, balloons, small toys, and other objects.
   a. If patient is stable (e.g., forcefully coughing, well oxygenated), removal of the foreign body by bronchoscopy or laryngoscopy should be attempted in a controlled environment.
   b. If patient is unable to speak, moves air poorly, or is cyanotic, intervene immediately.
      1) Infant: Straddle infant over arm or rest on lap. Give five back blows between the scapulae. If unsuccessful, turn infant over and give five chest thrusts (in the same location as external chest compressions). Use tongue-jaw lift to open mouth. Remove object *only if visualized.* Attempt to ventilate if unconscious. Repeat sequence as often as necessary.
      2) Child: Perform five abdominal thrusts (Heimlich maneuver) from behind a sitting or standing child or straddled over a child lying supine. Direct thrusts upward in the midline and not to either side of the abdomen.
      3) If back, chest, and/or abdominal thrusts have failed, open mouth and remove foreign body if visualized. Blind finger sweeps are not recommended. Magill forceps may allow removal of foreign bodies in the posterior pharynx.
      4) If the patient is unconscious, remove foreign body by direct visualization (use Magill forceps, if necessary) or laryngoscopy. If complete airway obstruction, consider needle cricothyrotomy.

VI. CARDIOVASCULAR EMERGENCIES
A. **Asystole and Pulseless Arrest Algorithm**
See inside back cover.
B. **Bradycardia Algorithm**
See inside back cover.
C. **Tachyarrythmias**
See Chapter 7.
D. **Bradyarrythmias**
See Chapter 7.

E. **Acute Hypertension**
  1. **Assessment**
      a. Width of bladder on blood pressure cuff should be at least 2/3 the length of the upper arm or the value may be falsely elevated.
      b. Patients with BP>95th percentile require further evaluation. Patients with evidence of target organ damage (e.g., headache, vomiting, epistaxis, decreased visual acuity, papilledema, retinal hemorrhage, congestive heart failure [CHF]) or BP significantly >95th percentile require **immediate** monitoring and treatment. This may be a rare circumstance in which treatment precedes full evaluation.
      c. Evaluate for underlying etiology: iatrogenic (e.g., over-the-counter medications), cardiovascular, renovascular, renal parenchymal, endocrine, CNS. **Rule out hypertension secondary to elevated intracranial pressure (ICP) before lowering BP!**
      d. Physical exam should include four-extremity BP, fundoscopy (papilledema, hemorrhage, exudate), visual acuity, thyroid exam, evidence of congestive heart failure (tachycardia, gallop rhythm, hepatomegaly, edema), abdominal exam (mass, bruit), thorough neurologic exam, evidence of virilization or cushingoid effect.
      e. Diagnostic evaluation should include urinalysis, blood urea nitrogen (BUN), creatinine, electrolytes, chest x-ray, ECG. Consider obtaining renin level before antihypertensive therapy.
      f. It is the presence or absence of acute end-organ dysfunction by history, exam, or lab that distinguishes **hypertensive emergency** from **hypertensive urgency.**
  2. **Management**
      a. **Hypertensive emergency:** IV, monitor, possible arterial line for continuous BP. Consultation with nephrology or cardiology. Goal is to lower BP *promptly* but gradually. Mean arterial pressure (MAP) should be lowered by 25% over several hours. After elevated ICP is ruled out, **do not delay treatment** because of diagnostic evaluation (Table 1.4).

TABLE 1.4.

Medications For Hypertensive Emergency

Drug	Onset (route)	Duration	Interval to repeat or increase dose	Comments
Nifedipine (Ca channel blocker)	10–15 min (PO, SL)	2–3 hr	30–60 min	May cause headache
Diazoxide (arteriole vasodilator)	1–5 min (IV)	Variable 2–12 hr	15–30 min	May cause edema, hyperglycemia
Hydralazine (arteriole vasodilator)	10–20 min (IV)	3–6 hr	10 min	Reflex tachycardia
Infusions				
Nitroprusside (arteriolar and venous vasodilator)	<30 sec	Very short	30–60 min	Requires ICU setting Follow thiocyanate level
Labetolol (alpha, beta blocker)	1–5 min	Variable, about 6 hr	10 min	May require ICU setting

PO, Per os; *SL,* sublingual; *IV,* intravenously. *ICU,* intensive care unit.

 b. **Hypertensive urgency:** Aim to lower MAP by 20%. Oral or sublingual routes may be adequate. Observe in emergency room for 4–6 hours. Close follow-up is mandatory. Many other medications are available; the two listed have been used frequently with success (Table 1.5).

TABLE 1.5.

Medications For Hypertensive Urgency

Drug (route)	Onset	Duration	Interval to repeat	Comments
Nifedipine (PO, SL)	15–30 min	6 hr	15 min	May cause headache
Captopril (PO)	15–30 min	8–12 hr		May cause cough, rash

PO, Per os; *SL,* sublingual.

F. **Hyperkalemia**
   1. **Assessment**
      a. For differential diagnosis, see Chapter 11.
      b. Symptoms and ECG changes (Table 1.6)
   2. **Treatment**
      a. Mild to moderate (K = 6.0–7.0): Goal is to enhance excretion of K+.
         1) Place patient on monitor.
         2) Kayexalate (sodium polysterene resin) 1–2 g/kg with 3 ml sorbitol/g resin given PO Q6 hr or with 5 ml sorbitol/g resin as retention enema over 4–6 hours
      b. Severe (K>7.0): Goal is to move K+ into cells acutely.

TABLE 1.6.

Serum K+	ECG changes	Other symptoms
~2.5	AV conduction defect, prominent U wave, ventricular arrhythmia, S-T segment depression	Apathy, weakness paresthesias
~7.5	Peaked T waves	Weakness, paresthesias
~8.0	Loss of P wave, widening of QRS	
~9.0	S-T depression, further widening of QRS	Tetany
~10	Bradycardia, sine-wave QRS-T, 1° AV block, ventricular arrythmias, cardiac arrest	

ECG, Electrocardiogram; *AV,* atrioventricular.
(From Feld et al: *Adv Pediatr* 35:497, 1988.)

1) Insulin, regular, 0.1 U/kg IV with 25% glucose as 0.5 g/kg (2 ml/kg) over 30 minutes. May repeat this dose in 30–60 minutes, or begin infusion of $D_{25}W$ 1–2 ml/kg/hr with regular insulin 0.1 U/kg/hr. Monitor glucose hourly.
2) $NaHCO_3$ 1–2 mEq/kg IV given over 5–10 minutes. (May be used in the absence of acidosis.)
3) With onset of arrythmias, urgent reversal of membrane effects is required. Calcium gluconate (10%) 100 mg/kg/dose (1 ml/kg/dose) over 3–5 minutes. May repeat in 10 minutes (does not lower serum K+ concentration).

Note: Ca gluconate solution is not compatible with NaHCO₃. Flush lines between infusions.

4) Dialysis if above measures are unsuccessful

VII. ENDOCRINE EMERGENCIES
A. Adrenal Crisis
1. **Assessment:** Characterized by hypoglycemia, hyponatremia, hyperkalemia, metabolic acidosis, and shock. If diagnosis is suspected, obtain blood for electrolytes and glucose. Serum cortisol, 17-hydroxyprogesterone, and adrenocorticotropic hormone (ACTH) should be obtained in infants with possible congenital adrenal hyperplasia before steroid administration, but *treatment should not be delayed.* The older patient should have serum cortisol, ACTH, renin, and aldosterone obtained before treatment.
2. **Management:** Includes rapid volume expansion and corticosteroid administration
   a. Give NS (20 ml/kg) to support blood pressure and D_5NS to maintain blood glucose.
   b. Give 4 times the daily maintenance dose of hydrocortisone IV bolus (4×12.5 mg/m²). (Rapid estimate: infants = 25 mg; children = 50–100 mg.) Follow bolus with 50–100 mg/m²/24 hr as continuous drip or divided Q4–6 hr. Only hydrocortisone and cortisone have some of the necessary mineralocorticoid effects. See Chapter 27 for details on steroid replacement therapy.

B. **Diabetic Ketoacidosis (DKA)**
    Defined by hyperglycemia, ketonemia, ketonuria, and
    metabolic acidosis (pH <7.30, HCO_3 <15 mEq/L)
    1. **Assessment**
       a. History: In known diabetic, determine usual insulin
          regimen, last dose, history of infection or inciting
          event. In suspected diabetic, history of polydypsia,
          polyuria, polyphagia, weight loss, vomiting, abdomi-
          nal pain.
       b. Exam: Assess for dehydration, Kussmaul's breath-
          ing, fruity breath, change in mental status, current
          weight.
    2. **Initial management**
       a. Fluids: Assume 10%–15% dehydration. Give 20
          ml/kg NS or LR over 1 hour, then start 0.45 NS as
          follows:
          1) First 8 hours: Replace 1/2 the remaining deficit
             plus insensible losses (approximately 40% of
             maintenance fluids for 8 hours) *plus* urine output.
          2) Next 16–24 hours: Replace remainder of deficit
             plus maintenance requirements (as hyperglyce-
             mia is corrected, urinary losses become minimal).
       b. Insulin: Begin insulin drip after first NS/LR bolus if
          hemodynamically stable.
          1) Insulin drip is preferred over IM or SC injec-
             tions.
          2) Give 0.1 U/kg regular insulin IV bolus, then 0.1
             U/kg/hr regular insulin as continuous drip.
       c. Glucose
          1) Measure hourly. Rate of glucose fall should not
             exceed 80–100 mg/dl/hr. See note on page 18.
          2) Increase insulin to 0.14–0.2 U/kg if glucose falls
             at less than 50 mg/dl/hr. If glucose falls faster
             than 100 mg/dl/hr, continue insulin infusion
             (0.1 U/kg/hr) and add D_5 to intravenous fluid
             (IVF). As glucose approaches 250–300 mg/dl,
             add D_5 to IVF.
       d. Electrolytes
          1) Potassium: Patients with DKA are potassium (K)
             depleted. Give maintenance plus deficit over 24
             hours (see Chapter 11). Give no K initially if K is
             elevated or patient is not urinating.

2) Phosphate (PO_4): Depleted in DKA and will drop further with insulin therapy. PO_4 improves release of oxygen to tissues. Consider replacing K as 1/2 KCl and 1/2 KPO_4 for the first 8 hours, then all as KCl. Excessive PO_4 may induce hypocalcemic tetany.

3) Bicarbonate: Use of bicarbonate is controversial. Consider in cases with initial pH <7.10.

e. Labs: Follow dextrostick hourly; blood gas and electrolytes Q2–3 hr. Check vital signs at least hourly.

3. **Further management**
   a. When blood pH >7.3, ketosis resolved, HCO_3 >15 mEq/L, and enteral nutrition is tolerated, start SC insulin and discontinue insulin drip 1 hour after SC dose.
   b. For previously diagnosed diabetics, begin their usual insulin regimen.
   c. For newly diagnosed diabetics
      1) For the first 24 hours after insulin drip is discontinued, give 0.1–0.25 U regular insulin/kg SC q6–8h.
      2) The next 24 hours, give 2/3 of the previous day's total insulin dose as a morning (AM) dose and 1/3 as an evening (PM) dose. For the AM dose, 2/3 should be NPH and 1/3 should be regular insulin. For the PM dose, 1/2 should be NPH and 1/2 should be regular. If needed, give additional regular insulin 0.1 U/kg before each meal (Fig. 1.2).
   d. Usual daily maintenance dose in children: 0.5–1 U/kg/24 hr. In adolescents during growth spurt: 0.8–1.2 U/kg/24 hr.

Note: Rapid correction of hyperglycemia may lead to the development of cerebral edema. Actual fluid and electrolyte requirements of patients in DKA may vary according to their clinical and nutritional status. Follow physical exam and lab data closely.

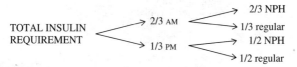

FIG. 1.2. Conversion to daily insulin dosing.

VIII. NEUROLOGIC EMERGENCIES
A. **Increased Intracranial Pressure**

See also Chapter 22 for evaluation and management of hydrocephalus.

1. Assessment
   a. History: Trauma, vomiting, fever, headache, neck pain, unsteadiness, visual change, gaze preference, change in mental status. In infants, irritability, poor feeding, lethargy, bulging fontanel.
   b. Exam: Assess for Cushing's response (hypertension, bradycardia, abnormal respiratory pattern), neck stiffness, photophobia, pupillary response, cranial nerve dysfunction (especially paralysis of upward gaze or abduction), papilledema, absence of venous pulsations on eye grounds, neurologic deficit, or abnormal posturing.

2. **Management: Do not lower BP if elevated ICP is suspected.**
   a. Stable child (not comatose, stable vital signs, no focal findings): Cardiac monitor. Elevate head of bed 30°. Obtain complete blood count (CBC), electrolytes, glucose, blood culture. Urgent head CT and neurosurgical consult. Give antibiotics early if meningitis is suspected.
   b. Unstable child: Emergent involvement of neurosurgery.
      1) Elevate head of bed 30°.
      2) Fluid restriction if hemodynamically stable
      3) Mannitol 0.25–1 g/kg IV and/or furosemide 1 mg/kg IV for temporary reduction of ICP.
      4) Hyperventilate to keep PCO_2 at 25–35 mm Hg. Controlled intubation as outlined on pages 4–6. (Consider lidocaine, atropine, thiopental, pancuronium. Avoid ketamine.) Continue paralysis and sedation.
      5) Emergent head CT
      6) Treat hyperthermia.

B. Coma

1. **Assessment**
   a. History: Trauma, ingestion, infection, fasting, drug use, diabetes, seizure or other neurologic disorder
   b. Exam: HR, BP, respiratory pattern, temperature, pupillary response, fundoscopy, rash, abnormal posturing, focal neurologic signs

2. **Management—"ABC DON'T"**
   a. *A*irway, *B*reathing, *C*irculation, *D*extrostick, *O*xygen, *N*aloxone, *T*hiamine
      1) Naloxone 0.1 mg/kg IV (max 2 mg/dose). May repeat as necessary.
      2) Thiamine 50 mg IV *and* 50 mg IM (before starting glucose). Consider in adolescents for deficiencies secondary to alcoholism or eating disorders.
      3) $D_{25}W$ 2–4 ml/kg IV bolus if hypoglycemia present
   b. Labs: CBC, electrolytes, LFTs, NH_3, lactate, toxicology screen (serum and urine), blood gas, blood culture. If infant or toddler, plasma amino acids, urine organic acids.
   c. Consider antibiotics and acyclovir if meningitis or encephalitis is suspected. Consider lumbar puncture if febrile and no evidence of elevated ICP.
   d. Emergent head CT, neurosurgical consult, electroencephalogram (EEG)
   e. If elevated ICP is suspected, see above management.
   f. If ingestion is suspected, airway must be protected before gastrointestinal (GI) decontamination. See Chapter 2.
   g. Monitor Glascow Coma Scale (Table 1.7)

B. Status Epilepticus

See also Chapter 22 for nonacute evaluation and management of seizures.

1. **Assessment**
   Common causes of childhood seizures include fever, subtherapeutic anticonvulsant levels, CNS infections, trauma, toxic ingestion, metabolic abnormalities. Less common causes include vascular, neoplastic, and endocrinologic diseases.

TABLE 1.7. Coma Scales

Glasgow coma scale		Modified coma scale for infants	
Activity	Best response	Activity	Best response
EYE OPENING			
Spontaneous	4	Spontaneous	4
To speech	3	To speech	3
To pain	2	To pain	2
None	1	None	1
VERBAL			
Oriented	5	Coos, babbles	5
Confused	4	Irritable	4
Inappropriate words	3	Cries to pain	3
Nonspecific sounds	2	Moans to pain	2
None	1	None	1
MOTOR			
Follows commands	6	Normal spontaneous movements	6
Localizes pain	5	Withdraws to touch	5
Withdraws to pain	4	Withdraws to pain	4
Abnormal flexion	3	Abnormal flexion	3
Abnormal extension	2	Abnormal extension	2
None	1	None	1

From Jennet B., Teasdale G: *Lancet* 1:878, 1977; James HE: *Pediatr Ann* 15:16, 1986.

2. **Management (Table 1.8)**
3. **Diagnostic work-up:** When stable, may include CT, EEG, lumbar puncture

TABLE 1.8. Initial Management Of Status Epilepticus

Time (min)	Intervention
0–5	Stabilize the patient
	Assess airway, breathing, circulation, and vital signs.
	Administer oxygen.
	Obtain intravenous access.
	Correct hypoglycemia if present.
	Obtain labs—glucose, electrolytes, calcium, magnesium, BUN, creatinine, liver function tests, CBC, toxicology screen, anticonvulsant levels, blood culture (if infection is suspected).
	Initial screening history and physical exam
5–15	Begin pharmacotherapy
	Lorazepam (Ativan), 0.05–0.1 mg/kg IV, up to 4–6 mg
	or
	Diazepam (Valium), 0.3 mg/kg IV (0.5 mg/kg rectally) up to 6–10 mg
	May repeat Lorazepam or Diazepam 5–10 minutes after initial dose.
15–35	If seizure persists, load with:
	Phenytoin,* 15–20 mg/kg IV, at 1 mg/kg/min, SLOWLY! (max rate 50mg/min)
	or
	Phenobarbital, 20 mg/kg IV, at 1 mg/kg/min, SLOWLY!
45	If seizure persists:
	Load with phenobarbital if phenytoin was previously used.
	Additional phenobarbital 10 mg/kg if previously loaded with this.
	Consider intubation.
60	If seizure persists,† consider pentobarbital or general anesthesia in intensive care unit.

*Phenytoin may be ineffective for seizures secondary to alcohol withdrawal or ingestion of theophylline or imipramine or carbamazepine.
†Pyridoxine 100mg IV in infant with persistent initial seizure.
BUN, Blood urea nitrogen; *CBC,* complete blood count; *CT,* computerized tomography; *EEG,* electroencephalogram. From Fischer P: Seizure disorders, *Child and Adol Psychiatric Clinics of N America,* 4:461, 1995.

IX. ONCOLOGIC EMERGENCIES
A. **Diagnosis of Acute Leukemia**
   See Chapter 15
B. **Tumor Lysis Syndrome**
   Massive cell lysis seen with chemotherapy, large tumor burdens, rapid doubling time. (May be seen before treatment.)
   1. **Assessment:** Characterized by hyperuricemia, hyperphosphatemia (with associated hypocalcemia), and hyperkalemia.
   2. **Management:** Frequent electrolyte monitoring (often q1–2h.). Involve nephrologist early.
      a. Hyperuricemia (>20 mg/dl may cause renal failure)
         1) Decrease production: Allopurinol 10 mg/kg/24 hr PO BID to QID (max 600 mg/24 hr).
         2) Promote solubility: Alkalinization with D_5 1/4 NS with 40 mEq/L $NaHCO_3$ solution. Goal: urine pH 7.0–7.5.
         3) Reduce concentration: Volume expansion with IVF at 2 × maintenance.
      b. Hyperkalemia (see p. 14)
      c. Hyperphosphatemia with associated hypocalcemia
         1) Hydration with 2 × maintenance IV fluid.
         2) Diuretics
         3) Aluminum hydroxide 50–150 mg/kg/24 hr PO q4–6hr (for PO_4 binding).
         4) Consider discontinuing alkalinization if PO_4 is elevated to greater degree than uric acid because PO_4 precipitation is enhanced in pH>6.0. Consider alkalinization for the first 24 hours of hydration, then discontinuation during the remainder of hydration and initiation of chemotherapy.
   3. Consider dialysis if K>7, uric acid>10–20, PO_4>10, hypertension, volume overload, or symptomatic ↓ Ca, ↓ Na, ↓ Mg.
C. **Spinal Cord Compression**
   1. **Assessment:** Back pain or radicular pain, motor deficit, sensory deficit, change in bowel or bladder function, tenderness to palpation, increased or absent reflexes

Magnetic resonance imaging (MRI) shows best detail for evaluation.

2. **Management:** *Do not delay treatment!* Urgent consultation with oncologist, radiation therapist, or neurosurgeon for possible chemotherapy, radiation therapy, or surgical decompression (especially if primary tumor is unknown). After consultation, by phone at a minimum, consider Dexamethasone 0.25–0.5 mg/kg IV Q6 hr.

D. **Fever and Neutropenia**

Usually defined by single temperature >38.4° C or >38.0° C × 3 with absolute neutrophil count < 500 cells/mm^3 or falling counts.

1. **Assessment**
   a. History: Date and type of last chemotherapy (nadir usually 10–14 days), previous documented infections, presence of central line, history of splenectomy, infectious exposure, thorough review of systems
   b. Exam: *Thorough* physical exam is essential with attention to oral mucosa, pharynx, pulmonary exam, perirectal area, entire skin surface, nailbeds, and central line sites if present.
   c. Studies: CBC with differential, blood cultures from peripheral site and all central line lumens if indwelling catheter is present, cultures of urine, throat, and stool, CXR. Consider electrolytes, chemistry panel, prothrombin time (PT), partial thromboplastin time (PTT), and type and cross. Lumbar puncture only if signs of meningitis present. Add other studies as clinically indicated.

2. **Management:** Antibiotic choice dependent upon the patient's history and the patterns of infection and antibiotic resistance in the area. Broad spectrum antibiotics to include gram negative bacilli, gram positive cocci, and Pseudomonas. Consider improved *Staphylococcus* coverage if central line site is suspected. Adjust antibiotic coverage by patient's history of previous infections if applicable. Do not delay antibiotic administration.

POISONINGS

2

The importance of local poison control centers must be emphasized. Early consultation with such centers allows physicians access to resources not normally found in emergency departments as well as guidance from expert personnel trained in the management of toxic ingestions.

I. **HISTORY**
A. **Corroborate histories from different family members to help in confirming the type and dose of the ingestion.**
B. **Obtain the bottle or container of the ingestant; access the police if necessary. Obtain all medicines from the household if there is any doubt as to which agent(s) have been ingested.**
C. **The following should be noted in the chart for each drug possibly ingested:**
   1. Exact name of the drug
   2. Preparation and concentration of the drug
   3. Weight of the child
   4. Probable dose (by history) in mg/kg, as well as the minimum and maximum possible doses
   5. Any pertinent medical history
   6. Medications that the patient is on and that are present at home

II. **SIGNS AND SYMPTOMS OF POISONING**
A. **Vital Signs**
   1. **Pulse**
      a. Bradycardia: Gasoline, digoxin, narcotics, organophosphates, cyanide, carbon monoxide, plants (lily of the valley, foxglove, oleander), clonidine, betablockers
      b. Tachycardia: Alcohol, amphetamines and sympathomimetics, atropinics, tricyclic antidepressants, theophylline, salicylates, phencyclidine, cocaine
   2. **Respiration**
      a. Slow, depressed: Alcohol, barbiturates (late), narcotics, clonidine, sedative/hypnotics

     b. Tachypnea: Amphetamines, barbiturates (early), methanol, salicylates, carbon monoxide

  3. **Blood pressure**

     a. Hypotension: Methemoglobinemia (nitrates, nitrites, phenacetin), cyanide, carbon monoxide, phenothiazines, tricyclic antidepressants, barbiturates, iron, theophylline, clonidine, narcotics, antihypertensives

     b. Hypertension: Amphetamines/sympathomimetics (especially phenylpropanolamine in over-the-counter [OTC] cold remedies, diet pills), tricyclic antidepressants, phencyclidine, phenothiazines, antihistamines, atropinics, clonidine (short-term effect at high doses)

  4. **Temperature**

     a. Hypothermia: Ethanol, barbiturates, sedative/hypnotics, narcotics, phenothiazines, antidepressants, clonidine, carbon monoxide

     b. Hyperpyrexia: Atropinics, quinine, salicylates, amphetamines, phenothiazines, tricyclic antidepressants, theophylline, cocaine

B. Neuromuscular

  1. **Coma:** Narcotic depressants, sedative/hypnotics, anticholinergics (antihistamines, antidepressants, phenothiazines, atropinics, OTC sleep preparations), alcohols, anticonvulsants, carbon monoxide, salicylates, organophosphate insecticides, clonidine

  2. **Delirium/psychosis:** Alcohol, phenothiazines, drugs of abuse (phencyclidine, LSD, peyote, mescaline, marijuana, cocaine, heroin, methaqualone), sympathomimetics and anticholinergics (including prescription and OTC cold remedies), steroids, heavy metals

  3. **Convulsions:** Alcohol, amphetamines, cocaine, phenothiazines, antidepressants, antihistamines, camphor, boric acid, lead, organophosphates, isoniazid, salicylates, plants (water hemlock), lindane, lidocaine, phencyclidine, strychnine, theophylline, carbamazepine

  4. **Ataxia:** Alcohol, barbiturates, carbon monoxide, phenytoin, heavy metals, organic solvents, sedative/hypnotics (especially benzodiazepines), hydrocarbons, hypoglycemics

  5. **Paralysis:** Botulism, heavy metals, plants (poison hemlock)

C. **Ophthalmologic**
   1. **Pupils**
      a. Miosis (constricted pupils): Narcotics, organophosphates, plants (mushrooms of the muscarinic type), ethanol, barbiturates, phenobarbital, phencyclidine, clonidine
      b. Mydriasis (dilated pupils): Amphetamines, anticholinergics, barbiturates (if comatose), cocaine, methanol, glutethamide, lysergic acid diethylamide (LSD), marijuana, phencyclidine, carbamazepine, theophylline
   2. **Nystagmus:** Phenytoin, sedative/hypnotics, carbamazepine, glutethimide, phencyclidine (both vertical and horizontal), barbiturates, ethanol
D. **Skin**
   1. **Jaundice:** Carbon tetrachloride, acetaminophen, napthalene, phenothiazines, plants (mushrooms, fava beans), heavy metals (iron, phosphorus, arsenic)
   2. **Cyanosis** (unresponsive to oxygen as a result of methemoglobinemia): Aniline dyes, nitrites, benzocaine, phenacetin, nitrobenzene, phenazopyridine
   3. **Pink to red:** Atropinics and antihistamines, alcohol, carbon monoxide, cyanide, boric acid
   4. **Dry:** Anticholinergics
E. **Odors**
   1. **Acetone:** Acetone, methyl and isopropyl alcohol, phenol and salicylates
   2. **Alcohol:** Ethanol
   3. **Bitter almond:** Cyanide
   4. **Garlic:** Heavy metal (arsenic, phosphorus, and thallium), organophosphates
   5. **Oil of wintergreen:** Methyl salicylates

III. GASTROINTESTINAL DECONTAMINATION

Note: Airway protection is the major concern with gastrointestinal (GI) decontamination procedures, since aspiration of charcoal and/or cathartic may cause a severe and potentially fatal pneumonitis. Insertion and inflation of a cuffed endotracheal tube is important in patients who have a depressed gag reflex or altered mental status, especially in those undergoing gastric lavage.

A. **Activated Charcoal**

   Activated charcoal is the treatment of choice for GI decontamination in the emergency department for substances that can adsorb onto charcoal. Numerous studies fail to show a clear benefit of treatment with ipecac or lavage plus activated charcoal over treatment with charcoal administered alone. An exception may be the seriously ill patient presenting within 1 hour of the ingestion where lavage may be indicated.

   1. **Mechanism of action:** Effectively adsorbs toxins and prevents their systemic absorption.
   2. **Initial dose**
      a. Children: 1 g/kg body weight activated charcoal PO or NG with a 70% sorbitol solution, or more ideally 10 g of charcoal/g of ingested drug.
      b. Adults: 50 to 60 g PO or NG with a 70% sorbitol solution.
      (The dose should be in a well-mixed slurry, diluted at least 1:4; also, it is better tolerated if cold.)
   3. **Contraindications**
      a. Increased risk of aspiration: Ileus, hydrocarbons, absent gag
      b. Ineffective for small molecules: Alcohols, iron, boric acid, cyanide, caustics, lithium
   4. **Multiple-dose activated charcoal**
      a. Consider multiple-dose charcoal regimen (cathartic only in first dose) for severe intoxication with theophylline, phenobarbital, tricyclic antidepressants, digoxin, carbamazepine, and salicylates.
      b. Give half the initial dose every 2–4 hours. End point is nontoxic blood levels or lack of signs or symptoms of clinical toxicity after 12–24 hours. Check for bowel sounds and abdominal distention.
      c. Tolerance can be improved using metaclopramide or ondansetron.

B. **Cathartics**

   1. Recommended in conjunction with activated charcoal therapy (with the first dose only). Give sorbitol administered as 70% solution with appropriate dose of charcoal (preferred) or magnesium citrate 4 ml/kg (max dose of 200 ml in adults).

2. **Contraindications:** Caustic ingestions, absent bowel sounds, recent bowel surgery. Avoid magnesium-containing cathartics in patients with compromised renal function.

C. **Gastric Lavage**
1. **Indications:** Orogastric lavage with a large-bore tube may still be useful in patients who arrive soon after (within 1 hour of) a life-threatening ingestion and/or are obtunded. *The decision to lavage should be made in consultation with a poison control center.*
2. **Contraindications:** Caustic or hydrocarbon ingestions, coingestion of sharp objects
3. **Airway protection:** In the patient with altered mental status or a depressed gag reflex, insertion and inflation of a cuffed endotracheal tube before gastric lavage protects against aspiration of gastric contents.
4. **Method**
   a. Position patient on left side, with the head slightly lower than the body. Insert large-bore orogastric tube (32 French in children, 40 French in adults).
   b. Lavage with normal saline, 15 ml/kg/cycle, to maximum of 200–400 ml/cycle in adults, until gastric contents are clear. This may require several liters. Save initial pass for toxicologic examination. Add activated charcoal to lavage solution to increase amount of poison removed.

D. **Emesis**
1. **Indications and contraindications:** Ipecac remains the drug of choice for home GI decontamination within 1 hour of an ingestion (under the guidance of a skilled provider or poison control center). It is rarely used in the ED.
   a. Contraindications: Ingestions with a potential for decreased or fluctuating level of consciousness (e.g., tricyclic antidepressant ingestions, caustic ingestions, hematemesis, and seizure risk)
   b. Relative contraindications: Under 6 months old, severe cardiorespiratory disease, late stage pregnancy, uncontrolled hypertension, bleeding diathesis, and most hydrocarbons
2. Syrup of ipecac dosages
   a. 6–12 months old: 10 ml with 15 ml clear fluid/kg PO

b. 1–12 years old: 15–30 ml with 240 ml clear fluid
c. > 12 years old: 30–60 ml with 240–480 ml clear fluid

Note: If no emesis occurs in 20 minutes, repeat dose with more fluids only once. Note also that ipecac can cause drowsiness and that children who have taken ipecac should be laid prone or on their side when falling asleep to avoid aspiration after emesis

E. **Whole Bowel Irrigation**
1. **Indications:** Polyethylene glycol solution via continuous NG infusion has been shown to be useful in certain instances when charcoal is not effective. Examples include toxic iron or lithium ingestions and ingestions of vials or whole packets of illicit substances. May also be useful in delayed therapy of sustained release preparations such as those of salicylates and calcium channel blockers.
2. **Contraindications:** GI hemorrhage or obstruction, use of ipecac, decreased level of consciousness, lack of cooperation
3. **Method**
   a. Children: Use polyethylene glycol electrolyte lavage solution (GOLYTELY, Braintree Laboratories) at a rate of 0.5 L/hr via NG until rectal effluent is clear.
   b. Adults: Same solution at a rate of 1–2 L/hr via NG until rectal effluent is clear

IV. **ENHANCED ELIMINATION**
A. **pH alteration**
1. Urinary alkalinization is helpful in elimination of weak acids such as salicylates, barbiturates, and methotrexate. Serum alkalinization is important in preventing tricyclic antidepressant toxicity (see p. 53).
2. IV bolus of 1–2 mEq/kg of $NaHCO_3$ is recommended, followed by continuous infusion of D_5W with 132 mEq/L of $NaHCO_3$ (3 ampules of $NaHCO_3$ added to D_5W to make 1 L, with each ampule containing 44 mEq of $NaHCO_3$) at 1.5–2 times maintenance. Goal is urinary pH of 7–8 or blood pH > 7.45.
B. **Hemodialysis**
Useful in low molecular weight substances that have a low volume of distribution and low binding to plasma proteins

C. **Charcoal Hemoperfusion**
Useful in dialyzable substances that can adsorb onto charcoal. Advantage over hemodialysis is that the level of protein binding is not a limitation.

From Kulig K: *N Engl J Med* 326(25):1677, 1992; Ellenhorn MJ, Barceloux DG: *Medical toxicology,* New York, 1988, Elsevier.

V. **TOXIDROMES (TABLE 2.1)**

VI. **SPECIFIC POISONINGS**
A. **Acetaminophen Poisoning**
   1. **Symptoms and signs:** Nausea, vomiting, and malaise for 24 hours, improvement over the next 48 hours, followed by clinical or laboratory evidence of hepatic dysfunction. AST is the earliest and most sensitive laboratory test of hepatotoxicity, usually being elevated by 24 to 36 hours. Death can occur from fulminant hepatic failure.
   2. **Hepatic toxicity:** Likelihood of hepatic toxicity related to the following:
      a. Dose: A single dose of 150 mg/kg in an otherwise healthy child requires intervention. Doses of greater than 150 mg/kg, but less than 200 mg/kg, may be managed with ipecac-induced emesis alone; consult your local poison control center for assistance.
      b. Plasma level: Draw level at 4 hours postingestion and plot on nomogram (Fig. 2.1).
      c. Initiation of therapy: *N*-acetylcysteine (NAC) is most effective if administered within 8 hours of ingestion. Efficacy is unchanged whether NAC is given at 2, 4, 6, or 8 hours postingestion but is definitely lowered when given between 8 and 16 hours postingestion. Few deaths have been reported when NAC is used within 24 hours. However, NAC should be used even in patients presenting after 24 hours.

TABLE 2.1.

Toxic Syndromes

Syndrome	Manifestations	Examples
Anticholinergic	**Parasympatholytic:** Dry skin/mucous membranes, thirst/dysphagia, blurred vision (near objects), fixed dilated pupils, tachycardia, hypertension, flushing, scarlatiniform rash, hyperthermia, abdominal distention, urinary urgency and retention **Central:** Lethargy, confusion, delirium, hallucinations, delusions, ataxia, respiratory failure, cardiovascular collapse, extrapyramidal movements	Belladonna alkaloids, atropine, scopolamine Synthetic: Glycopyrrolate Other: Antihistamines, tricyclic antidepressants
Anticholinesterase	**Muscarinic:** Sweating, constricted pupils, lacrimation, wheezing, cramps, vomiting, diarrhea, tenesmus, bradycardia, hypotension, blurred vision, urinary incontinence, excessive salivation **Nicotinic:** Striated muscle: fasciculations, cramps, weakness, twitching, paralysis, respiratory compromise, cyanosis, cardiac arrest **Sympathetic ganglia:** Tachycardia, hypertension **Central:** Anxiety, restlessness, ataxia, convulsions, insomnia, coma, absent reflexes, Cheyne-Stokes breathing, respiratory/circulatory depression	Organophosphates, carbamate insecticides

(Continued.)

TABLE 2.1. (cont.)

Syndrome	Manifestations	Examples
Cholinergic	See anticholinesterases: Nicotinic and Muscarinic	Acetylcholine, betel nut, bethanecol, muscarine, pilocarpine
Extrapyramidal	**Parkinsonian:** Dysphonia, dysphagia, oculogyric crisis, rigidity, tremor, torticollis, opisthotonos, shrieking, trismus	Chlorpromazine, haloperidol, perphenazine, promazine, thioridazine, trifluoperazine
Hemoglobinopathy	Disorientation, headache, coma, dyspnea, cyanosis, cutaneous bullae, gastroenteritis	Carboxyhemoglobin (carbon monoxide), methemoglobin, sulfhemoglobin
Metal Fume Fever	Chills, fever, nausea, vomiting, muscular pain, throat dryness, headache, fatigue, weakness, leukocytosis, respiratory distress	Fumes of oxides: brass, cadmium, copper, iron, magnesium, mercury, nickel, titanium, tungsten, and zinc.
Narcotic	CNS depression, pinpoint pupils, slowed respirations, hypotension. Response to naloxone: pupils may dilate and excitement may predominate.	Codeine diphenoxylate (Lomotil), fentanyl, heroin, morphine, opium, oxycodone
Sympathomimetic	CNS excitation, convulsions, hypertension, tachycardia	Aminophylline, amphetamines, caffeine, cocaine, dopamine, ephedrine, epinephrine, fenfluramine, levarterenol, methylphenidate, pemoline, phencyclidine
Narcotic withdrawal	Diarrhea, mydriasis, goose bumps, hypertension, tachycardia, insomnia, lacrimation, muscle cramps, restlessness, yawning, hallucinosis	Cessation of alcohol, barbiturates, benzodiazepines, chloral hydrate, glutethimide, meprobamate, methaqualone, narcotics, opioids, paraldehyde

From Done AK: Poisoning: a systematic approach for the emergency department physician. In Tintihalli et al. editors: *Emergency Medicine*, 1985, McGraw-Hill.

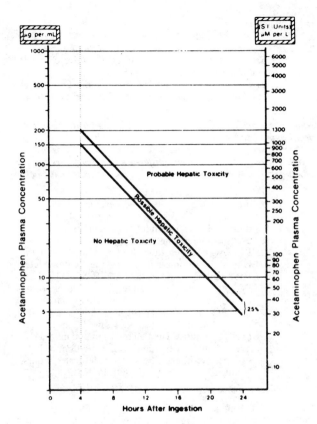

FIG. 2.1. Semilogarithmic plot of plasma acetaminophen levels vs. time, for use after single ingestions of acetaminophen. *(From* Pediatrics *55: 871, 1975, and* Micromedex.)

Note: This nomogram is invalid with chronic overdosing, where toxicity can be seen with much lower plasma levels. This is especially true in situations of relative glutathione-deficiency (such as in AIDS and alcoholism) and use of certain anticonvulsants (carbamazepine, phenytoin, phenobarbital).

3. **Therapy**
   a. Treatment under 1 hour of ingestion: +/− Lavage; give charcoal; draw plasma level at 4 hours.
   b. Treatment 1–4 hours after ingestion: Give charcoal and draw acetaminophen level at 4 hours.
   c. Treatment over 4 hours after ingestion: Draw level and treat with NAC orally or IV if level is in toxic range.

Note: Although charcoal adsorbs oral NAC, and ideally simultaneous administration should be avoided (an interval of 1 hr between doses is recommended), NAC and charcoal can be given together without any measurable difference in efficacy. See pp. 28, 29 for details of gastric lavage and use of activated charcoal.

   1) Oral NAC regimen (PO or NG): Give 20% NAC diluted 1:4 in a carbonated beverage as a loading dose of 140 mg/kg, then 70 mg/kg Q4 hr for 17 doses. Metoclopramide or ondansetron can be used if there is emesis.
   2) IV NAC regimen (approved in Canada and the United Kingdom, but not by the United States Food and Drug Administration [USFDA]; to use IV NAC in the United States, contact local poison control center): Indicated when patient is unable to take PO and presents within 8 hours. Use 20% NAC solution. Give 150 mg/kg in 200 ml of D_5W over 15 minutes. Then 50 mg/kg in 500 ml of D_5W over 4 hours. Then 100 mg/kg in 1000 ml of D_5W over next 16 hours. Check plasma level at 24 hours. Small risk of anaphylaxis with IV NAC.

Note: Do not use oral preparation of NAC IV unless pyrogen free.

From Anker AL, Smilkstein MJ: *Emerg Med Clin North Am* 12(2):335, 1994.

B. **Alcohols**
   1. **Agents:** Ethanol (often greater than 50% in mouthwashes, colognes, aftershaves), isopropanol, methanol, ethylene glycol (antifreeze)
   2. **Symptoms and signs:** Blindness (methanol), inebriation, central nervous system (CNS) depression, seizures, coma. CNS effects are primarily the result of the metabolites of these alcohols.

3. **Evaluation**
   a. A high anion gap acidosis is common in significant ingestions (except for isopropanol) and is usually due to the alcohol itself or its metabolites. Sometimes, however, the acidosis is due to accumulated lactic acid or ketones.
   b. An osmolar gap is also common, with the alcohols and their metabolites accounting for the increased actual osmolarity.

Note: The osmolar gap is the difference between the actual measured osmolality and the calculated value from the Na, glucose, and blood urea nitrogen (BUN) (see Chapter 11). Be sure that the laboratory measures the osmolality directly (by the freezing point depression method), or else a significant gap will be missed.

   c. Children who have ingested a significant quantity of ethanol are particularly prone to hypoglycemia.
   d. Blood volatile toxicology screens and specific levels are useful in confirming the diagnosis.
4. **Treatment:** Charcoal is generally not useful since it poorly adsorbs alcohols, and most alcohols are so rapidly absorbed through the GI tract.
   a. Ethanol: Support blood glucose as necessary with IV dextrose.
   b. Methanol, ethylene glycol
      1) Give 100% ethanol at 800 mg/kg IV or PO for a loading dose, then give 130 mg/kg/hr. The goal is to attain a blood alcohol level of 100–150 mg/dl. Maintain adequate urine output. Commercially available ethanol can be used, but always consider the absolute ethanol content of each product (i.e., 80 proof = 40% ethanol).
      2) Alkalinization aids in urinary excretion.
      3) Consider hemodialysis in severe cases.

From Goldfrank LR: *Toxicologic emergencies,* Norwalk, 1994, Appleton and Lange.

C.   Anticholinergic Toxicity
1. **Agents:** Antihistamines, antiparkinsonians, scopolamine, belladonna, plants (jimson weed, nightshade, mushrooms, Jerusalem cherries), ophthalmic mydriatics, atropine (e.g., Lomotil), phenothiazines, glycopyrrolate (Robinul)

Note: Tricyclics and carbamazepine have anticholinergic properties that can be treated with similar measures as described below; however, they have numerous other effects that need to be addressed as well (see pp. 39, 53)

2. **Symptoms:** "Mad as a hatter, red as a beet, blind as a bat, hot as a hare, dry as a bone": Oral dryness and burning, speech and swallowing difficulties, decreased GI motility, thirst, blurred vision, photophobia, mydriasis, skin flushing, tachycardia, fever, urinary urgency, delirium, hallucinations, cardiovascular collapse
3. **Treatment**
   a. Activated charcoal and cathartic; see p. 27
   b. Observation is all that is necessary in mild cases.
   c. In life-threatening emergencies (dysrhythmias, hypertension, myoclonic seizures, severe hallucinations), physostigmine will reverse symptoms.

Note: Neostigmine and pyridostigmine will not affect the CNS symptoms. Do not use physostigmine simply to maintain an alert state in an otherwise stable patient in coma. Also, do not use physostigmine for tricyclic related anticholinergic toxicity (see p. 53). Do not use phenytoin for seizures.

   1) Dose: Physostigmine 0.02 mg/kg/dose IV Q5 minutes until a therapeutic effect is seen (max dose 2 mg). Note that each dose should be given over 5 minutes.
   2) Reversal: Atropine should be available to reverse excess cholinergic side effects; these include dysrhythmias and bronchconstriction. Give 0.5 mg for every mg of physostigmine just given.

From Goldfrank LR: *Toxicologic emergencies,* Norwalk, 1994, Appleton and Lange.

D.   Barbiturates
1. **Agents:** Pentobarbital, phenobarbital, secobarbital, amobarbital, street "downers"

2. **Diagnosis**
   a. Symptoms
      1) CNS: Ataxia, lethargy, headache, vertigo, coma
      2) Respiratory: Pulmonary edema, respiratory depression
      3) Cardiovascular (CVS): Shock, hypothermia
      4) Skin: Bullae
   b. Electroencephalogram (EEG) may correlate with progression of coma.

3. **Treatment**
   a. Assure ventilation.
   b. Give 10 times ingested dose or 1 g/kg of body weight of charcoal followed by a cathartic. May use multiple doses of activated charcoal. See p. 27.
   c. Urinary alkalinization can increase phenobarbital excretion; consider hemodialysis or hemoperfusion in severe cases.

From Ellenhorn MJ, Barceloux DG: *Medical toxicology,* New York, 1988, Elsevier.

E. **Benzodiazepines**
   1. **Agents:** Lorazepam (Ativan), diazepam (Valium), chlordiazepoxide (Librium), midazolam (Versed), clonazepam (Klonopin), temazepam (Restoril), triazolam (Halcion), alprazolam (Xanax), flurazepam (Dalmane)
   2. **Symptoms:** Dizziness, ataxia, slurred speech, respiratory depression, coma, hypotension
   3. **Treatment**
      a. Assure ventilation; if airway and breathing are secured, there is rarely any need for other interventions.
      b. Activated charcoal as on p. 27.
      c. In rare cases, flumazenil may be used, in 0.1 to 0.3 mg increments up to 1 mg. Resedation occurs within 20–120 minutes.

Note: Flumazenil may precipitate difficult to control seizures in patients who have a seizure disorder, who have chronically been taking benzodiazepines, or who may have coingested any substances that can cause seizures (including tricyclics, theophylline, chloral hydrate, and carbamazepine).

F. **Beta-blockers**
   1. **Symptoms:** Bronchospasm (in those with preexisting bronchospastic disease), respiratory depression, brady-dysrhythmias, hypotension, hypoglycemia, altered mental status, hallucinations, and seizures
   2. **Treatment**
      a. Establish airway, assure ventilation, and support circulation with isotonic fluids.
      b. +/− Lavage, give activated charcoal; consider whole bowel irrigation for sustained release preparations (see p. 29).
      c. Glucagon (0.05 mg/kg bolus, followed by 2–5 mg/hr) is useful in reversing bradycardia and hypotension in beta-blocker overdoses. Atropine, beta-agonists, and amrinone can be used if bradycardia or hypotension persists after using glucagon.
      d. In cases of arrest, may need to give massive doses of epinephrine, titrated to clinical effect (sometimes 10–20 times the standard dose).
G. **Calcium Channel Blockers**
   1. **Agents:** Nifedipine (Procardia), verapamil (Calan), nicardipine (Cardene), diltiazem (Cardizem)
   2. **Diagnosis**
      a. Symptoms: Altered mental status, seizures, coma, hypotension
      b. Electrocardiogram (ECG) can show atrioventricular (AV) conduction abnormalities, sinoatrial (SA) node abnormalities, idioventricular rhythms, or asystole.
   3. **Treatment**
      a. Establish airway, assure ventilation, and support circulation with isotonic fluids.
      b. +/− Lavage, give activated charcoal. Consider whole bowel irrigation for sustained release preparations (see p. 29).
      c. Use calcium chloride (10–25 mg/kg of 10% CaCl) or calcium gluconate (100 mg/kg of 10% Ca gluconate) for hypotension and bradydysrhythmias. Give glucagon, amrinone, or beta-agonists for hypotension unresponsive to fluids and calcium.

From Goldfrank LR: *Toxicologic emergencies,* Norwalk, 1994, Appleton and Lange

H. **Carbamazepine (Tegretol)**
1. **Diagnosis**
   a. Symptoms: Nausea, vomiting, bradycardia, AV block, hypotension or hypertension, respiratory depression, lethargy, coma, dystonic posturing, anticholinergic symptoms, syndrome of inappropriate antidiuretic hormone (SIADH), abnormal DTRs, seizures, ataxia
   b. Serum levels poorly correlate with toxicity; treatment should proceed based on clinical status with respiratory depression, coma, and seizures being the most worrisome.
   c. ECG may show prolonged PR, QRS, or QT intervals, but malignant dysrhythmias are rare.
2. **Treatment**
   a. Maintain airway and cardiovascular status.
   b. Activated charcoal and cathartics for significant ingestions; multiple doses of charcoal can be used as needed (see p. 27).
   c. With prolonged coma, consider use of charcoal hemoperfusion.
   d. Limited use of physostigmine for dystonic/athetoid posturing.
   e. Seizures should be treated with benzodiazepines and phenobarbital. Phenytoin is discouraged.

From Goldfrank LR: *Toxicologic emergencies,* Norwalk, 1994, Appleton and Lange; Weaver DF et al, *Neurology* 38:755, 1988.

I. **Carbon Monoxide Poisoning**
1. **Diagnosis**
   a. Symptoms: Mild to moderate exposures can cause headache, dizziness, nausea, confusion, chest pain, dyspnea, gastroenteritis, weakness. Severe exposures can cause syncope, seizures, coma, myocardial ischemia, dysrhythmias, pulmonary edema, skin bullae, and myoglobinuria.
   b. Sources: Fire, automobile exhaust, gasoline or propane engines operating in enclosed spaces, faulty furnaces or gas stoves, charcoal burners, paint remover with methylene chloride
   c. Obtain carboxyhemoglobin (COHb) level in blood; however, toxicity does not necessarily correlate with levels.

      d. Pulse oximetry may be misleadingly normal.

      e. In fires, consider the possibility of concomitant cyanide poisoning.

  2. **Treatment**

      a. Administer 100% O_2.

      b. Ensure adequate airway, prevent hypercapnea.

      c. Consider hyperbaric O_2 therapy if the COHb level >25%, there is evidence of myocardial ischemia or dysrhythmias, the patient has any neurologic or neuropsychiatric impairment, the patient is pregnant with a COHb >15% or has fetal distress, or the patient has persistent symptoms after 4 hours of 100% O_2.

      d. If hyperbaric O_2 is unavailable, administer 100% O_2 until COHb level decreases below 10%.

From Goldfrank LR: *Toxicologic emergencies,* Norwalk, 1994, Appleton and Lange.

J. Caustic Ingestions (Strong Acids and Alkalis)

  1. Determining the significance of the injury

      a. Substances that have a pH < 2.0 or > 12.0 have the potential for airway swelling or esophageal perforation, even if there are no symptoms initially.

      b. Symptoms include stridor, hoarseness, dyspnea, aphonia, chest pain, abdominal pain, vomiting (often with blood or tissue), drooling, persistent salivation.

Note: The absence of oropharyngeal burns or symptoms does not exclude esophageal or airway pathology.

      c. Asymptomatic patients who have ingested substances with a pH between 2.0 and 12.0 (e.g., household bleaches) and who can demonstrate good oral intake need not be hospitalized. These patients should be given PO fluids as a diluent (10–15 ml/kg of water, milk, etc.) and followed as an outpatient.

  2. Management of significant ingestions

      a. Stabilize airway. Flexible fiberoptic intubation over an endoscope is preferable to a standard orotracheal intubation. Intubation may further traumatize damaged areas or perforate the pharynx; therefore blind nasotracheal intubation is contraindicated. Emergent cricothyrotomy may be necessary.

b. Obtain IV access and start isotonic fluids. Obtain blood count, chest x-ray exam, blood type, and cross-match. Chest x-ray exam may demonstrate esophageal perforation or free intraperitoneal air.
c. Provide tetanus as needed.
d. Maintain NPO. Attempts to neutralize the burn are ineffective and obscure and delay endoscopy. Ipecac or lavage is contraindicated.
e. Obtain surgical consultation; proceed to endoscopy. Do **not** pass NG tube. Discontinue endoscopy immediately if esophageal burn identified.
f. Consider IV steroid therapy (methylprednisolone at 2 mg/kg/24 hr divided Q6 hr or Q8 hr); may be of benefit for some patients (e.g., 2nd degree circumferential burns). If steroids are used, then begin IV ampicillin 100–200 mg/kg/24 hr for infection prophylaxis.

Note: Ingestion of alkaline button batteries can lead to esophageal and gastric burns. If initial x-ray exam shows battery to be lodged in esophagus, immediate endoscopic retrieval is indicated. If the disc is beyond the esophagus, patient is discharged and follow up x-ray exams performed only if battery has not passed in 4–7 days. For batteries >23 mm diameter a 48 hour x-ray exam should be performed to exclude persistent gastric position and need for endoscopic retrieval.

From Rothstein FC: *Ped Clin North Am* 33:665, 1986; Moore WR: *Clin Pediatr* 25:192, 1986; Wason S: *Emerg Med* 2:175, 1985; Goldfrank LR: *Toxicologic emergencies,* Norwalk, 1994, Appleton and Lange.

K. **Digoxin Intoxication**
1. **Symptoms:** Major manifestations include the following:
   a. Cardiac: Any new rhythm, especially with those exhibiting induction of ectopic pacemakers and impaired conduction
   b. GI: Anorexia, nausea, vomiting
   c. CNS: Headache, disorientation, somnolence, seizures
   d. Other: Fatigue, weakness, blurry vision, and aberrations of color vision, such as yellow halos around light

2. **Evaluation**
    a. Determine serum digoxin level. Therapeutic level is between 0.5 and 2 ng/ml. Toxic symptoms predict a serum level >2 ng/ml, but toxicity can develop in initially asymptomatic patients and can occur at therapeutic levels, especially in chronic users. Quinidine, amiodarone, or poor renal function increase the digoxin level.
    b. Determine electrolytes. Low potassium (K), magnesium (Mg), or T_4 will increase digoxin toxicity at a given level, as will high calcium (Ca). Initial hyperkalemia results from release of intracellular K and indicates serious toxicity.
    c. Continuous ECG monitoring
3. **Treatment**
    a. Give ipecac, charcoal (even several hours after ingestion), and cathartic. Multiple doses of charcoal are often useful (see p. 27).
    b. Correct electrolyte abnormalities.
        1) Hypokalemia: If any dysrhythmias are present, then give K^+ IV at 0.5 to 1 mEq/min; do not give K^+ if AV block is present.
        2) Hyperkalemia: If K^+ >5, then give insulin and dextrose, sodium bicarbonate, or Kayexelate; do not give calcium chloride or calcium gluconate since these can potentiate ventricular dysrhythmias.
        3) Hypomagnesemia: May result in refractory hypokalemia if not treated. Give Mg cautiously, since high levels can cause AV block; Mg replacement is therefore contraindicated in AV block.
    c. Digoxin specific Fab: In the event of ventricular dysrhythmias, supraventricular bradydysrhythmias unresponsive to atropine, hyperkalemia (K^+ >5), or hypotension, administer purified digoxin specific Fab fragments. Since this therapy can be life-saving, continue CPR for prolonged periods if Fab fragments are available. Dose (based on total body load of digoxin): Digoxin immune Fab (Digibind) is available in 40 mg vial. Each vial will bind approximately 0.5 mg digoxin. Estimate body load in milligrams using either of the following methods:

1) Use the known acutely ingested dose in milligrams for IV doses as well as liquid filled capsules. For PO tablets or elixir, multiply dose by 0.8 to correct for incomplete absorption.
2) Serum drug concentration (ng/ml) × 5.6 × weight in kg/1000. (The volume of distribution of digoxin is approximately 6 L/kg; for digitoxin, it is 0.6 L/kg)

Then, number of vials to be given equals the body load (mg)/0.5 mg of digoxin neutralized per vial. Administer IV over 30 minutes. If cardiac arrest is imminent, give as bolus injection.

Note: If ingested dose is unknown, and level is not available, then give 10 vials of Fab (i.e., 400 mg).

d. In cardiac rhythm disturbances, if digoxin Fab is not immediately available, refer to the following:
1) Bradydysrhythmias: **Atropine** alone 0.01–0.02 mg/kg IV may reverse sinus bradycardia or AV block and may be used before digoxin Fab. **Phenytoin** improves AV conduction. Dose is 1.25 mg/kg, no faster than 0.5 mg/kg/min. **Transvenous ventricular pacing** is usually effective if atropine, digoxin Fab, and phenytoin fail. Avoid propranolol, quinidine, procainamide, isoproterenol, or disopyramide if AV block is present.
2) Tachydysrhythmias: Phenytoin and lidocaine are effective for ventricular dysrhythmias; propranolol is useful for both ventricular and supraventricular tachydysrhythmias. Cardioversion is indicated when pharmacotherapy fails in the hemodynamically unstable patient.

From Goldfrank LR: *Toxicologic emergencies,* Norwalk, 1994, Appleton and Lange.

L. **Hydrocarbon Ingestions**
1. **Symptoms**
a. Pulmonary: Tachypnea, dyspnea, tachycardia, cyanosis, grunting, cough
b. CNS: lethargy, seizures, coma
2. **Evaluation**
a. Aliphatic hydrocarbons have the greatest aspiration hazard and pulmonary toxicity. They include gasoline, kerosene, mineral seal oil, lighter fluid, tar, mineral oil, lubricating oils, and turpentine.

b. Hydrocarbons that are aromatic (benzene, toluene, camphor), halogenated (carbon tetrachloride, chloral hydrate), attached to heavy metals, or that have anti-cholinergic properties, such as pesticides, have systemic toxicity. This includes hepatic, CNS, renal, and cardiac toxicity.

3. **Therapy**
    a. Decontamination
        1) Avoid emesis or lavage if possible since these increase the risk of aspiration.
        2) If the hydrocarbon contains a potentially toxic substance (e.g., insecticide, heavy metal, camphor) and a toxic amount has been ingested, induce emesis with ipecac in the fully conscious patient. In lethargic patients, consider intubation with a cuffed endotracheal tube (ETT) followed by lavage.
        3) Avoid charcoal. It does not bind aliphatics and will increase the risk of aspiration.
    b. Obtain CXR and arterial blood gases on patients with pulmonary symptoms.
    c. Observe patient for 6 hours.
        1) If child is asymptomatic for 6 hours and CXR is normal—discharge home.
        2) If child becomes symptomatic in 6 hour period—admit.
        3) If asymptomatic but CXR abnormal—consider admission for further observation. Discharge only if close follow up can be ensured.
    d. Treat pneumonitis with oxygen and positive end-expiratory pressure (PEEP). Antibiotics and steroids are not routinely warranted.

From Tenenbein M: *Curr Probl Pediatr* 16:185, 1986; Klein BL: *Ped Clin North Am* 33:411, 1986.

M. **Iron Poisoning**
    1. **Diagnosis**
        a. Symptoms
            1) First stage: GI toxicity (30 minutes to 12 hours after ingestion): Nausea, vomiting, diarrhea, abdominal pain, hematemesis, melena. Rarely, this phase may progress to shock, seizures, coma.

    2) Second stage: Latent period (8–36 hours after ingestion): Improvement but not resolution in clinical symptoms

    3) Third stage: Systemic toxicity (12–48 hours after ingestion): Hepatic injury or failure, hypoglycemia, metabolic acidosis, bleeding, shock, coma, convulsions, death

    4) Fourth stage: Late complications (4–8 weeks after ingestion): Pyloric or antral stenosis, CNS sequelae

  b. Determine serum iron concentration 2–6 hours after ingestion (time of peak concentration varies with iron product ingested). A level >350 mcg/dl is frequently associated with systemic toxicity.

Note: However, serum iron levels obtained at any time after ingestion may be normal even in the presence of severe poisoning. Treatment should be determined by clinical symptoms.

2. **Treatment**

  a. If dose < 20 mg/kg, then no treatment is needed.

  b. For all ingestions of unknown dose or those >20 mg/kg, if the patient does not develop symptoms in the first 6 hours, then no further treatment is needed.

    1) Induce emesis and observe if dose >20 mg/kg, but < 60 mg/kg and patient is asymptomatic.

    2) Perform gastric lavage if dose >60 mg/kg and patient presents within 6 hours of the ingestion or is symptomatic. Abdominal x-ray (AXR) exams are helpful in the decision to lavage since most iron tablets are radiopaque (except children's chewable vitamins). If iron tablets are present in the stomach despite lavage, consider whole bowel irrigation (see p. 30), especially if AXR reveals iron tablets distal to the pylorus.

  c. Give deferoxamine IV at 15 mg/kg/hr in all cases of serious poisoning (the presence of signs or symptoms, a positive AXR, or elevated iron [Fe] level). When traditional "vin rose" (red-colored) urine is noted *before* therapy is started, continue chelation until 24 hours after the child is producing an adequate volume of normally colored urine. Chelation therapy may be discontinued when a repeat AXR is negative and all symptoms and signs of toxicity have resolved.

d. Above all, supportive care is the most important therapy. Large IV fluid volumes may be needed in first 24 hours to avoid hypovolemic shock and acidemia. Urine output should be maintained at >2 ml/kg/hr.

From Schauben JL et al: *J Emerg Med* 8: 309, 1990; Mills KC, Curry SC: *Emerg Med Clin North Am* 12(2): 397, 1994.

N. Lead (Pb) Poisoning

See Chapter 15 for risk classification and diagnostic criteria.

1. **Signs and symptoms:** Vomiting, constipation, ataxia, gross irritability, anemia, seizures, or alteration in state of consciousness. X-ray exams may show opacities in the GI tract and lead lines in the metaphyseal regions.

2. **Treatment (Lead [Pb] level >70–100 mcg/dl or encephalopathy present)**

   a. Establish urine output with 10–20 ml/kg IV $D_{10}W$ if necessary. Saline can cause hypernatremia in severe Pb poisoning. Then adjust fluid therapy to maintain urine output of 350–500 ml/m²/24 hr.

   b. Control seizures initially with benzodiazepines. Phenobarbital and/or phenytoin may be necessary for long-term seizure control.

   c. Chelate with British antilewisite (BAL) and edetate calcium disodium (CaEDTA).

      1) Dosage: Dimercaprol (BAL) 75 mg/m²/dose IM Q4 hr, CaEDTA 1000 to 1500 mg/m²/day, either as IM Q4 hr or as continuous infusion IV. If using IM injections, use lidocaine added directly to the injection fluid (to make 0.05% concentration of lidocaine) so that pain associated with injection is reduced. Note that CaEDTA can reduce the ionized calcium and ultimately cause myocardial depression.

      2) Administration: For first dose inject BAL (IM) only. 4 hours later, start either IV or IM CaEDTA.

Note: Usual 5-day course may be extended to 7 days cautiously if clinical evidence of encephalopathy persists beyond 4 days or if Pb level >50 mcg/dl.

    d. Serial Pb measurements should be made after the last doses of BAL and CaEDTA and at days 4, 11, and 18 thereafter. If Pb rebounds to 35 mcg/dl or more, use dimercaptosuccinic acid (DMSA) at the dosage and administration outlined below.

3. **Treatment (Pb level >45 and no encephalopathy)**
   a. DMSA should be given at 1050 mg/m²/day PO Q8 hr for 5–7 days, then 700 mg/m²/day PO Q8 hr for 14–21 days.
   b. CaEDTA at the doses noted above may be given along with the DMSA for the first 5 days.

Note: BAL contraindicated in acute hepatocellular injury, glucose-6-phosphate dehydrogenase (G6PD) deficiency, and peanut allergy. Medicinal iron should not be given concomitantly with BAL.

From Chisholm JJ, Gellis SS, Kagen BM: *Current pediatric therapy,* ed 12, Philadelphia, 1986, WB Saunders; Personal communication with Dr. Chisholm, Professor of Pediatrics, Johns Hopkins University School of Medicine, October 11, 1995.

O. **Narcotics, Opiates, and Morphine Analogs**
1. **Diagnosis**
   a. Suspect in any patient with depressed mental status of unknown etiology. Pinpoint pupils and respiratory depression are classically seen; hypotension may be noted as well.
   b. Administer naloxone (Narcan) 2 mg IV to anyone with CNS depression. This may be repeated every 2 minutes up to a total of 10–20 mg of naloxone, after which (if there is no response) the diagnosis of narcotic overdose is unlikely. Note that naloxone can potentiate acute withdrawal in patients with narcotic addiction.
2. **Withdrawal response:** Nausea, vomiting, hyperactive bowel sounds (BS), yawning, piloerection, pupillary dilatation
3. **Treatment of narcotic overdose**
   a. Administer naloxone 2 mg IV (regardless of weight or age) if there is respiratory or CNS depression. Repeat every 2 minutes as needed to improve respiratory and mental status.
   b. Careful inpatient monitoring is required because of the short half-life of naloxone compared with most opiates. Indications for continuous naloxone infusion include the following:

opiates. Indications for continuous naloxone infusion include the following:

1) Requirement for repeat bolus therapy
2) Ingestion of large amount of opiate or long-acting opiate
3) Decreased opiate metabolism (as in renal or hepatic failure)

c. Suggested regimen is as follows:

1) Repeat the previously successful bolus as a loading dose.
2) Administer two thirds of the above loading dose as an hourly infusion dose.
3) Wean naloxone drip in 50% decrements as tolerated over 6–12 hours depending on the half-life of the narcotic ingested. For methadone, may require infusion up to 48 hours.

From Goldfrank LR: *Toxicologic emergencies,* Norwalk, 1994, Appleton and Lange; Moore R et al: *Am J Dis Child* 134:156, 1980; Tenebein M: *J Pediatr* 105:645, 1984.

P. Phenothiazine and Butyrophenone Intoxication

1. **Agents:** Chloropromazine (Thorazine), thioridazine (Mellaril), trifluoperazine (Stelazine), perphenazine (Trilafon), prochlorperazine (Compazine), fluphenazine (Prolixin), haloperidol (Haldol)

2. **Diagnosis**

a. Symptoms (may be delayed 6–24 hours postingestion): Depressed neurologic status, miosis, hypotension, dysrhythmias (including increased PR, QRS, and QT_C intervals), extrapyramidal signs (dysphonia, dysphagia, tremor, torticollis, opisthotonus, trismus), neuroleptic malignant syndrome (fever, diaphoresis, rigidity, tachycardia, coma), anticholinergic symptoms

b. Blood levels confirm ingestion but do not correlate with clinical effects.

3. **Treatment**

a. Support and monitoring of respiratory and cardiovascular status.

b. +/− Lavage; activated charcoal. Dialysis is of limited benefit because of a large volume of distribution.

c. Extrapyramidal Signs: IV diphenhydramine 2 mg/kg (up to 50 mg) slowly over 2–5 minutes, or IV benztropine (Cogentin) 0.5 mg/kg.

d. Dysrhythmias
　　1) Ventricular: Lidocaine 1 mg/kg IV push; bicarbonate may also be useful. Procainamide and disopyramide are contraindicated. Cardioversion is indicated if hemodynamically unstable.
　　2) Supraventricular: If hemodynamically stable and tachycardic, use adenosine; however, if hemodynamically unstable proceed to cardioversion.
e. Neuroleptic malignant syndrome: Hyperthermia, muscle rigidity, autonomic disturbances of heart rate and blood pressure, and altered consciousness
　　1) Reduce hyperthermia with lavage and cooling blankets. Antipyretics are not helpful.
　　2) Support respiratory and cardiovascular status; monitor neurologic and fluid status.
　　3) Both dantrolene (1 mg/kg IV) and benzodiazepines are useful in reducing muscle rigidity.

From Goldfrank LR: *Toxicologic emergencies,* Norwalk, 1994, Appleton and Lange.

Q. Phenytoin (Dilantin)
　1. **Diagnosis**
　　a. Symptoms include ataxia, dysarthria, drowsiness, tremor, nystagmus, seizures, and hyperglycemic nonketotic coma. IV preparations may cause bradycardia and hypotension.
　　b. Symptoms seen with blood levels >20 mcg/ml
　2. **Treatment**
　　a. Supportive care: If seizures, discontinue phenytoin and use benzodiazepines and/or phenobarbital. Use insulin for hyperglycemic nonketotic coma. Give fluids and monitor glucose.
　　b. +/− Lavage; activated charcoal. Consider multiple dose activated charcoal (see p. 27).

From Larsen LS et al: *Clin Toxicol* 24:37, 1986.

R. Salicylate Poisoning
　1. **Symptoms:** Hyperpnea, hyperthermia, lethargy, nausea, vomiting, tinnitus, dehydration, primary respiratory alkalosis and/or metabolic acidosis, coma
　2. **Dosages:** Establish the severity of ingestion.
　　a. The acute toxic dose (single-dose ingestion): 150 mg/kg

    b. Chronic overdosage can produce toxicity at much lower doses.

    c. Preparations (mg of salicylate)

      1) Children's aspirin: 1.25 grain (80 mg) tablets (36 tablets per bottle)

      2) Adult aspirin: 5 grain (325 mg) tablets

      3) Methyl salicylate (oil of wintergreen): 1.4 g/ml

      4) Pepto Bismol: 8.77 mg/ml

3. **Evaluation**

    a. Urine ferric chloride ($FeCl_3$): Mix 1 ml of urine with 1 ml 10% $FeCl_3$ solution. Purple color change indicates a positive test. However, even an insignificant amount of salicylate will produce a positive test. Urinary ketones also will produce a false positive test; these can be removed by first boiling the urine.

    b. Serum salicylate level

      1) Serial salicylate levels, along with the signs and symptoms, are useful in guiding the length of therapy; however, the institution of therapy must be based upon clinical symptoms. Therapy should not be based on the actual serum level or on the Done nomogram.

      2) Salicylate levels are less useful in chronic ingestions. In ingestions of enteric-coated and sustained-release preparations, levels may peak anywhere from 10–60 hours

4. **Treatment**

    a. Administer multiple dose activated charcoal and cathartic. Consider whole bowel irrigation in ingestions of enteric coated preparations (see p. 29).

    b. Monitor serum electrolytes, calcium, arterial blood gases, glucose, urine pH and SG, and coagulation studies as needed.

    c. Treat fluid and solute deficits; alkalinization is important in increasing the excretion of salicylate as well as decreasing the entry of salicylate into the CNS.

      1) Replenish intravascular volume with D_5 LR at 20 ml/kg/hr for 1–2 hr until adequate urine output is established. Also give 1–2 mEq/kg $NaHCO_3$ by IV.

      2) Then begin infusing D_5W with 132 mEq $NaHCO_3$ (3 ampules of 44 mEq $NaHCO_3$ each)/L and 20–40

mEq K/L at rates of 2–3 L/m^2/24 hr (i.e., 1.5–2 times maintenance fluids). Aim for a urine output of 2 ml/kg/hr. Adjust concentrations of the electrolytes as needed to correct serum electrolyte abnormalities (especially hypokalemia, which inhibits salicylate excretion), and to maintain a urinary pH >7.5.

3) Note that CNS glucose levels can be low despite normal serum glucose levels; thus increasing glucose delivery is indicated in the presence of hypoglycemic symptoms.

d. Administer parenteral vitamin K as indicated by coagulation studies (especially in chronic intoxications).

e. Continue fluid therapy until the patient is asymptomatic for several hours, regardless of the serum salicylate level.

f. Proceed to hemodialysis in the presence of unresponsive acidosis, renal or hepatic failure, persistent CNS impairment, pulmonary edema, or progressive clinical deterioration despite adequate therapy.

From Yip L, Dart RC, Gabow PA: *Emerg Med Clin North Am* 12(2):351, 1994.

S. Theophylline Toxicity

1. **Symptoms**
   a. GI: Vomiting, hematemesis, abdominal pain, bloody diarrhea
   b. CV: Tachycardia, dysrhythmias, hypotension, cardiac arrest
   c. CNS: Seizures, agitation, coma, hallucinations

2. **Evaluation**
   a. Obtain a theophylline level immediately and again in 1–4 hours to see the pattern of absorption. Peak absorption has been reported to be delayed as long as 13–17 hours after ingestion.
   b. Levels >20 mcg/ml are associated with increasing toxicity, especially if >40 mcg/ml.
   c. Levels >40 mcg/ml or patients with neurotoxicity require admission and careful monitoring.
   d. Hypokalemia, hyperglycemia, and metabolic acidosis are often seen.

3. **Therapy**
   a. Charcoal followed by cathartic, regardless of the length of time after ingestion. For severe intoxication consider multiple dose charcoal. If there is persistent vomiting, give metoclopramide or ondansetron, and instill charcoal by NG/OG tube (see p. 27).
   b. Establish IV access and treat dehydration.
   c. Cardiac monitor until level falls below 20 mcg/ml. Treat dysrhythmias by correcting electrolytes and administering appropriate antiarrhythmics.
   d. Monitor serum K, Mg, P, Ca, acid base balance in moderate to severe intoxication until trends are reassuring.
   e. Treat seizures aggressively with benzodiazepines and phenobarbital. Do not use phenytoin.
   f. Charcoal hemoperfusion: An effective and safe method of rapidly lowering theophylline levels. Indicated in the following circumstances:
      1) The patient has or has had seizures, hypotension, ventricular dysrhythmias, or protracted vomiting unresponsive to antiemetics.
      2) The theophylline level is >90 mcg/ml at any time, or >70 mcg/ml 4 hours after the ingestion of a sustained release preparation.

From Goldfrank LR: *Toxicologic emergencies,* Norwalk, 1994, Appleton and Lange.

T. **Tricyclic Antidepressant Overdose**
   1. **Agents:** Imipramine, desipramine, amitriptyline, nortriptyline, doxepin, maprotiline

Note: Serotonin reuptake inhibitors such as fluoxetine (Prozac) and sertraline (Zoloft) have minimal toxicity in overdoses. Contact the local poison control center for these ingestions.

   2. **Symptoms:** Symptoms of anticholinergic toxicity
      a. CNS: Agitation, seizures, myoclonus, lethargy, coma, choreoathetosis
      b. CV: Hypotension or hypertension, conduction abnormalities, dysrhythmias, respiratory depression
   3. **Evaluation**
      a. Signs of toxicity usually appear within 4 hours of ingestion. Any ingestion should be observed for at least 6 hours.

    b. ECG (acute overdose): QRS duration >0.10 seconds predicts risk of seizures, and QRS duration >0.16 seconds predicts ventricular dysrhythmia in acute overdose. ECG must be monitored for at least 24 hours if there is any QRS prolongation in the first 6 hours.

    c. Serum drug levels are not of predictive value.

4. **Therapy**

    a. Assure adequate airway, ventilation, and circulation. Establish IV access, and start continuous ECG monitoring, even in the patient who is asymptomatic at presentation. If the patient remains asymptomatic and has no ECG abnormalities in the 6-hour period after the ingestion, then no further medical intervention is necessary.

    b. If altered mental status, stabilize with dextrose, oxygen, and naloxone.

    c. Treat seizures with benzodiazepines, then phenobarbital if seizures persist. Do not use phenytoin since this can precipitate ventricular dysrhythmias.

    d. For cardiac symptoms, give $NaHCO_3$ $1-2$ mEq/kg to keep pH >7.45 (lessens risk of dysrhythmia). Alternatively, give continuous infusion of D_5W with 132 mEq/L of $NaHCO_3$ at $1.5-2$ times maintenance. Monitor alkalinization by following electrolytes and arterial blood gases (ABGs).

    e. Give charcoal and cathartic. For severe intoxication consider multiple dose charcoal regimen (see p. 27).

    f. Physostigmine is **contraindicated** for anticholinergic toxicity in TCA ingestions; its use can cause serious complications, including death.

    g. Admit if any signs of major toxicity; cardiac monitor until symptom-free for 24 hours.

From Boehnert MT, Lovejoy FH: *N Engl J Med* 313:474, 1985; Pimentel L, Trommer L: *Emerg Med Clin North Am* 12(2) 533, 1994.

The authors would like to thank Dr. Bruce Anderson and his associates at the Maryland Poison Control Center for proivding information critical to the development of this chapter.

PROCEDURES 3

"See one, do one, teach one"

I. **BLOOD SAMPLING AND VASCULAR ACCESS (Fig. 3.1)**
A. **External Jugular Puncture**
    1. **Indications:** Blood sampling in patients with inadequate peripheral vascular access or during resuscitation
    2. **Complications**
       a. Hematoma
       b. Pneumothorax
       c. Infection
    3. **Procedure** (Fig. 3.2)
       a. Restrain infant securely.
       b. Position infant with towel roll under shoulders or with head over side of bed to extend neck and accentuate the posterior margin of contralateral sternocleidomastoid muscle.
       c. Prepare area carefully with povidone-iodine and alcohol.
       d. To distend the external jugular vein, occlude its most proximal segment, or provoke child to cry. The vein runs from angle of mandible to posterior border of lower third of sternocleidomastoid muscle.
       e. With continual negative suction on the syringe, insert the needle at about a 30° angle to the skin. Continue as with any peripheral venipuncture.
       f. Apply sterile dressing and pressure of site for 5 minutes.
B. **Femoral Artery and Femoral Vein Puncture**
    1. **Indications:** Venous or arterial blood sampling of patients with inadequate vascular access or during resuscitation
    2. **Contraindications:** Femoral puncture is particularly hazardous in neonates and is not recommended in this age group. Avoid femoral punctures in children who have thrombocytopenia, have coagulation disorders, or are scheduled for cardiac catheterization.

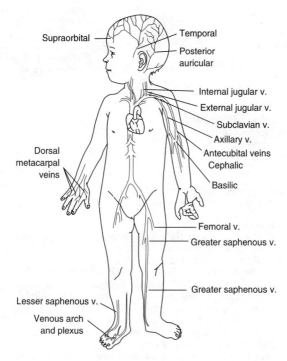

FIG. 3.1. Venous access sites. *(Courtesy of Josie Pirro, RN, Johns Hopkins Children's Center.) Modified from Levin DL, Morriss F:* Essentials of pediatric intensive care, *St Louis, 1990, Quality Medical Publishers.*

3. **Complications**
    a. Hematoma at femoral triangle
    b. Thrombosis of vessel
    c. Infection
    d. Osteomyelitis
    e. Septic arthritis of femur or hip

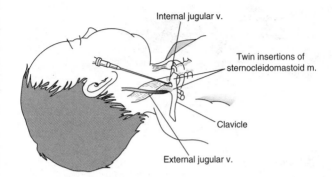

FIG. 3.2. Approach for external and internal jugular puncture. *(Courtesy of Josie Pirro, RN, Johns Hopkins Children's Center.)*

   4. **Procedure** (Fig. 3.3)
      a. Hold child securely in frog leg position with the hips flexed and abducted.
      b. Prep area with povidone-iodine and alcohol.
      c. Locate femoral pulse just distal to inguinal crease, then insert needle 2 cm distal to inguinal ligament and 0.5–0.75 cm into the groin. **Note that vein is medial to pulse.** Continually aspirate while maneuvering the needle until blood is obtained.
      d. Apply direct pressure for minimum of 5 minutes.
C. **Radial Artery Puncture and Catheterization**
   1. **Indications:** Arterial blood sampling or for frequent blood gases and blood pressure monitoring in an intensive care setting
   2. **Complications**
      a. Occlusion of artery by hematoma or thrombosis
      b. Infection—thrombophlebitis
      c. Ischemia if ulnar circulation inadequate
   3. **Procedure**
      a. Before procedure, test the adequacy of ulnar blood flow with the **Allen test.** Clench the hand while simultaneously compressing ulnar and radial arteries. The hand will blanch. Release pressure from the ulnar

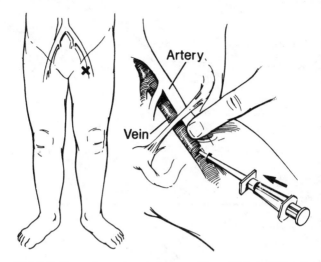

FIG. 3.3. Femoral puncture technique. *(From Nichols DG et al: Golden hour: the handbook of advanced pediatric life support, ed 2, St Louis, 1996, Mosby).*

artery and observe the flushing response. Procedure is safe to perform if entire hand flushes.
  b. Secure the hand to an arm board with the wrist extended. Leave the fingers exposed to observe any color changes.
  c. Locate the radial pulse. It is optional to infiltrate area over point of maximal impulse with lidocaine. Cleanse site with povidone-iodine.
    1) Puncture: Insert needle attached to a syringe at a 30°–60° angle over point of maximal impulse; blood should flow freely into syringe in pulsatile fashion; suction may be required for plastic tubes. Once sample obtained apply firm constant pressure for 5 minutes and then place pressure dressing.
    2) Catheter placement (Fig. 3.4): Secure hand to arm board. Prep wrist with sterile technique and infiltrate over point of maximal impulse with 1% lido-

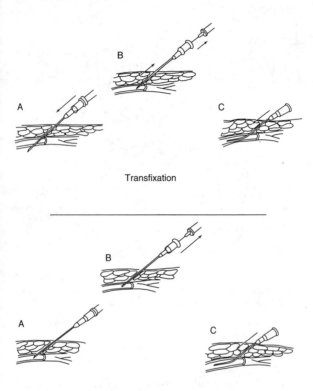

Transfixation

Direct

FIG. 3.4. Radial artery catheterization by transfixation and direct technique. *(Courtesy of Josie Pirro, RN, Johns Hopkins Children's Center.)*

caine. Make a small skin puncture over point of maximal impulse with a needle. Insert intravenous catheter through the puncture site at a 30° angle to the horizontal, and pass the needle through the artery to transfix it. Withdraw the inner needle. Very slowly withdraw the catheter until free flow of blood is noted, then advance the catheter. Secure catheter in place via sutures or tape. Apply antibiotic ointment dressing. Infuse isotonic heparinized saline (1 unit heparin/ml saline) at 1 ml/hr. A pressure transducer may be attached to monitor blood pressure.

Note: Do not infuse any medications, blood products, or hypertonic solutions through arterial line.

D. **Central Venous Catheter Placement**
   1. **Indications:** To obtain emergency access to central venous circulation, to monitor central venous pressure, to deliver high concentration parenteral nutrition or prolonged IV therapy, to infuse blood products or large volumes of fluid
   2. **Complications**
      a. Arterial or venous laceration
      b. Infection of hemothorax, pneumothorax
      c. Catheter fragment in circulation
      d. Air embolism
      e. Atrioventricular (AV) fistula
      f. Hematoma
   3. **Access sites**
      a. External jugular vein
      b. Internal jugular vein
      c. Subclavian vein
      d. Femoral vein

Note: Femoral vein catheterization is contraindicated in severe abdominal trauma, and the internal jugular is contraindicated in patients with elevated intracranial pressure (ICP).

   4. **Procedure:** The Seldinger technique (Fig. 3.5)
      a. Secure patient, choose vessel for catheteriztion, prep, and drape in sterile fashion.

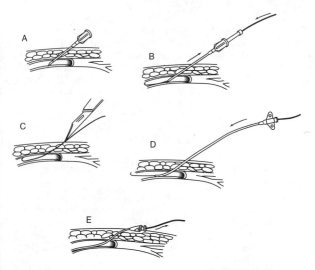

FIG. 3.5. The Seldinger technique. *(Courtesy of Josie Pirro, RN, Johns Hopkins Children's Center.)*

  b. Insert needle applying negative pressure to locate vessel.
  c. When there is blood return, insert a guidewire through needle into vein to approximately 1/4 to 1/3 length of wire.
  d. Remove needle, *holding guidewire firmly.*
  e. Slip catheter that has been preflushed with sterile saline over wire into vein in a twisting motion. Entry site may be enlarged with a small skin incision or dilator. Pass entire catheter over wire until hub is at skin surface. Slowly remove wire and secure catheter by suture and attach IV infusion.
  f. Apply sterile dressing over site.
  g. For neck vessels, obtain chest x-ray results to rule out pneumothorax.

5. **Approach**
    a. External jugular (see p. 56 and Fig. 3.2)
    b. Internal jugular (Fig. 3.2): Place patient in 15°–20° Trendelenburg. Hyperextend the neck to tense the sternocleidomastoid muscle. Palpate sternal and clavicular heads of the muscle and enter at the apex of the triangle formed. Aim needle toward the ipsilateral nipple. When blood flow is obtained continue with Seldinger technique.
    c. Subclavian vein (Fig. 3.6): Position child in Trendelenburg with towel roll under thoracic spine to hyperextend the back. Aim needle as indicated in Fig. 3.6 under the distal third of clavicle.
    d. Femoral vein (see Fig. 3.3)

E. Intraosseous Infusion
    1. **Indications:** Obtain emergency access in children less than 6 years old. This is very useful during circulatory collapse and/or cardiac arrest. Optimally the needle should be removed after 3–4 hours once adequate vascular access has been established.
    2. **Complications**
        a. Osteomyelitis
        b. Fat embolism
        c. Extravasation of fluid into subcutaneous tissue
        d. Subcutaneous abscess
        e. Fracture, epiphyseal injury

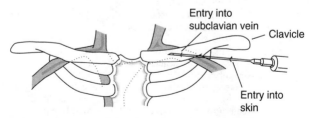

FIG. 3.6. Approach for catheterization of subclavian vein. *(Courtesy of Josie Pirro, RN, Johns Hopkins Children's Center.)*

3. **Sites of entry**
   a. Anteromedial surface of proximal tibia, 2 cm below and 1–2 cm medial to the tibial tuberosity on the flat part of bone
   b. Distal femur 3 cm above lateral condyle in the midline
   c. Medial surface of the distal tibia above the medial malleolus

4. **Procedure**
   a. Prepare and drape the patient for a sterile procedure.
   b. Anesthetize the puncture site down to the periosteum with 1% lidocaine (optional in emergency situations).
   c. Insert an intraosseous needle perpendicular to the skin and advance to the periosteum. Then, with a boring rotary motion, penetrate through cortex into the marrow. Needle should stand firm without support.
   d. Remove stylet and attempt to flush saline (note that it is not necessary to aspirate marrow). Observe for fluid extravasation.
   e. Attach standard IV tubing. Any crystalloid, blood product, or drug that may be infused into a peripheral vein may also be infused into the intraosseus space.

F. **Umbilical Artery and Umbilical Vein Catheterization**
   1. **Indications:** Vascular access, blood pressure and blood gas monitoring in critically ill neonates
   2. **Complications**
      a. Hemorrhage from displacement of line or perforation of artery
      b. Thrombosis with distal embolization of iliac, renal, or inferior mesenteric arteries
      c. Infection
      d. Ischemia/infarction of lower extremities, bowel
      e. Arrhythmias if catheter enters heart
      f. Air embolization
   3. **Line placement: Umbilical artery (UA) catheters** may be placed in either of two positions: low-line position, between lumbar vertebrae 3 and 5; or high-line position, between thoracic vertebrae 6 and 9. The tip of a low-line is below the renal and mesenteric arteries, perhaps decreasing the incidence of clots. However, a high-line may be recommended in infants less than 750 g when a low-

line could easily slip out. The length of catheter required to achieve either position may be determined using a standardized graph or a regression formula.

Umbilical vein (UV) catheters should be placed in the inferior vena cava above the level of the ductus venosus and the hepatic veins and below the level of the left atrium. The length of the catheter necessary to achieve the position can be determined using the graph or regression formula below.

a. Graphic representation
  1) Determine the shoulder-umbilical length by measuring the perpendicular line dropped from the tip of the shoulder to the level of the umbilicus.
  2) For UA: Use the graph in Fig. 3.7 to determine catheter length. For a low-line, the tip of the catheter should lie just above the aortic bifurcation (to avoid renal artery orifice, around L_1). With a high-line, the tip should be above the diaphragm. Add length for the height of the umbilical stump.
  3) For UV: Use the graph in Fig. 3.8 to determine the catheter length needed to place the tip between the diaphragm and left atrium. Add length for the height of the umbilical stump.
b. Birthweight (BW) regression formula
  1) For UA

HIGH LINE: UA catheter length (cm) = [3 × BW (kg)] + 9

LOW LINE: UA catheter length (cm) ≈ BW + 7

Note: Formula may not be appropriate for SGA or LGA infants.

  2) For UV

UV catheter length (cm) = [0.5 × UA (cm)] + 1

Note: May not be appropriate for SGA of LGA infants.

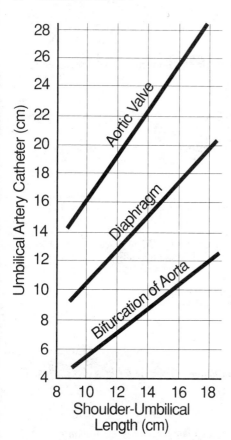

FIG. 3.7. Umbilicial artery catheter length.

4. **Procedure for UA line** (Fig. 3.9)
   a. Restrain infant. Prepare and drape umbilical cord and adjacent skin using sterile technique. Infant's warmth is critical.

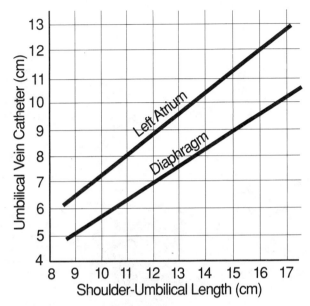

FIG. 3.8. Umbilical vein catheter length.

- b. Determine the length of catheter to be inserted for either high (T_6 to T_9) or low (L_3 to L_5) position (see Fig. 3.7)
- c. Flush catheter with sterile saline solution before insertion.
- d. Place sterile umbilical tape around base of cord. Cut through cord horizontally approximately 1.5–2.0 cm from skin; tighten umbilical tape to prevent bleeding.
- e. Identify the 1 large, thin-walled umbilical vein and 2 smaller, thick-walled arteries. Use one tip of open curved forceps to gently probe and dilate one artery. Gently probe with both points of closed forceps and dilate artery by allowing forceps to open gently.

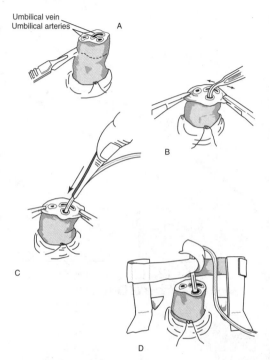

FIG. 3.9. Technique for placing umbilical catheters. *(Courtesy of Josie Pirro, RN, Johns Hopkins Children's Center.)*

    f. Grasp catheter 1 cm from tip with toothless forceps and insert catheter into lumen of artery. Aim the tip toward the feet, and gently advance catheter to desired distance determined above. **DO NOT FORCE.** If resistance is encountered, try loosening umbilical tape, applying steady gentle pressure, or manipulating angle of umbilical cord to skin. Often catheter cannot be advanced because of creation of a "false luminal tract."

g. Secure catheter with both a suture through the cord and marker tape and a tape bridge. Confirm the position of the catheter tip radiologically. Line may be pulled back but not advanced once sterile field broken.

h. Observe for complications: Blanching or cyanosis of lower extremities; perforation; thrombosis; embolism or infection.

Note: Infants remain NPO until 24 hours after catheter removed. Never run hyposmolar fluids through UA line. Isotonic fluids should contain 0.5 unit heparin per ml.

5. **Procedure for UV line** (see Fig. 3.9)

a. Follow steps a–d above. However, determine length via Fig. 3.8.

b. Isolate thin-walled umbilical vein, clear thrombi with forceps, and insert catheter, aiming the tip toward the right shoulder. Gently advance catheter to desired distance. **DO NOT FORCE.** If resistance is encountered, try loosening umbilical tape, applying steady gentle pressure, or manipulating angle of umbilical cord to skin.

c. Secure catheter as described for UA catheter. Confirm position of the catheter tip radiologically.

II. BODY FLUID SAMPLING
A. Lumbar Puncture

1. **Indications:** Examination of spinal fluid for suspected infection or malignancy, instillation of intrathecal chemotherapy, or measurement of opening pressure

2. **Complications**
   a. Headache
   b. Subarachnoid epidermal cyst caused by foreign body reaction
   c. Local back pain
   d. Infection or bleeding
   e. Herniation associated with increased ICP
   f. Paralysis

3. **Cautions**
   a. Increased ICP: Before lumbar puncture (LP), perform fundiscopic examination. The presence of papilledema, retinal hemorrhage, or clinical suspicion of in-

creased ICP may be contraindications to the procedure. A sudden drop in intraspinal pressure by rapid release of cerebrospinal fluid (CSF) may cause fatal herniation. If LP is to be performed, proceed with extreme caution. A computerized tomography (CT) scan may be indicated before LP.

b. Bleeding diathesis: A platelet count of $>50,000/mm^3$ is desirable before LP, and correction of any clotting factor deficiencies is in order to prevent spinal cord hemorrhage and potential paralysis.

c. Overlying skin infection: May result in inoculation of CSF with organisms.

4. **Procedure** (Fig. 3.10)

a. Position the child in either the sitting position or lateral recumbent position with hips, knees, and neck flexed. Ensure that small infants' cardiorespiratory status is not compromised by positioning.

b. Locate the desired interspace (either L_3–L_4 or L_4–L_5) by drawing an imaginary line between the top of the iliac crests.

c. Clean the skin with povidone-iodine and 70% alcohol. Drape conservatively so as to be able to monitor the infant. Use a spinal needle with stylet. (Epidermoid tumors from introduced epithelial tissue have been reported.)

d. Anesthetize overlying skin with lidocaine or eutectic mixture of local anesthetics (EMLA) (optional).

e. Puncture skin in midline just caudad to palpated spinous process, angling slightly cephalad. Advance several millimeters at a time, and withdraw stylet frequently to check for CSF flow. The needle may be advanced without the stylet once through the skin completely. In small infants, one may not feel a change in resistance or "pop" as the dura is penetrated.

f. If resistance is met initially (you hit bone), withdraw needle to skin surface and redirect angle slightly.

g. Send CSF for appropriate studies (see Chapter 6 for normal values).

h. Accurate measurement of CSF pressure can only be made with the patient lying quietly on the side. Once free flow of spinal fluid is obtained, attach the manometer and measure CSF.

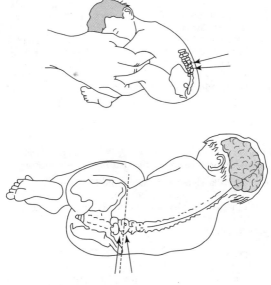

FIG. 3.10. Lumbar pucture. *(Courtesy of Josie Pirro, RN, Johns Hopkins Children's Center.)*

B. **Bone Marrow Aspiration**
   1. **Indications:** Examination of bone marrow in a hematologic or oncologic workup
   2. **Complications**
      a. Bleeding/hematoma
      b. Infection
      c. Bone spur formation (if biopsy is performed)
   3. **Procedure**
      a. Identify site for aspiration. For most children the posterior iliac crest is superior, however anterior iliac crest may be used. For some children less than 3 months of age the tibia can be used.
      b. Position patient in prone position with pillow elevating pelvis.

    c. Prep the site with povidone-iodine and anesthetize skin, soft tissue, and periosteum with 1% lidocaine.

    d. Insert needle (16- or 18-gauge) with steady pressure in a boring motion. Needle should be directed perpendicular to the surface of the bone. Enter the ileum at the posterior superior iliac spine, which is a visible and palpable bony prominence superior and lateral to the intergluteal cleft. Needle will enter cortex and will "pop" into marrow space; needle should be firmly anchored in the bone.

    e. Remove stylet and aspirate marrow with at least 20 ml syringe.

Note: In young infants and infiltrated leukemic, marrow aspiration may be impossible and thus bone marrow biopsy necessary.

C. Chest Tube Placement and Thoracentesis

   1. **Indications:** Evacuation of a pneumothorax, hemothorax, chylothorax, large pleural effusion or empyema for diagnostic or therapeutic purposes

   2. **Complications**

    a. Pneumothorax or hemothorax

    b. Bleeding or infection

    c. Pulmonary contusion or laceration

    d. Puncture of diaphragm, liver, or spleen

   3. **Procedure**

    a. For small pneumothoraces it may be possible to decompress by sterilely inserting a 23-gauge butterfly or 22-gauge angiocatheter at the anterior 2nd intercostal space in the midclavicular line.

    b. Attach to 3-way stopcock and syringe and aspirate air. *Chest tube may still be necessary.*

    c. Chest tube insertion (Fig. 3.11)

      1) Position child supine or with affected side up.

      2) Point of entry is the 3rd to 5th intercostal space in the mid to anterior axillary line. Usually at level of nipple (avoid breast tissue).

      3) Sterilely prep and drape with providone and alcohol.

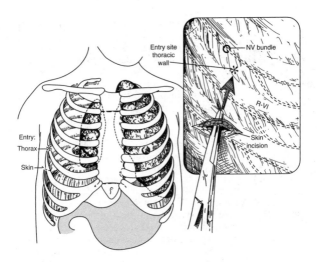

FIG. 3.11. Technique for insertion of chest tube.

   4) Patient may require IV sedation (see Chapter 27).
      Anesthetize locally the skin, subcutaneous tissue,
      periosteum of rib, chest wall muscles, and pleura
      with lidocaine.
   5) Make sterile incision one intercostal space below
      desired insertion point and bluntly dissect
      through tissue layers until the superior portion of
      the rib is reached.
   6) Push hemostat over top of rib, through the pleura,
      and into the pleural space. Enter pleural space
      cautiously, not > 1 cm. Spread hemostat to open,
      place chest tube in clamp, and guide through
      entry site to desired distance.
   7) For a pneumothorax insert the tube anteriorly
      toward the apex. For a pleural effusion direct the
      tube inferiorly and posteriorly.
   8) Secure tube with purse string sutures through
      incision and wrapped around the tube.

  9) Attach to drainage system with -20 to -30 cm H_2O pressure.
  10) Apply sterile dressing.
  11) Confirm position and function with chest x-ray exam.
d. Thoracentesis (Fig. 3.12)
  1) Confirm fluid in pleural space via clinical exam, radiographs, or sonography.
  2) If possible, place child in sitting position leaning over table.
  3) Point of entry usually is in the 7th intercostal space and posterior axillary line.
  4) Sterilely prep and drape area.
  5) Anesthetize skin, subcutaneous tissue, rib periosteum, chest wall, and pleura with lidocaine.
  6) Advance an IV catheter or large bore needle attached to a syringe onto rib and then "walk" over superior aspect into pleural space while providing steady negative pressure; often a "popping" sensation is generated. Be careful not to advance too far into the pleural cavity. If an IV catheter is used the soft catheter may be advanced into the pleural space aiming downward.
  7) Attach syringe and stopcock device to remove fluid for diagnostic studies and for symptomatic relief as well. See Chapter 6 for evaluation of pleural fluid.
  8) After removing needle or catheter, place occlusive dressing and obtain chest x-ray results to rule out pneumothorax.

D. Pericardiocentesis
  1. **Indications:** To emergently obtain pericardial fluid for diagnostic or therapeutic purposes
  2. **Complications**
     a. Puncture of cardiac chamber
     b. Hemopericardium/pneumopericardium
     c. Cardiac arrhythmias
     d. Pneumothorax
  3. **Procedure** (Fig. 3.13)
     a. Unless contraindicated, sedate the patient. Monitor ECG.
     b. Place patient at a 30° angle. Have patient secured.

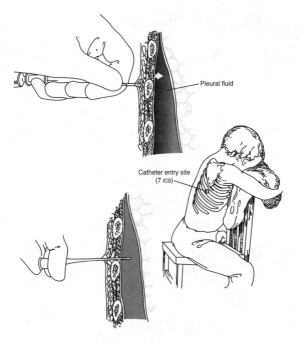

FIG. 3.12. Thoracentesis.

    c. Prepare and drape puncture site. A drape across the upper chest is unnecessary and may obscure important landmarks.

    d. Anesthetize the puncture site with 1% lidocaine.

    e. Insert an 18- or 20-gauge needle just to the left of the xiphoid process, 1 cm inferior to the bottom rib at approximately a 60° angle to the skin.

    f. While gently aspirating, advance needle toward the patient's left shoulder until pericardial fluid is obtained.

    g. Upon entering the pericardial space, clamp the needle at the skin edge to prevent further penetration. Attach a 30 ml syringe with a stopcock.

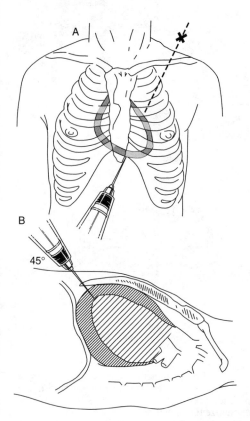

FIG. 3.13. Pericardiocentesis. *(From Nichols DG et al:* Golden hour: the handbook of advanced pediatric life support, *ed 2, St Louis, 1996, Mosby.)*

      h. Gently and slowly remove the fluid. Rapid withdrawal of the pericardial fluid can result in shock or myocardial insufficiency.

      i. Send fluid for appropriate laboratory studies (see Chapter 6).

E. **Paracentesis**
1. **Indications:** Removal of intraperitoneal fluid for diagnostic or therapeutic purposes
2. **Complications**
   a. Bleeding or infection
   b. Puncture of internal organs
3. **Cautions**
   a. Do not remove a large amount of fluid too rapidly since hypovolemia and hypotension may result from rapid fluid shifts.
   b. Avoid scars from previous surgery; localized bowel adhesions increase the chances of entering a viscus in these areas.
   c. The bladder should be empty to avoid perforation.
4. **Procedure**
   a. Prepare and drape the abdomen as for a surgical procedure. Anesthetize puncture site.
   b. With patient in supine position, insert IV catheter attached to a syringe just lateral to the rectus muscle in either the right or left lower quadrants, a few centimeters above the inguinal ligament. If patient is placed in semi-Fowler or cardiac position, place needle midline approximately midway between the umbilicus and pubis.
   c. Puncture skin, then move needle parallel a short distance and then enter the peritoneal cavity. This creates a Z tract. Apply continuous negative pressure.
   d. Once fluid appears in the syringe, remove introducer needle and leave catheter in place. Attach a stopcock and aspirate slowly until an adequate amount of fluid has been obtained for studies.
   e. If, upon entering the peritoneal cavity, air is aspirated, withdraw the needle immediately. Aspirated air indicates entrance into a hollow viscus. (In general, penetration of a hollow viscus during paracentesis does not lead to complications.) Then repeat paracentesis with sterile equipment.
   f. Send fluid for appropriate lab studies (see Chapter 6).

F. **Urinary Bladder Catheterization**
1. **Indications:** To sterilely obtain urine for urinalysis and culture and to monitor hydration status
2. **Complications**
   a. Trauma to urethra or bladder
   b. Vaginal catheterization
   c. Infection
   d. Intravesical knot of catheter (rarely occurs)

Note: Infant/child should not have voided within one hour of technique. Catheterization is contraindicated in pelvic fractures.

3. **Procedure**
   a. Prepare the urethral opening using sterile technique.
   b. In the male, apply gentle traction to the penis in a caudal direction to straighten the urethra.
   c. Gently insert a lubricated catheter into the urethra. Slowly advance the catheter until resistance is met at the external sphincter. Continued pressure will overcome this resistance, and the catheter will enter the bladder. In the female only a few centimeters of advancement is required to reach the bladder.
   d. Carefully remove the catheter once the specimen is obtained.
   e. Cleanse skin of providone-iodine.
G. **Suprapubic Bladder Aspiration**
1. **Indications:** To sterilely obtain urine for urinalysis and culture in children less than 2 years of age (avoid in children with genitourinary tract anomalies)
2. **Complications**
   a. Hematuria; usually microscopic in all cases
   b. Intestinal perforation
   c. Infection of abdominal wall
   d. Bleeding
3. **Procedure**
   a. Anterior rectal pressure in females or gentle penile pressure in males may be used to prevent urination during the procedure. Child should not have voided within one hour of procedure.
   b. Restrain the infant in the supine, frog-leg position. Clean the suprapubic area with povidone-iodine and alcohol.

    c. The site for puncture is 1 to 2 cm above the symphysis pubis in the midline. Use a syringe with a 22-gauge, 1-inch needle and puncture at 10° to 20° angle to the perpendicular, aiming slightly caudad.

    d. Exert suction gently as the needle is advanced until urine enters syringe. The needle should not be advanced more than 2.5 cm. Aspirate the urine with gentle suction.

H. Knee Joint Aspiration

1. **Indications:** Removal of joint effusion causing severe pain or limitations of function and to obtain fluid for diagnosis of systemic illness (collagen vascular disease) or septic arthritis

2. **Complicated**
   a. Bleeding
   b. Infection

3. **Procedure** (Fig. 3.14)
   a. Secure the child with knee actively extended.
   b. Prepare and drape for a sterile procedure.
   c. Anesthetize the aspiration site with 1% lidocaine/bicarbonate. Anesthetize the subcutaneous tissue down to the joint capsule.
   d. Localize the under surface of patella. You may slightly flex the knee to create space for the injection. Insert an 18-gauge or larger bore needle into the joint space at a 60° angle to the skin.
   e. Aspiration of joint contents confirms an intraarticular placement.
   f. Collect fluid for appropriate studies (see Chapter 6).
   g. Place a dry, sterile dressing over aspiration site when done.

I. Tympanocentesis

1. **Indications:** Removal of middle ear fluid for diagnostic or therapeutic purposes

2. **Complications**
   a. Bleeding
   b. Contamination with bacteria from canal
   c. Damage to ossicles
   d. Laceration of membrane

3. **Procedure**
   a. Restrain patient securely. Typically sedation is not required; however, an anxiolytic may be considered.

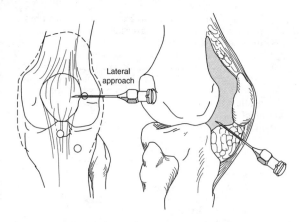

FIG. 3.14. Knee joint aspiration.

     b. Remove all cerumen from canal with loop.
     c. Attach 22-gauge, 3-inch spinal needle to 1 ml syringe with 0.2 ml of nonbacteriostatic saline.
     d. Bend spinal needle to allow for visualization.
     e. Sterilize canal by filling with 70% alcohol or povidone-iodine for 60 seconds, and then allow ear to drain.
     f. Visualize the posterior inferior quadrant of tympanic membrane with an otoscope fitted with an operating head.
     g. Perforate membrane while applying negative pressure to remove fluid in 1–2 seconds. Remove needle avoiding contamination in canal.
     h. Send fluid for appropriate cultures and gram stain.

III. BASIC LACERATION REPAIR

Note: Lacerations of the face, lips, hands, genitalia, mouth, or periorbital area may require consultation with a specialist.

A. Securely restrain child.
B. Forcefully irrigate wound with copious amounts of sterile normal saline. Use at least 250 ml for smaller, superficial

wounds; more for larger wounds. This is the most important step in preventing infection.

C. Prep and drape the patient for a sterile procedure.

D. Anesthetize the wound with lidocaine/bicarbonate by infusing the anesthetic into the subcutaneous tissues.

E. Debride the wound and probe for foreign bodies. Consider x-ray exam if a foreign body was involved in injury.

F. Select suture type for percutaneous closure (see Table 3.1).

G. When suturing is complete, apply topical antibiotic and sterile dressing. Splinting of the affected area to limit mobility often speeds healing.

H. Check wounds at 48–72 hours for patients with wounds of questionable viability, if wound was packed, or for patients prescribed prophylactic antibiotics. Change dressing at check.

I. For hand lacerations, close skin only; do not use subcutaneous stitches. Elevate and immobilize the hand.

J. Consider the child's need for tetanus prophylaxis.

IV. BASIC SPLINTING OF MUSCULOSKELETAL INJURIES

A. Basic Splinting

1. **Indications:** To provide short term stabilization of limb injuries
2. **Complications**
   a. Pressure sores
   b. Dermatitis
   c. Neurovascular impairment
3. **Procedure**
   a. Determine style of splint needed.
   b. Measure and cut plaster to appropriate length noting that upper extremity splints require 8–10 layers and lower extremity splints require 12–14 layers.
   c. Pad extremity with cotton webrile taking care to overlap each turn by 50%. Place cotton in between digits if they are in splint.
   d. Immerse plaster slab into room temperature water.

WARNING: Plaster becomes hot upon drying.

   e. Smooth out wet plaster slab avoiding any wrinkles.

TABLE 3.1.

Guidelines for Suture Material, Size, and Removal

Body region	Monofilament* (for superficial lacerations)	Absorbable† (for deep lacerations)	Duration time‡ (days)
Scalp	5–0/4–0	4–0	5–7
Face	6–0	5–0	3–5
Eyelid	7–0/6–0	—	3–5
Eyebrow	6–0/5–0	5–0	3–5
Trunk	5–0/4–0	3–0	5–7
Extremities	5–0/4–0	4–0	7
Joint surface	4–0	—	10–14
Hand	5–0	5–0	7
Foot sole	4–0/3–0	4–0	7–10

*Examples of monofilament nonabsorable sutures: nylon, polypropylene
†Examples of absorbable sutures: polyglycolic acid and polyglactin 910 (Vicryl)
‡As a general rule, the longer sutures are left in place, the more scarring and
  potential for infection. Sutures in cosmetically sensitive areas should be removed
  as soon as possible, whereas sutures in high-tension areas such as exterior
  surfaces should stay in longer.

    f. Position splint over extremity and wrap externally
       with gauze. When dry, an ace wrap can be added.
    g. Use crutches or slings as indicated.
B. Long Arm Posterior Splint (Fig. 3.15)
    1. **Indications:** Immobilization of elbow and forearm injuries
C. Posterior Ankle Splint
    1. Immobilization of ankle sprains and fractures of the foot,
       ankle, and distal fibula. Measure leg for appropriate
       length of plaster. The splint should extend to base of toes
       and the upper portion of calf.
D. Sugar Tong Forearm Splint (Fig. 3.16)
    1. Distal radius and wrist fractures; to immobilize the
       elbow and minimize pronation and supination

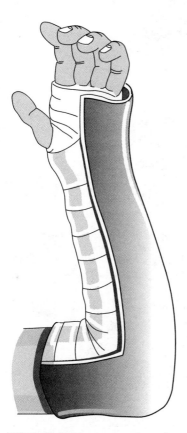

FIG. 3.15. Long arm posterior splint. *(From Fliesher G, Ludwig S:* Pediatric emergency medicine, *Baltimore, 1993, Williams and Wilkins.)*

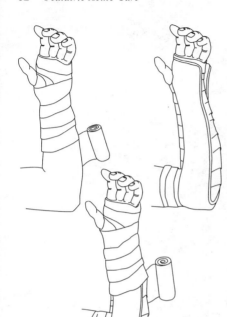

FIG. 3.16. Sugar tong forearm splint. *(From Fliesher G, Ludwig S:* Pediatric emergency medicine, *Baltimore, 1993, Williams and Wilkins.)*

REFERENCES:

Baldwin G: *Handbook of pediatric emergencies,* Boston, 1989, Little, Brown and Company.

Fleisher G, Ludwig S: *Textbook of pediatric emergency medicine,* ed 3, Baltimore, 1993, Williams and Wilkins.

Levin D: *Essentials of pediatric intensive care,* St Louis, 1990, Quality Medical.

Trott A: *Wounds and lacerations: emergency care and closure,* St Louis, 1991, Mosby.

TRAUMA AND BURNS

4

I. EVALUATION AND MANAGEMENT OF PEDIATRIC TRAUMA

Trauma remains the leading cause of death and disability in children. Timely resuscitation is paramount since there is often significant potential for full recovery. Initial assessment begins with evaluation of cardiopulmonary function while simultaneously performing a rapid thoracoabdominal examination to identify the highest priority life-threatening injuries such as airway obstruction, tension pneumothorax, open pneumothorax, hemothorax, flail chest, cardiac tamponade, and massive hemorrhage. Children with multi-system trauma or significant mortality risk should be transported to a pediatric trauma center if possible.

A. Airway

1. Immobilize cervical spine with a semi-rigid cervical collar (consider placing firm padding beneath the torso to facilitate a neutral position of the head since a child's prominent occiput predisposes the neck to slight flexion when on a completely flat board).
2. Inspect for foreign body, blood, mucus, or broken teeth.
3. Administer 100% oxygen.
4. Suction secretions with large bore (Yankhauer) suction catheter.
5. Jaw thrust/spinal stabilization maneuver (head tilt-chin lift is contraindicated for risk of converting an incomplete spinal cord injury to complete).
6. Bag-valve-mask assisted ventilation if needed
7. Consider oral airway in unconscious child.
8. Indications for intubation include the following:
   a. Respiratory arrest

        b. Respiratory failure (hypoventilation, arterial hypoxemia despite supplemental oxygen, and/or respiratory acidosis)

        c. Airway obstruction

        d. Coma

        e. Need for prolonged ventilatory support (e.g., thoracic injuries or need for diagnostic studies)

    9. Cricothyrotomy may be required in the presence of severe orofacial trauma and occasionally in the care of a patient with an unstable cervical spine injury.

B. Breathing

    1. If airway is patent and respiratory effort effective, then administer 100% oxygen by nonrebreather.

    2. If respiratory effort is ineffective then administer bag-valve-mask ventilatory assistance. Hyperventilation will eliminate excess carbon dioxide, provide hypocarbia, which can buffer metabolic acidosis associated with shock and hypovolemia, and reduce excessive cerebral blood flow (CBF) following closed head trauma. However, over-ventilation may reduce CBF to ischemic levels and should be avoided.

    3. An orogastric tube should be considered for gastric decompression, since distention may compromise ventilation and increase the risk of vomiting and aspiration.

    4. Inspect chest for open wounds, abrasions, contusions, and overall color.

    5. Note abnormal breathing pattern.

    6. Assess adequacy of ventilation.

    7. **Tension pneumothorax** presents as severe respiratory distress, distended neck veins, contralateral tracheal deviation, diminished breath sounds, and compromising systemic perfusion by obstructing venous return. Treatment involves needle decompression followed by chest tube placement. A 20-gauge over-the-needle catheter is inserted into the 2nd intercostal space in the mid-clavicular line. The chest tube should be directed toward the lung apex.

    8. **Open pneumothorax,** or sucking chest wound, is rare but allows free flow of air between atmosphere and hemithorax. Treatment consists of covering the defect with an occlusive dressing, such as petroleum jelly gauze, and

positive pressure ventilation followed by insertion of a chest tube.

9. **Hemothorax** treatment consists of fluid resuscitation followed by placement of a thoracostomy tube directed posterior and inferior.

C. **Circulation**

1. Direct pressure to external bleeding with thin sterile gauze dressings. Tourniquets should be avoided except in cases of traumatic amputation associated with uncontrolled bleeding from a large vessel.

2. Hypotension will not be present until 25%–30% of the child's blood volume is lost acutely. Heart rate is a better indicator of circulatory status.

3. Intravenous catheter access with two large bore catheters. Allow 3 attempts or 90 seconds.

4. Consider intraosseous needle in patient <6 years old if access is delayed, or consider percutaneous cannulation of the femoral vein or a saphenous vein cutdown.

5. Fluid therapy should be geared toward rapid volume replacement with isotonic crystalloid such as lactated Ringer's solution or normal saline. Initial treatment of shock should include hemostasis and a 20 ml/kg bolus of fluid. A response should be assessed by monitoring urine output, skin perfusion, heart rate, and blood pressure. Another 20 ml/kg bolus may be given, and systemic perfusion should be reassessed. If signs of shock persist, then 10 ml/kg packed red blood cells or 20 ml/kg whole blood should be considered. If type specific crossmatched blood is not readily available, O negative blood should be given. If shock persists despite fluid resuscitation and hemostasis, then internal bleeding is likely. Medical anti-shock trousers (MAST) have not been shown to be efficacious in pediatric hemorrhagic shock except in cases involving unstable pelvic fractures.

6. When patient is hemodynamically stable, begin maintenance fluids.

7. If increased intracranial pressure (ICP) is suspected, see Chapter 1.

D. **Examination**

Remove all patient's clothing, and perform thorough head to toe examination with special emphasis on the following:

1. **Head:** Scalp/skull injury, raccoon eyes (periorbital ecchymoses, which suggest orbital roof fracture), Battle's sign (ecchymosis behind pinna, which suggests mastoid fracture), cervical spine injury, cerebrospinal fluid (CSF) leak from ears or nose suggests basilar skull fracture, pupillary equality, size, and reaction to light (unilateral dilation of one pupil suggest compression of cranial nerve III (CNIII) and possibly impending herniation, whereas bilateral dilation of pupils is ominous and suggests bilateral CNIII compression or severe anoxia and ischemia), corneal reflex, fundoscopic exam, hyphema, hemotympanum.
2. **Neck:** Cervical spine tenderness, trachea midline, subcutaneous emphysema
3. **Chest:** Breath sounds, heart sounds, symmetry, paradoxical movement, rib fracture
4. **Abdomen:** Tenderness, ecchymoses, distention, shoulder pain (suggests referred subdiaphragmatic process), serial exams. Orogastric aspirates that are blood or bile stained suggest possible intraabdominal injury.
5. **Pelvis:** Tenderness, stability
6. **Genitourinary:** Meatal blood, scrotal hematoma
7. **Rectal:** Tone, blood, displaced prostate
8. **Back:** Step-off along spinal column, tenderness, penetrating wound
9. **Extremities:** Deformity, pulses, perfusion, crepitus, sensation, clinical signs of compartment syndrome including pain out of proportion to the expected, paresthesias, pallor distally, and pulselessness and paralysis (very late signs)
10. **Neurologic:** Thorough exam (see Chapter 22)
11. **Skin:** Capillary refill, perfusion, lacerations, abrasions
    Relationship between color and age of contusions
    Reddish-blue purple: <1 day
    Blue purple: 1–5 days
    Green: 5–7 days
    Yellow: 7–10 days
    Brown: 10–14 days
    Resolution: 2–4 weeks

Wilson EF: *Pediatrics* 60:750, 1977.

E. Lab Evaluation
   1. Hemoglobin/hematocrit
   2. Liver function enzymes if suspect hepatic injury
   3. Type and cross
   4. Urinalysis (any hematuria requires evaluation)
   5. Consider toxicology screen
   6. Review tetanus status (see Chapter 17)

F. Radiologic Evaluation
   1. Cervical spine anteroposterior (AP) and lateral (including the 7th cervical vertebra). Cervical spine injury is more likely to occur in children with an acceleration-deceleration injury such as a motor vehicle accident or falls. In infants and toddlers, subluxation at the atlanto-occipital (base of skull-C1) or atlantoaxial (C1–C2) joints is more likely, whereas in school age children the lower cervical spine is involved (C5–C7). Spinal cord injury without radiologic abnormality (SCIWORA) has been recognized as an important cause of pediatric spinal cord injury and is a functional cervical spine injury that cannot be excluded by radiographic studies. SCIWORA is thought to be attributable to the increased elasticity and mobility of the pediatric spine. Thus cervical spine injuries must be assumed to be present in the child with multiple injuries. Neurologic recovery after acute spinal cord injury is improved with prompt administration of methylprednisolone 30 mg/kg IV loading dose followed by 5.4 mg/kg/hr IV infusion. (Bracken: *N Engl J Med* 322:20, 1990)
   2. CXR rib fractures indicate severe chest trauma and are associated with visceral injury
   3. AXR
   4. Pelvis
   5. Extremities as indicated
      a. Unique fracture patterns seen rarely in adults include **greenstick fracture,** a fracture of one cortex under tension while the contralateral cortex remains intact; **plastic deformation,** a bend in the bone without a fracture; and **torus fracture,** a fracture with buckling of one cortex in compression while the contralateral cortex is undamaged. Keep in mind that ligaments are stronger than bone or growth plate in children; thus

FRACTURE TYPES

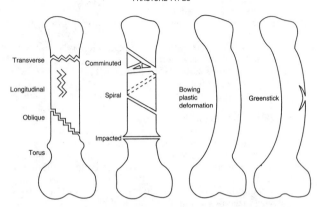

FIG. 4.1. Fracture patterns in children.

  dislocations and sprains are relatively uncommon,
  whereas growth plate disruption and bone avulsion are
  more common (Fig. 4.1).
  b. Salter classification of growth plate injuries
    1) Fracture along but not across plate
    2) Fracture along plate with metaphyseal extension
    3) Fracture along plate with epiphyseal extension
    4) Fractures across plate and joint
    5) Crush injury to plate without obvious fracture (Fig
       4.2.)
  6. Consider skeletal survey or bone scan if suspect child
     abuse.
G. Special Exams
  1. **CT of head** is indicated for loss of consciousness, change
     in mental status, seizures, amnesia; focal neurologic defi-
     cit, or persistent emesis.
  2. **CT of abdomen** with IV contrast to evaluate abdominal
     trauma.

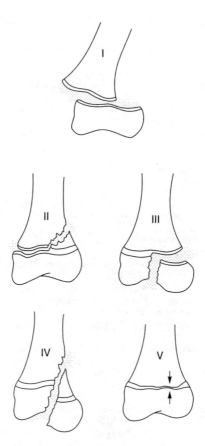

FIG. 4.2. Salter classification of growth plate fractures. *(From Nichols DG et al:* Golden hour: the handbook of advanced pediatric life support, *ed 2, St Louis, 1996, Mosby.)*

3. **Intravenous pyelography (IVP)** if suspect renal trauma (or abdominal CT with IV contrast). Blood at urethral meatus indicates the need for **urethrocystography** to exclude lower urinary tract injury before the insertion of a Foley catheter.
4. Measurement of **compartment pressures**
5. **Echocardiography** to detect cardiac contusion and wall motion abnormalities
6. **Diagnostic peritoneal lavage (DPL)** is good at evaluating intraabdominal hemorrhage; however, children can often be managed nonoperatively because bleeding from blunt injuries to the liver and spleen will usually stop.

H. **Monitoring**
1. Place on cardiac monitor
2. Frequent vital signs with oxygen saturation
3. Body temperature
4. Vital signs (Cushing's response of bradycardia, increased BP, and abnormal respiratory pattern is a late finding in increased ICP)
5. Repeated assessments of Glasgow Coma Scale (GCS) (See Chapter 1)
6. Assess AVPU (**A**lert, responsive to **V**erbal stimuli, responsive to **P**ainful stimuli, or **U**nresponsive)
7. Foley catheter to follow urine output (contraindicated if blood at meatus or displaced prostate
8. Orogastric tube for decompression (consider nonparticulate antacid to reduce pulmonary consequences if gastric contents aspirated)

I. **Obtain detailed history from family or witnessess and obtain AMPLE history including A**llergies, **M**edications, **P**ast illnesses, **L**ast meal, and **E**vents preceding the injury. For head trauma ask "Was there LOC?", "Does the child remember events preceding, during, and following the injury?", "What have been the levels of consciousness and activity since the injury?", and "Has there been vomiting, headache, or diplopia?" Explore the possibility of intentional injury if indicated.

II. BURNS
A. **Epidemiology**
In the United States, burns are the second most common cause of accidental death in children less than 5 years of age.

Burns result in 600,000 ER visits and 30,000 hospitalizations per year. In certain patterns of burns, child abuse must be considered.

1. **Types of Burns**
   a. Flame: Approximately 75% of those patients treated in a burn care facility have injuries secondary to fire. When clothing burns, the exposure to heat is prolonged, and the severity of the burn is worse.
   b. Scald/contact: Mortality is similar to that in flame burns when total body surface area (BSA) involved is equal. Circumferential scald burns of hands or feet that are uniform and clearly demarcated with no additional splash burn wounds suggest that a child may have been forcibly submerged in hot water. A burn limited to the buttocks and genitalia is often suggestive of inflicted injury. Contact burns that show a uniform depth of injury, as opposed to a burn that is deeper on one edge than on another, suggest that a hot object was held against the child. Additional criteria that suggest intentional injury include delay in seeking medical attention, other injuries, malnutrition, or history inconsistent with injury.
   c. Chemical: Tissue is damaged by protein coagulation or liquefaction rather than hyperthermic activity.
   d. Electrical: Injury is often extensive, involving skeletal muscle and other tissues in excess to the skin damage. The tissues that have the least resistance are the most heat sensitive. Bone has the greatest resistance and nerve tissue has the least. A cardiac arrest may occur from passage of the current through the heart.
   e. Cold injury (frostbite): Freezing results in direct tissue injury. Toes, fingers, ears, and nose are commonly involved. Initial treatment includes rapidly rewarming in tepid (105°–110° F) water for 20–40 min. Excision of tissue should not be done until complete demarcation of nonviable tissue has occurred.

B. **Burn Assessment**

Calculate body surface area. See BSA nomogram in Chapter 14.

1. **Burn depth**
   a. First-degree: Only epidermis involved, painful and erythematous. May or may not blister.

b. Second-degree: Epidermis and dermis involved, but dermal appendages spared. Superficial second-degree burns are blistered and painful. Deep second-degree burns may be white and painless, may require grafting, and may progress to full-thickness burns with wound sepsis.

c. Third-degree: Full-thickness burns involve epidermis and all of dermis (including dermal appendages), are painless, and require grafting.

Note: The extent and severity of burn injury may change over the first several days after injury; therefore be cautious in discussing prognosis with the victim's family.

2. **Burn assessment chart:** Use burn assessment chart to map areas of second- and third-degree burn and to calculate the total BSA burned. Extent of tissue damage with electrical burns may not be apparent initially (Fig. 4.3).

C. **Initial Assessment**

1. **Vital signs**

a. Assess and establish adequate airway, breathing, and circulation. Intubate if necessary for pulmonary toilet or if evidence of inhalation injury is present. This evidence can include the following:

- History of fire in enclosed space
- Singed nares
- Facial burns
- Charred lips
- Carbonaceous secretions
- Edema of posterior pharynx
- Hoarseness
- Cough
- Wheezing

Neuromuscular blockade with succinylcholine for intubation is contraindicated because of risk of worsening hyperkalemia. Assess and maintain an adequate core temperature; patients with extensive burns are at risk for hypothermia.

b. Inhalation injury is present in >30% of victims of major burns. All patients with large burns should be assumed to have carbon monoxide (CO) poisoning until examination and evaluation of blood carboxyhe-

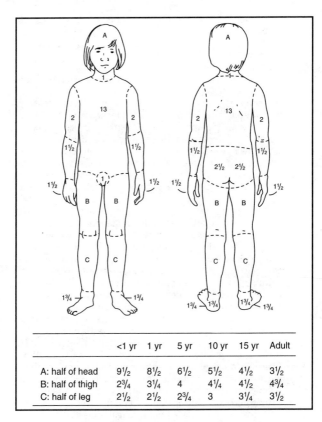

	<1 yr	1 yr	5 yr	10 yr	15 yr	Adult
A: half of head	9½	8½	6½	5½	4½	3½
B: half of thigh	2¾	3¼	4	4¼	4½	4¾
C: half of leg	2½	2½	2¾	3	3¼	3½

FIG. 4.3. Burn assessment chart. *(From Barkin RM, Rosen P: Emergency pediatrics: a guide to ambulatory care, ed 4, St Louis, 1994, Mosby.)*

moglobin is undertaken. Humidified 100% O_2 should be administered during the initial assessment. The presence of inhalation injury increases the risk of mortality.

2. **Pulmonary status**
   a. Monitor pulmonary status with serial arterial blood gases (ABG).
   b. Increasing tachypnea may be seen in patients with pulmonary insufficiency caused by acute asphyxia and CO toxicity, upper airway obstruction secondary to edema, or overwhelming parenchymal damage.
   c. Delivery of 100% O_2 counteracts the effects of CO and speeds its clearance. Chest x-ray exam may not show changes for 24–72 hours. Carboxyhemoglobin falsely elevates oxygen saturation as determined by pulse oximetry.

3. **Other injuries:** One must always remember to maintain the basic principles of any trauma evaluation. Always do a primary and secondary survey to avoid missing associated injuries. Include ECG. Electrical injuries, for example, can produce extensive deep tissue damage, intravascular thrombosis, cardiac and respiratory arrest, fractures resulting from muscle contractions, and cardiac arrhythmias. Motor vehicle accidents, falls, or explosions may result in associated head, visceral, or bone injuries.

4. **Intravenous access:** Establish IV access and begin fluid resuscitation immediately on infants with burns greater than 10% of BSA, children with greater than 15% BSA burned, or children with evidence of smoke inhalation. Consider bolus of 20 ml/kg Ringer's lactate and continue at approximately 500 ml/m² of total BSA per hour (enough to maintain a urine output of 0.5–2 ml/kg/hr).

5. **Initial labs:** Consider complete blood count (CBC), type and cross, carboxyhemoglobin, coagulation studies, chemistry panel, arterial blood gas (ABG), and chest x-ray exam.

6. **Stomach and bladder decompression:** Insert nasogastric (NG) tube (ileus common in major burns) and Foley catheter (monitor urine output). Make NPO initially. Use sucralfate or H_2-blockers/antacids for stress ulcer prophylaxis.

7. **Tetanus toxoid:** Give tetanus toxoid if last vaccine was in excess of 5 years ago. If patient has not received a tetanus vaccine, then administer tetanus immunoglobulin and begin a series of tetanus immunizations. (See Chapter 17 for details.)

8. **Analgesia:** IV analgesia is often necessary to treat pain. Do not attribute combativeness or anxiety to pain until adequate perfusion and oxygenation are established. Consider morphine 0.1 mg/kg IV or demerol 1 mg/kg IV/PO (see Chapter 27).

D. Treatment

1. **Triage/management:** Cooling decreases the severity of the burn if administered within 30 minutes of the time of injury, and it also helps to relieve pain. If burn is <10% of BSA, apply clean towels soaked in cold water to help prevent burn progression. If burn is >10% of BSA, use clean dry towels to avoid heat loss. Do not use grease, butter, etc. With regard to chemical burns it is important to either wash the chemical away or neutralize it. Except in rare circumstances, the most efficacious first aid treatment for chemical burns is lavaging with copious volumes of water for approximately 20 minutes.

2. **Triage**

   a. If burn is <10% (infants) or <15% (children) and involves no full-thickness areas, may treat as outpatient.

   b. Consider inpatient management for the following:
      1) More extensive burn
      2) Electrical or chemical burns (full extent of burn may not be apparent initially)
      3) Burns of critical areas such as face, hands, feet, perineum, or joint surfaces
      4) Suspected child abuse or home situation inadequate to assure good care and follow up
      5) Child with underlying chronic illness
      6) Smoke inhalation or CO poisoning

   c. After stabilization, consider transfer to a burn center if any of the following conditions are satisfied:
      1) Burns of at least 20%–30% BSA
      2) Major burns to hand, face, joints, or perineum
      3) Electrical burns
      4) Burns with associated injuries

3. **Outpatient management**
   a. Cleanse with warm saline or mild soap and water. Consider debridement with forceps or sterile gauze to pick up the edges and peel it off of the base of the burn. Leave intact blisters.
   b. Apply topical antibacterial agent (Table 4.1).
   c. Follow up daily or every other day.
   d. Have patient cleanse burn at home twice daily with mild soap followed by application of an antibacterial agent and sterile dressing as above. Once epithelialization is under way, may be reduced to daily dressing change.
   e. Consider tetanus immunoprophylaxis (see Chapter 17 for details).

4. **Inpatient management:** Fluid therapy: Goal is to provide sufficient fluid to prevent shock and renal failure from excessive fluid losses and "third spacing." The two formulas listed below are only guidelines. Any resuscitation formula provides only an estimate of fluid need. Assess adequacy of perfusion using urine output (0.5–2 ml/kg/hr), BP, peripheral circulation, and sensorium. Check electrolytes and ABG to monitor acidosis. Consider central venous access in burns >25% BSA.
   a. Galveston formula
      1) Based on BSA, since weight and surface area relationships are not constant in a growing child
      2) First 24 hours: Give 5000 ml/m^2 of burned area (burn losses) plus 2000 ml/m^2 of total BSA (maintenance fluids) over the first 24 hours; infuse half over the first 8 hours after burn injury. Include fluid already given enroute to referral center. For children older than 1 year, use LR plus 12.5 g of 25% albumin/L. For infants younger than 1 year, prepare a 1 L solution of 930 ml of 1/3 NS, 20 ml NaHCO$_3$ (1 mEq/ml), and 50 ml of 25% albumin.
      3) Second and subsequent days: Give 3750 ml/m^2 burned area/24 hr (burn losses) plus 1500 ml/m^2 of total BSA/24 hr (maintenance fluids). Since sodium requirements after the first 24 hours are less, use D$_5$, 1/3 NS with 20–30 mEq/L of potassium phosphate (phosphate is used because of frequent hypophosphatemia).

TABLE 4.1.

Topical Antibacterial Agents

Agent	Action	Side Effects	Use
Silver sulfadiazine (silvadene)	Broad antibacterial, painless, fair eschar penetration	Sulfonamide sensitivity, occasional leukopenia, contraindicated in pregnancy	BID; cover with light dressings; leave face and chest open
Bacitracin ointment	Limited antibacterial action, poor eschar penetration, transparent, easy to apply	Rapid development of resistance, conjunctivitis if contact with eye	BID, apply to small areas
Mafenide sulfamylon	Excellent antibacterial for gram positive and gram negative and costridium, rapid eschar penetration	Painful, sulfonamide sensitivity, carbonic anhydrase inhibition may lead to acidosis	BID: cover with light dressings; leave face, chest, abdomen open
Aqueous silver nitrate solution	Universal antibacterial action, poor eschar penetration	Strong tissue staining, hypochloremic alkalosis	BID, light gauze dressing
Iodophors (efodine)	Universal antibacterial action, poor eschar penetration	Strong tissue staining, iodine absorption	BID, light gauze dressing

BID, Twice a day.

      4) Reevaluate fluid requirements as wounds heal. Map wounds weekly.

  b. Parkland formula: This is a simple formula. It is useful for replacement of deficits and ongoing losses; however, it does not provide maintenance fluids.

      1) First 24 hours: Give Ringer's lactate 3 ml/kg/% BSA burned (if <30% BSA) or 4 ml/kg/% BSA burned (if >30% BSA) over the first 24 hours; give half of total over the first 8 hours calculated from the time of injury. Give the remaining half over the next 16 hours.

      2) Second 24 hours: Fluid requirements average 50%–75% of first day's requirement. Determine concentrations and rates by monitoring weight, serum electrolytes, urine output, NG losses, etc.

      3) Consider adding colloid after 18–24 hours (1g/kg/day of albumin) to maintain serum albumin greater 2 g/dl.

      4) Withhold potassium generally for the first 48 hours because of large release of potassium from damaged tissues. To most effectively manage electrolytes monitor urine electrolytes biweekly and replace urine losses accordingly.

E. Prevention: The best treatment is prevention!

Measures include child-proofing the home, installing smoke detectors, turning hot water tap temperature down to 49°–52° C (it takes 2 minutes of immersion at 52° C to cause a full-thickness burn, compared to 5 seconds of immersion at 60° C).

PART II

Diagnostic and Therapeutic Information

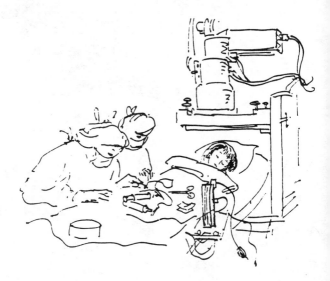

ADOLESCENT MEDICINE

5

I. ABBREVIATED RECOMMENDED CONTENT FOR ROUTINE ADOLESCENT HEALTH VISIT (TABLE 5.1)

TABLE 5.1.

MEDICAL HISTORY

Immunizations
Chronic illness, chronic medications, dental care

FAMILY HISTORY

Psychiatric disorders, suicide
Alcoholism/substance abuse

REVIEW OF SYSTEMS

Dietary habits: typical foods consumed, types and frequency of meals skipped, use of laxatives or other weight loss methods
Recent weight gain or loss

PSYCHOSOCIAL/MEDICOSOCIAL HISTORY (HEADSS)

H(OME)

Household composition
Family dynamics and relationships with adolescent
Living/sleeping arrangements
Guns in the home

E(DUCATION)

School attendance/absences
Ever failed a grade(s)
Attitude towards school
Favorite, most difficult, best subjects
Special education needs

A(CTIVITIES)

Physical activity, exercise, hobbies
Sports participation
Job

(Continued.)

TABLE 5.1. (cont.)

D(RUGS)

Cigarettes/smokeless tobacco: age at first use, packs or cans per day
Alcohol (beer, wine coolers): use at school or parties; use by friends, self
If yes, **CAGE:** Have you ever felt the need to **C**ut down; have others **A**nnoyed you
by commenting on your use; have you ever felt **G**uilty about your use; have you
ever needed an **E**yeopener (alcohol first thing in morning)?

S(EXUALITY)

Sexual feelings: opposite or same sex
Sexual intercourse: age at first intercourse, number of lifetime partners
Contraception/sexually transmitted disease (STD) prevention
History of STDs
Prior pregnancies, abortions; ever fathered a child?

S(UICIDE)/DEPRESSION

Feelings about self: positive and negative
History of depression or other mental health problems, prior suicidal thoughts,
prior suicide attempts
Sleep problems: difficulty getting to sleep, early waking

PHYSICAL EXAMINATION (MOST PERTINENT ASPECTS)

Skin: acne (type and distribution of lesions)
Spine (scoliosis)
Breasts: Tanner stage, masses
External genitalia: pubic hair distribution, Tanner stage
Testicular exam, Tanner stage

LAB

Purified protein derivative (PPD) (if high risk)
Hemoglobin/hematocrit (once during puberty for males, once after menarche for
females)
Sexually active adolescents: serologic tests for syphilis annually, offer HIV testing
Males: first part voided urinalysis (FPVU); gonorrhea and chlamydia cultures (or
other detection tests) if FPVU positive
Females: gonorrhea and chlamydia cultures (or other detection tests), wet prep,
KOH, cervical gram stain, PAP smear, midvaginal pH

IMMUNIZATIONS

Tetanus and diphtheria (Td) booster age 11–12 years
Measles: two doses of live attenuated vaccine are required after first birthday. Use
measles-mumps-rubella vaccine if not previously vaccinated for mumps or
rubella. Assess pregnancy status, and do not administer rubella vaccine to
woman anticipating pregnancy within 90 days
Hepatitis B vaccine: recommended for adolescents (3 doses)
Varicella vaccine: recommended for seronegative adolescents

(Continued.)

TABLE 5.1. (cont.)

ANTICIPATORY GUIDANCE

Sexuality issues   Nutrition   Coping Skills
Safety: driving/seat belts, guns/bicycle helmets   Substance abuse prevention

Adapted from Oski FA et al: *Principles and practice of pediatrics,* Philadelphia 1994, JB Lippincott; Adger H et al: *Lancet* 8409:944, 1984.

II. PUBERTAL EVENTS AND TANNER STAGE DIAGRAMS (SEE FIGS. 5.1 TO 5.3)

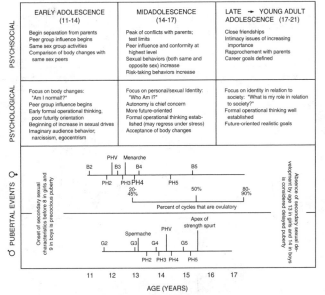

The temporal relation between the biologic, psychologic, and psychosocial events of adolescence. Age limits for the events and stages are approximations and may differ from those used by other authors. The mean age of onset of pubic hair development for males (=13.4) is likely too high due to bias in the data collection method. These limits and the points indicating the attainment of individual stages of puberty were chosen for consistency and to reflect the earlier maturation of American versus British adolescents. PH2, 3, 4, 5—pubic hair stage2, 3, etc; B2, 3, 4, 5—breast stage 2, 3, etc; PHV—peak height velocity; G2, 3, 4, 5—genital stage2, 3, etc.

FIG. 5.1. *(From Oski FA et al:* Principles and practice of pediatrics, *Philadelphia, 1994, JB Lippincott.)*

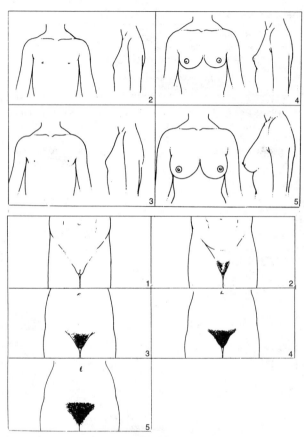

FIG. 5.2.

A, Breast development in girls, Tanner Stages 2–5. (Stage 1 not shown)

B, Pubic hair development in girls, Tanner stages 1–5. *(From Neinstein LS: Adolescent health care: a practical guide, ed 2, Baltimore, 1991, Urban & Schwarzenberg.)*

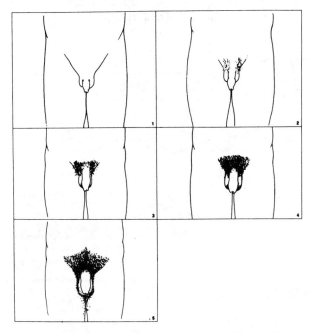

FIG. 5.3. Pubic hair and genital development in boys, Tanner Stages 1–5. *(From Neinstein LS:* Adolescent health care: a practical guide, *ed 2, Baltimore, 1991, Urban & Schwarzenberg.)*

III. METHODS OF CONTRACEPTION (SEE TABLES 5.2 AND 5.3)

TABLE 5.2.

Methods of Contraception

Method	Failure rate in typical user (%)	Benefits	Risk/disadvantages
Combined oral contraceptives (refer to OCP information chart)*	3.0 (May be increased among adolescents)	Intercourse independent, decreased risk of dysmenorrhea, breast disorders, arthritis, iron deficiency anemia, ovarian and uterine cancers, ovarian cysts, symptomatic PID	Thromboembolic phenomena, cerebrovascular accident, coronary artery disease, hypertension, worsening of migraines, breakthrough bleeding, amenorrhea, nausea, weight gain, acne, depression, glucose intolerance
Injectable contraceptives (Depo-Provera)*	0.3	Intercourse independent, long-acting (3 months), can be used when breast feeding, no estrogen, decreased risk of endometrial/ovarian cancer, no drug interactions	Injection every 3 months, delayed return to fertility, menstrual irregularity/amenorrhea, expensive, weight gain
Progestin-only pill (mini pill)*	1.1	Fewer metabolic complications, used for patients with hypertension, diabetes, sickle cell disease	Menstrual irregularities (generally not recommended for adolescents)

(Continued.)

TABLE 5.2. (cont.)

Norplant*	0.04	Intercourse independent, highly effective, long-lasting protection	Requires minor surgical procedure for insertion, removal; menstrual irregularities, headaches, nervousness, nausea, dizziness, dermatitis, acne, change in appetite, weight gain, breast tenderness, hirsutism, hair loss
Condom	12.0	No major risks, low cost, nonprescription, male involvement, protects against STD and cervical cancer	Allergy to materials (rare), loss of sensation, use with each act of coitus
Diaphragm with contraceptive cream or jelly	18.0	Protects against STD, no major risks	Allergy (rare), toxic shock syndrome (rare), increases incidence of urinary tract infection, vaginal ulceration, requires motivation
Spermicide	21.0	Nonprescription, no major medical risks, some STD protection	Allergy (rare), use related to coitus
Intrauterine device	3.0	Minimal demands after insertion, secrecy	Generally not recommended for adolescents, increased risk of pelvic inflammatory disease, ectopic pregnancy, infertility, dysmenorrhea, menorrhagia

(Continued.)

TABLE 5.2. (cont.)

Natural family planning	20.0	Natural, no risks, nonprescription	Not very effective with irregular menses, requires highly motivated partners

Adapted from Oski FA et al: *Principles and practice of pediatrics.* Philadelphia, 1994, JB Lippincott.
*Hormonal methods of birth control do not afford protection against acquisition of STDs and HIV.
STD, Sexually transmitted disease; *HIV,* human imunodeficiency virus; *PID,* pelvic inflammatory disease.

TABLE 5.3.

OCP Information

	Contraindications	Use	Side effects: ACHES
ABSOLUTE	History of thrombophlebitis/ thromboembolic disease, stroke, ischemic heart disease, breast/liver cancer, estrogen dependent neoplasia, acute liver disease, benign hepatic adenoma, uncontrolled hypertension	1. Sunday start most common method 2. Start with low dose estrogen pill (less than or equal to 35 mcg) 3. 21 days hormonal pills, 7 days inactive pills 4. Advise patient about need for back-up methods during first month of use/STD, HIV prevention 5. Pelvic exam recommended at baseline or during first 3–6 months of use; then annually 6. 2–3 visits a year to monitor compliance, BP, side effects	**A**bdominal pain (pelvic vein/mesenteric vein thrombosis, pancreatitis) **C**hest pain (pulmonary embolism) **H**eadaches (thrombotic/ hemorrhagic stroke, retinal vein thrombosis) **E**ye symptoms (thrombotic/ hemorrhagic stroke, retinal vein thrombosis) **S**evere leg pain (thrombophlebitis of the lower extremity)
RELATIVE	Diabetes, heavy smoking (10–15 cigarettes per day), breast feeding, hypertension, sickle cell disease, active gallbladder disease, family history of hyperlipidemia		

From Bruner A: *Pediatric trends,* 1995, Johns Hopkins Hospital.

IV. VAGINAL INFECTIONS, GENITAL ULCERS, AND WARTS

A. Diagnostic Features and Management of Vaginal Infection in Premenopausal Adults (see Table 5.4 and Chapter 18 for discussion of chlamydia, gonorrhea, and PID)

TABLE 5.4.

	Normal vaginal exam	Yeast vaginitis	Trichomonal vaginitis	Bacterial vaginosis (NSV)
Etiology	Uninfected; *Lactobacillus* predominant	*Candida albicans* and other yeasts	*Trichomonas vaginalis*	Associated with *G. vaginalis,* various anaerobic bacteria, and mycoplasma
Typical symptoms	None	Vulvar itching and/or irritation, increased discharge	Profuse purulent discharge, vulvar itching	Malodorous, slightly increased discharge
Discharge:				
Amount	Variable; usually scant	Scant to moderate	Profuse	Moderate
Color*	Clear or white	White	Yellow	Usually white or gray
Consistency	Nonhomo-geneous, floccular	Clumped; adherent plaques	Homogeneous	Homogeneous, low viscosity; uniformly coating vaginal walls
Inflammation of vulvar or vaginal epithelium	None	Erythema of vaginal epithelium, introitus; vulvar dermatitis common	Erythema of vaginal and vulvar epithelium; colpitis macularis	None
pH of vaginal fluid†	Usually ≤4.5	Usually ≤4.5	Usually ≥5.0	Usually ≥4.7

(Continued.)

TABLE 5.4. (cont.)

Amine ("fishy") odor with 10% KOH	None	None	May be present	Present
Microscopy‡	Normal epithelial cells; lactobacilli predominate	Leukocytes, epithelial cells; yeast, mycelia, or pseudomycelia in up to 80%	Leukocytes; motile trichomonads seen in 80%–90% of symptomatic patients, less often in the absence of symptoms	Clue cells; few leukocytes; lactobacilli outnumbered by profuse mixed flora, nearly always including G. vaginalis plus anaerobic species, on Gram's stain
Usual treatment	None	Miconazole or clotrimazole intravaginally each 100 mg daily for 7 days Nystatin, 100,000 units intravaginally twice daily for 7–14 days	Metronidazole or tinidazole 2.0 g orally (single dose) *or* Metronidazole 500 mg orally twice daily for 7 days	Metronidazole 500 mg orally twice daily for 7 days *or* Metronidazole 2 g PO × 1
Usual management of sex partners	None	None; topical treatment if candidal dermatitis of penis is present	Examine for STD; treat with metronidazole, 2 g PO × 1	Examine for STD; no treatment if normal

From Holmes KK et al: *Sexually transmitted diseases,* New York, 1990, McGraw-Hill.
*Color of discharge is determined by examining vaginal discharge against the white background of a swab.
†pH determination is not useful if blood is present.
‡To detect fungal elements, vaginal fluid is digested with 10% KOH before microscopic examination; to examine for other features, fluid is mixed (1:1) with physiologic saline. Gram's stain also is excellent for detecting yeasts and pseudomycelia and for distinguishing normal flora from the mixed flora seen in bacterial vaginosis but is less sensitive than the saline preparation for detection of *T. vaginalis*.

B. **Diagnostic Features and Management of Genital Ulcers and Warts (see Table 5.5 and Formulary for additional information and comments regarding medications.)**
TABLE 5.5.

Infection	Appearance	Inguinal adenopathy	Presumptive diagnosis	Definitive diagnosis	Treatment/management of sex partners
Genital herpes	Grouped vesicles, painful shallow ulcers	Tender	Tzanck smear	Viral culture	No known cure. Prompt initiation of acyclovir therapy shortens duration of first episode. For severe recurrent disease, start therapy with Acyclovir at beginning of prodrome or within 2 days of onset of lesions (see Formulary for dose). Abstain from sex while lesions are present. Transmission can occur during asymptomatic periods. Women of child bearing age should inform providers during pregnancy about their HSV infection.

(Continued.) |

TABLE 5.5. (cont.)

Infection	Appearance	Inguinal adenopathy	Presumptive diagnosis	Definitive diagnosis	Treatment/management of sex partners
Primary syphilis	Indurated, well defined usually single painless ulcer. "Chancre"	Nontender	Darkfield microscopy	Darkfield microscopy, RPR/FTA	See Chapter 18 for antimicrobial therapy and indications. Abstain from sex during therapy.
Chancroid	Multiple, ragged, painful, nonindurated ulcer(s)	Painful, suppurative	Bipolar staining of gram-negative coccobacilli	Culture of *H. ducreyi*	Azithromycin 1 g PO × 1. or Ceftriaxone 250 mg IM in a single dose or Erythromycin 500 mg PO QID for 7 days. Sexual contacts within 10 days before onset of symptoms should be examined and treated. This should occur even in the absence of symptoms.

Lymphogranuloma venereum (LGV)	Transient, small ulcers, often multiple	Tender, most prominent feature, commonly unilateral	Complement fixation, Frie test, Serology	Culture of LGV specific *Chlamydia trachomatis*	Doxycycline 100 mg PO BID × 3–6 weeks. Sexual contacts within 30 days before onset of symptoms should be examined, tested for urethral or cervical chlamydial infection, and treated.
Granuloma inguinale (donovanosis)	Granulomatous painless nodules progressing to ulceration with sharply defined border	Not present, although lesions may mimic adenopathy	Giemsa or Wright stain demonstrating Donovan's bodies. History of travel to the tropics substantiates clinical impression	Biopsy of lesion. The dx agent is *Calymmatobacterium granulomatis*	Doxycycline 100 mg PO BID × 21 days or until lesion completely heals. Return weekly or biweekly for evaluation until infection is healed. Examine patient and partners for other STDs.

TABLE 5.5. (cont.)

Infection	Appearance	Inguinal adenopathy	Presumptive diagnosis	Definitive diagnosis	Treatment/management of sex partners
Genital warts (Human papillomavirus infection)	Single or multiple soft, fleshy papillary or sessile, painless growth around the anus, vulvovaginal area, penis, urethra, or perineum	Not present	Typical clinical presentation	Pap smear reveals typical cytologic changes	Treatment does not eradicate infection. Goal: removal of exophytic warts. Exclude cervical dysplasia before treatment. Cryotherapy with liquid nitrogen or cryoprobe (not for vaginal warts). Alternative: Podophyllin 10%–25% in compound tincture of benzoin (contraindicated in pregnancy). See package insert for more detailed information. Examine sex partners. Abstain during therapy. Period of communicability is unknown.

From Oski FA: *Principles and practice of pediatrics*, Philadelphia, 1994, JB Lippincott; and MMWR 42: i, 1993.

BLOOD CHEMISTRIES/ BODY FLUIDS

6

These values are compiled from the published literature and from the Johns Hopkins Hospital Department of Laboratory Medicine. Normal values vary with the analytic method used. If any doubt exists, consult your laboratory for its analytic method and range of normal values. Hematologic values may be found at the end of Chapter 15, and endocrine values may be found in Chapter 10.

From Meites S, editor: *Pediatric clinical chemistry* ed 2 and 3, 1981, The American Association for Clinical Chemistry; Tietz NW: *Textbook of clinical chemistry,* 1986; Lundberg GD et al: *JAMA* 260:73; 1988, Wallach, J: *Interpretation of diagnostic tests,* Boston 1992, Little Brown and Co.

I. TABLE 6.1.

	Conventional units	SI units
ACID PHOSPHATASE		
Newborn	7.4–19.4 U/L	7.4–19.4 U/L
2–13 yr	6.4–15.2 U/L	6.4–15.2 U/L
Adult male	0.5–11.0 U/L	0.5–11.0 U/L
Adult female	0.2–9.5 U/L	0.2–9.5 U/L
ALANINE AMINOTRANSFERASE (ALT)		
Infant	<54 U/L	<54 U/L
Child/adult	1–30 U/L	1–30 U/L
ALDOLASE		
Newborn	<32 U/L	<32 U/L
Child	<16 U/L	<8 U/L
Adult	<8 U/L	<8 U/L

(Continued.)

TABLE 6.1. (cont.)

	Conventional units	SI units
ALKALINE PHOSPHATASE		
Infant	150–420 U/L	150–420 U/L
2–10 yr	100–320 U/L	100–320 U/L
11–18 yr male	100–390 U/L	100–390 U/L
11–18 yr female	100–320 U/L	100–320 U/L
Adult	30–120 U/L	30–100 U/L
ALPHA-1 ANTITRYPSIN	93–224 mg/dl	0.93–2.24 g/L
ALPHA FETOPROTEIN		
Fetal (1st trimester)	200–400 mg/dl	Peak 2–4 g/L
Cord	<5 mg/dl	<0.05 g/L
>1yr–adult	<30 ng/ml	<30 mcg/L
Tumor marker	0–10 mg/ml	

AMMONIA NITROGEN (HEPARINIZED VENOUS SPECIMEN ON ICE WATER ANALYZED WITHIN 30 MINUTES)

	Conventional units	SI units
Newborn	90–150 mcg/dl	64–107 mcmol N/L
0–2 wk	79–129 mcg/dl	56–92 mcmol N/L
>1 mo	29–70 mcg/dl	21–50 mcmol N/L
Adult	0–50 mcg/dl	0–35.7 mcmol N/L
AMYLASE		
Newborn	0–44 U/L	5–65 U/L
Adult	0–88 U/L	0–130 U/L
ANTI-HYALURONIDASE ANTIBODY	<1:256	
ANTINUCLEAR ANTIBODY	<1:160	

ANTI-STREPTOLYSIN O TITER (4X RISE AT WEEKLY INTERVAL IS SIGNIFICANT)

Preschool	<1:85
School age	<1:170
Older adult	<1:85

Note: Alternatively, values up to 200 Todd units is normal.

ARSENIC

	Conventional units	SI units
Normal	<3 mcg/dl	<0.39 mcmol/L
Acute poisoning	60–930 mcg/dl	7.98–124 mcmol/L
Chronic poisoning	10–50 mcg/dl	1.33–6.65 mcmol/L

(Continued.)

TABLE 6.1. (cont.)

		Conventional units	SI units
ASPARTATE AMINOTRANSFERASE (AST)			
Newborn/infant		20–65 U/L	20–65 U/L
Child/adult		0–35 U/L	0–4350 U/L
BICARBONATE			
Premature		18–26 mEq/L	18–26 mmol/L
Full term		20–25 mEq/L	20–25 mmol/L
>2 yr		22–26 mEq/L	22–26 mmol/L
BILIRUBIN (TOTAL)			
Cord	Preterm	<1.8 mg/dl	<30 mcmol/L
	Term	<1.8 mg/dl	<30 mcmol/L
0–1 day	Preterm	<8 mg/dl	<137 mcmol/L
	Term	<6 mg/dl	<103 mcmol/L
1–2 days	Preterm	<12 mg/dl	<205 mcmol/L
	Term	<8 mg/dl	<137 mcmol/L
3–7 days	Preterm	<16 mg/dl	<274 mcmol/L
	Term	<12 mg/dl	<205 mcmol/L
7–30 days	Preterm	<12 mg/dl	<205 mcmol/L
	Term	<7 mg/dl	<120 mcmol/L
Thereafter	Preterm	<2 mg/dl	<34 mcmol/L
	Term	1.2 mg/dl	<20.5 mcmol/L
Adult		0.1–1.2 mg/dl	1.7–20.5 mcmol/L
BILIRUBIN (CONJUGATED)		0–0.4 mg/dl	0–8 mcmol/L
CALCIUM (TOTAL)			
Premature <1 wk		6–10 mg/dl	1.5–2.5 mmol/L
Full term <1 wk		7.0–12.0 mg/dl	1.75–3.0 mmol/L
Child		8.0–10.5 mg/dl	2–2.6 mmol/L
Adult		8.5–10.5 mg/dl	2.1–2.6 mmol/L
CALCIUM (IONIZED)			
Newborn <48 hr		4.0–4.7 mg/dl	1.00–1.18 mmol/L
Adult		4.52–5.28 mg/dl	1.13–1.32 mmol/L
CARBON DIOXIDE (CO_2 CONTENT)			
Cord blood		14–22 mEq/L	14–22 mmol/L
Infant/child		20–24 mEq/L	20–24 mmol/L
Adult		24–30 mEq/L	24–30 mmol/L

(Continued.)

TABLE 6.1. (cont.)

	Conventional units	SI units
CARBON MONOXIDE (CARBOXYHEMOGLOBIN)		
Nonsmoker	0%–2% of total hemoglobin	
Smoker	2%–10% of total hemoglobin	
Toxic	20%–60% of total hemoglobin	
Lethal	>60% of total hemoglobin	
CAROTENOIDS (CAROTENES)		
Infant	20–70 mcg/dl	0.37–1.30 mcmol/L
Child	40–130 mcg/dl	0.74–2.42 mcmol/L
Adult	50–250 mcg/dl	0.95–4.69 mcmol/L
CERULOPLASMIN	21–53 mg/dl	210–530 mg/L
CHLORIDE		
Pediatric	99–111 mEq/L	99–111 mmol/L
Adult	96–109 mEq/L	96–109 mEq/L
CHOLESTEROL	See Lipids	
COPPER		
0–6 mo	20–70 mcg/dl	3.1–11 mcmol/L
6 yr	90–190 mcg/dl	14–30 mmol/L
12 yr	80–160 mcg/dl	12.6–25 mcmol/L
Adult male	70–140 mcg/dl	11–22 mcmol/L
Adult female	80–155 mcg/dl	12.6–24.3 mcmol/L
C-REACTIVE PROTEIN		
	Negative	
CREATINE KINASE (CREATINE PHOSPHOKINASE)		
Newborn	10–200 U/L	10–200 U/L
Adult male	12–80 U/L	12–80 U/L
Adult female	10–55 U/L	10–55 U/L
CREATININE (SERUM)		
Cord	0.6–1.2 mg/dl	53–106 mcmol/L
Newborn	0.3–1.0 mg/dl	27–88 mcmol/L
Infant	0.2–0.4 mg/dl	18–35 mcmol/L
Child	0.3–0.7 mg/dl	27–62 mcmol/L
Adolescent	0.5–1.0 mg/dl	44–88 mcmol/L
Adult male	0.6–1.3 mg/dl	53–115 mcmol/L
Adult female	0.5–1.2 mg/dl	44–106 mcmol/L

(Continued.)

TABLE 6.1. (cont.)

	Conventional units	SI units
FERRITIN		
Newborn	25–200 ng/ml	25–200 mcg/L
1 mo	200–600 ng/ml	200–600 mcg/L
6 mo	50–200 ng/ml	50–200 mcg/L
6 mo–15 yr	7–140 ng/ml	7–140 mcg/L
Adult male	15–200 ng/ml	15–200 mcg/L
Adult female	12–150 ng/ml	12–150 mcg/L
FIBRINOGEN	200–400 mg/dl	2–4 g/L
FOLIC ACID (FOLATE)	>3 ng/ml	4.0–20.0 nmol/L
FOLIC ACID (RBCS)	153–605 mcg/ml RBC	
GALACTOSE		
Newborn	0–20 mg/dl	0–1.11 mmol/L
Thereafter	<5 mg/dl	<0.28 mmol/L
GAMMA-GLUTAMYL TRANSFERASE (GGT)		
Cord	19–270 U/L	19–270 U/L
Premature	56–233 U/L	56–233 U/L
0–3 wk	0–130 U/L	0–130 U/L
3 wk–3 mo	4–120 U/L	4–120 U/L
>3 mo male	5–65 U/L	5–65 U/L
>3 mo female	5–35 U/L	5–35 U/L
1–15 yr	0–23 U/L	0–23 U/L
Adult male	11–50 U/L	11–50 U/L
Adult female	7–32 U/L	7–32 U/L
GASTRIN	<100 pg/ml	100 ng/L
GLUCOSE (SERUM)		
Premature	45–100 mg/dl	1.1–3.6 mmol/L
Full term	45–120 mg/dl	1.1–6.4 mmol/L
1 wk–16 yr	60–105 mg/dl	3.3–5.8 mmol/L
>16 yr	70–115 mg/dl	3.9–6.4 mmol/L
IRON		
Newborn	100–250 mcg/dl	18–45 mcmol/L
Infant	40–100 mcg/dl	7–18 mcmol/L
Child	50–120 mcg/dl	9–22 mcmol/L

(Continued.)

TABLE 6.1. (cont.)

	Conventional units	SI units
Adult male	65–170 mcg/dl	12–30 mcmol/L
Adult female	50–170 mcg/dl	9–30 mcmol/L
KETONES		
Qualitative	Negative	
Quantitative	0.5–3.0 mg/dl	5–30 mg/L
LACTATE		
Capillary blood		
Newborn	<27 mg/dl	0.0–3.0 mmol/L
Child	5–20 mg/dl	0.56–2.25 mmol/L
Venous	5–20 mg/dl	0.5–2.2 mmol/L
Arterial	5–14 mg/dl	0.5–1.6 mmol/L
LACTATE DEHYDROGENASE (AT 37° C)		
Neonate	160–1500 U/L	160–1500 U/L
Infant	150–360 U/L	150–360 U/L
Child	150–300 U/L	150–300 U/L
Adult	0–220 U/L	0–220 U/L
LACTATE DEHYDROGENASE ISOENZYMES (% TOTAL)		
LD_1 heart	24%–34%	
LD_2 heart, erythrocytes	35%–45%	
LD_3 muscle	15%–25%	
LD_4 liver, trace muscle	4%–10%	
LD_5 liver, muscle	1%–9%	
LEAD (SEE CHAPTER 2)		
Child	<10 mcg/dl	<48 mcmol/L
LIPASE	4–24 U/dl	
LIPIDS		

	Cholesterol (mg/dl)			LDL (mg/dl)		
	Desirable	Borderline	High	Desirable	Borderline	High
Child/adolescent	<170	170–199	≥200	<110	110–129	≥130
Adults	<200	200–239	≥240	<130	130–159	≥160
Desirable HDL:	<35 mg/dl					

From Summary of the NCEP Adult Treatment Panel II Report, *JAMA*, 269:1993. Highlights of the report of the expert panel on blood and cholesterol levels in children and adolescents, 1991, US Dept. of Health and Human Services

TABLE 6.1. (cont.)

	Conventional units	SI units
MAGNESIUM	1.3–2.0 mEq/L	0.65–1.0 mmol/L
MANGANESE (BLOOD)		
Newborn	2.4–9.6 mcg/dl	2.44–1.75 mcmol/L
2–18 yr	0.8–2.1 mcg/dl	0.15–0.38 mcmol/L
METHEMOGLOBIN	0–1.3% of total hg	
OSMOLALITY	285–295 mOsm/kg	285–295 mmol/kg
PHENYLALANINE		
Premature	2.0–7.5 mg/dl	0.12–0.45 mmol/L
Newborn	1.2–3.4 mg/dl	0.07–0.21 mmol/L
Adult	0.8–1.8 mg/dl	0.05–0.11 mmol/L
PHOSPHOROUS		
Newborn	4.2–9.0 mg/dl	1.36–2.91 mmol/L
0–15 yr	3.2–6.3 mg/dl	1.03–2.1 mmol/L
Adult	2.7–4.5 mg/dl	0.87–1.45 mmol/L
PORCELAIN	10–25 mg/dl	2.67–8.01 mmol/L
POTASSIUM		
<10 days of age	4.0–6.0 mEq/L	4.0–6.0 mmol/L
>10 days of age	3.5–5.0 mEq/L	3.5–5.0 mmol/L
PREALBUMIN		
Newborn–6 wk	4–36 mg/dl	
6 wk–16 yr	13–27 mg/dl	
Adult	18–45 mg/dl	

TABLE 6.1 (cont.)

PROTEINS

Age	TP	Alb.	A-1	A-2	Beta	Gamma
			Protein electrophoresis g/dl (100ml)			
Cord	4.8–8.0	2.2–4.0	0.3–0.7	0.4–0.9	0.4–1.6	0.8–1.6
Newborn	4.4–7.6	3.2–4.8	0.1–0.3	0.2–0.3	0.3–0.6	0.6–1.2
1d–1 mo	4.4–7.6	2.5–5.5	0.1–0.3	0.3–1.0	0.2–1.1	0.4–1.3
1–3 mo	3.6–7.4	2.1–4.8	0.1–0.4	0.3–1.1	0.3–1.1	0.2–1.1
4–6 mo	4.2–7.4	2.8–5.0	0.1–0.4	0.3–0.8	0.3–0.8	0.1–0.9
7–12 mo	5.1–7.5	3.2–5.7	0.1–0.6	0.3–1.5	0.4–1.0	0.2–1.2
13–24 mo	3.7–7.5	1.9–5.0	0.1–0.6	0.4–1.4	0.4–1.4	0.4–1.6
25–36 mo	5.3–8.1	3.3–5.8	0.1–0.3	0.4–1.1	0.3–1.2	0.4–1.5
3–5 yr	4.9–8.1	2.9–5.8	0.1–0.4	0.4–1.0	0.5–1.0	0.4–1.7
6–8 yr	6.0–7.9	3.3–5.0	0.1–0.5	0.5–0.8	0.5–0.9	0.7–2.0
9–11 yr	6.0–7.9	3.2–5.0	0.1–0.4	0.7–0.9	0.6–1.0	0.8–2.0
12–16 yr	6.0–7.9	3.2–5.1	0.1–0.4	0.5–1.1	0.5–1.1	0.6–2.0
Adult	6.0–8.0	3.1–5.4	0.1–0.4	0.4–1.1	0.5–1.2	0.7–1.7

	Conventional units	SI units
PYRUVATE	0.3–0.9 mg/dl	0.03–0.10 mmol/L

RHEUMATOID FACTOR
<20

RHEUMATON TITER (MODIFIED WAALER-ROSE SLIDE TEST)
<10

SODIUM

Premature	130–140 mEq/L	130–140 mmol/L
Older	135–148 mEq/L	135–148 mmol/L

TRANSAMINASE (SGOT)
 See AST (aspartate aminotransferase)

TRANSAMINASE (SGPT)
 See ALT (alanine aminotransferase)

TRANSFERRIN

Newborn	130–275 mg/dl	1.3–2.75 g/L
Adult	200–400 mg/dl	2.0–4.0 g/L

UREA NITROGEN	7–22 mg/dl	2.5–7.9 mmol/L

TABLE 6.1. (cont.)

	Conventional units	SI units
URIC ACID		
0–2 yr	2.4–6.4 mg/dl	0.14–0.38 mmol/L
2–12 yr	2.4–5.9 mg/dl	0.14–0.35 mmol/L
12–14 yr	2.4–6.4 mg/dl	0.14–0.38 mmol/L
Adult male	3.5–7.2 mg/dl	0.20–0.43 mmol/L
Adult female	2.4–6.4 mg/dl	0.14–0.38 mmol/L
VITAMIN A (RETINOL)		
Newborn	35–75 mcg/dl	1.22–2.62 mcmol/L
Child	30–80 mcg/dl	1.05–2.79 mcmol/L
Adult	30–65 mcg/dl	1.05–2.27 mcmol/L
VITAMIN B$_1$ (THIAMINE)	5.3–7.9 mcg/dl	0.16–0.23 mcmol/L
VITAMIN B$_2$ (RIBOFLAVIN)	3.7–13.7 mcg/dl	98–363 mcmol/L
VITAMIN B$_{12}$ (COBALAMIN)	130–785 pg/ml	96–579 pmol/L
VITAMIN C (ASCORBIC ACID)	0.2–2.0 mg/dl	11.4–113.6 mcmol/L
VITAMIN D$_3$ (1,25 DIHYDROXY)	25–45 pg/ml	60–108 pmol/L
VITAMIN E	5–20 mg/dl	11.6–46.4 mcmol/L
ZINC	70–150 mcg/dl	10.7–22.9 mcmol/L

II. EVALUATION OF PLEURAL, PERICARDIAL, AND AS-CITIC FLUID
A. Transudate vs. Exudate (Table 6.2)
B. Other Information
1. For pleural fluid, amylase >500 U/ml or fluid: serum ratio >1 suggests pancreatitis.
2. For ascitic fluid, white blood cells (WBCs) >800 cells/mm^3 suggests peritonitis.

From Wallach J: *Interpretation of diagnostic tests,* Boston, 1992, Little Brown and Co.

TABLE 6.2.

Measurement†	Transudate	Exudate
Specific gravity	< 1.016	> 1.016
Protein (g/dL)	< 3.0	> 3.0
Fluid: serum ratio	< 0.5	> 0.5
LDH (IU)	< 200	> 200
Fluid: serum ratio (isoenzymes not useful)	< 0.6	> 0.6
WBC	< 1000/mm^3 (lymphs)	> 1000/mm^3
RBC	< 10,000	Variable
Glucose	Same as serum	Decreased
pH*	7.4–7.5	< 7.4

*Collect anaerobically in a heparinized syringe.
†Always get serum for glucose, LDH, protein, amylase, etc.
LDH, Lactate dehydrogenase; *WBC*, white blood cell; *RBC*, red blood cell.

III. EVALUATION OF CEREBROSPINAL FLUID
   For normal valves, see Table 6.3.

IV. EVALUATION OF SYNOVIAL FLUID (Table 6.4)

TABLE 6.3.

Evaluation of Cerebrospinal Fluid

CELL COUNT

Preterm mean	9.0 (0–25.4 WBC/mm³)	57% PMNs
Term mean	8.2 (0–22.4 WBC/mm³)	61% PMNs
Child	0–7 WBC/mm³	0% PMNs

GLUCOSE

Preterm	24–63 mg/dl (mean 50)
Term	34–119 mg/dl (mean 52)
Child	40–80 mg/dl

CSF GLUCOSE/BLOOD GLUCOSE

Preterm	55%–105%
Term	44%–128%
Child	50%

LACTIC ACID DEHYDROGENASE

Mean	20 (5–30 U/L), or about 10% of serum value

MYELIN BASIC PROTEIN <4 ng/ml

OPENING PRESSURE

Newborn	80–110 (<110 mm H_2O)
Infant/child	<200 mm H_2O (lateral recumbent)
Respirations	5–10 mm H_2O

PROTEIN

Preterm	Mean 115 (65–150 mg/dl)
Term	Mean 90 (20–170 mg/dl)
Child	5–40 mg/dl

From Oski FA: *Principles and practice of pediatrics,* ed 2, Philadelphia, 1994, JB Lippincott.

TABLE 6.4.

Evaluation of Synovial Fluid

Group	Condition	Synovial complement	Viscosity	Color/clarity	Mucin clot	WBC count	PMN (%)	Miscellaneous findings
Noninflammatory	Normal	N	VH	Yellow Clear	G	<200	<25	
	Traumatic arthritis	N	H	Xanthochromic Turbid	F–G	<2,000	<25	Debris
	Osteoarthritis	N	H	Yellow Clear	F–G	1,000	<25	
Inflammatory	SLE	→	N	Yellow Clear	N	5,000	10	LE cells
	Rheumatic fever	N – ↑	→	Yellow Cloudy	F	5,000	10–50	
	Juvenile rheumatoid arthritis	N – →	→	Yellow Cloudy	Poor	15,000–20,000	75	
	Reiter's syndrome	↑	→	Yellow Opaque	Poor	20,000	80	Reiter's cells
Pyogenic	Tuberculous arthritis	N – ↑	→	Yellow-white Cloudy	Poor	25,000	50–60	Acid-fast bacteria
	Septic arthritis	↑	→	Serosanguinous Turbid	Poor	50,000–300,000	>75	Low glucose, bacteria

N, Normal; VH, very high; H, high; G, good; F, fair; ↓, decreased; ↑, increased.
From Cassidy JT, Petty RE: *Textbook of pediatric rheumatology*, ed 3, Philadelphia, 1995, WB Saunders.

126

CARDIOLOGY 7

I. CARDIAC CYCLE (FIG. 7.1)

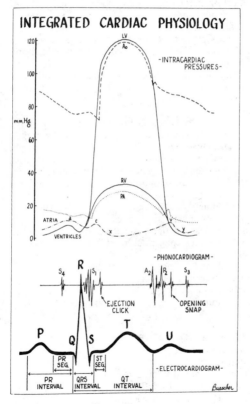

FIG. 7.1. The cardiac cycle.

II. USE OF THE CHEST X-RAY EXAM
A. Heart
  1. Size
  2. Situs (levocardia, mesocardia, dextrocardia)
  3. Although there are classic shapes for several well-known lesions (e.g., the "boot" for tetralogy of Fallot, or the "egg on a shoestring" for transposition of the great arteries), the shapes vary widely enough that they are often not useful.
B. Lung Fields
  1. Pulmonary blood flow: Decreased in pulmonary stenosis, tetralogy of Fallot, increased in left-to-right shunting lesions
  2. Evidence of venous congestion in patients with total anomalous pulmonary venous return or mitral valve stenosis or regurgitation
C. Airway
  The trachea usually bends slightly to the right above the carina in normal patients with a left-sided aortic arch; a perfectly straight or left-bending trachea suggests a right aortic arch, which is usually associated with other defects. Also, asplenia and polysplenia syndromes usually have anomalies of the mainstem bronchial branching and lobation.
D. Abdominal Situs
  1. Asplenia/polysplenia syndromes
  2. Abnormalities of abdominal situs are usually associated with complex congenital heart disease.
E. Skeletal Anomalies
  1. Rib notching (e.g., coarctation of the aorta)
  2. Sternal abnormalities (e.g., Down syndrome)
  3. Vertebral anomalies (e.g., VATER association)
  4. Limb anomalies (e.g., Holt-Oram syndrome) (Fig. 7.2.)

III. ELECTROCARDIOGRAPHY
A. Lead Placement
  1. Bipolar leads
    a. Lead I: Right arm-left arm
    b. Lead II: Right arm-left leg
    c. Lead III: Left arm-left leg

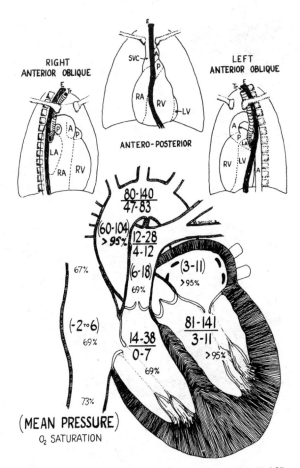

FIG. 7.2. X-ray contour of the heart, which includes normal pressures and saturations. Plain films of the chest are a valuable part of the initial workup of congenital heart disease.

2. Unipolar leads
   a. aVR: Right arm
   b. aVL: Left arm
   c. aVF: Left foot
3. Precordial leads (Fig. 7.3)

B.   Terminology
1. P wave: Atrial depolarization
2. QRS complex: Ventricular depolarization
   a. Q wave: The first negative deflection before a positive deflection
   b. R wave: The first positive deflection

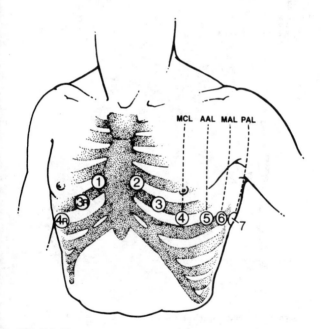

FIG. 7.3. Placement of precordial leads.

      c. S wave: The negative deflection following the R wave
      d. QS wave: A monophasic negative complex
      e. R′ wave: The second positive deflection
      f. S′ wave: The second negative deflection
   3. T wave: Ventricular repolarization
   4. U wave: May follow the T wave

C.   **Rate**
   1. Determination
     a. Standard ECG paper speed is 25 mm/sec.
     b. 1 mm = one small square = 0.04 sec; 5 mm = one
        large square = 0.2 sec
     c. Heart rate = 60 divided by (average R-R interval in
        seconds)
     d. Record both atrial and ventricular rates when AV
        block is present.
     e. Fig. 7.4 summarizes the method for estimating the
        rate based on the R-R interval in 0.2 second incre-
        ments.

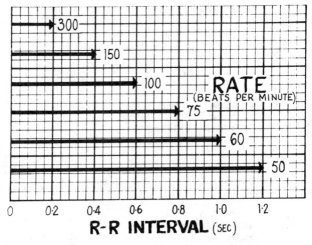

FIG. 7.4. Estimation of the rate based on the R-R interval.

2. Age-specific heart rates (beats/min) (Table 7.1)

TABLE 7.1.

Age	2%	Mean	98%
<1 day	93	123	154
1–2 days	91	123	159
3–6 days	91	129	166
1–3 wk	107	148	182
1–2 mo	121	149	179
3–5 mo	106	141	186
6–11 mo	109	134	169
1–2 yr	89	119	151
3–4 yr	73	108	137
5–7 yr	65	100	133
8–11 yr	62	91	130
12–15 yr	60	85	119

D. **Intervals**
   1. P-R Interval with rate and age (and upper limits of normal) (Table 7.2)
   2. QTc (corrected QT interval): QT interval varies with and should be corrected for rate.
      a. Equation

$$QTc = \frac{\text{measured QT(sec)}}{\sqrt{\text{R-R interval (sec)}}}$$

      b. Normal values: QTc should not exceed the following:
         1) 0.45 in infants <6 mo,
         2) 0.44 in children,
         3) 0.425 in adolescents and adults.
E. **Axis** (Fig. 7.5)
   1. P wave axis: The normal frontal P wave axis in sinus rhythm is 0–90°.
   2. QRS axis: The normal frontal QRS axis is age specific (Table 7.3)
   3. T wave axis (see Table 7.4)
F. **Atrial Enlargement**
   1. Right atrial enlargement (RAE): Peaked P wave, >3 mm (normal standardization = 10 mv/mm) in any lead (best seen in II, III, V_3R, and V_1)

TABLE 7.2.

Rate	0–1 mo	1–6 mo	6 mo–1 yr	1–3 yr	3–8 yr	8–12 yr	12–16 yr	Adult
<60						0.16(0.18)	0.16(0.19)	0.17(0.21)
60–80	0.10(0.12)				0.15(0.17)	0.15(0.17)	0.15(0.18)	0.16(0.21)
80–100	0.10(0.12)				0.14(0.16)	0.15(0.16)	0.15(0.17)	0.15(0.20)
100–120	0.10(0.11)	0.11(0.14)		(0.15)	0.13(0.16)	0.14(0.15)	0.15(0.16)	0.15(0.19)
120–140		0.10(0.13)	0.11(0.14)	0.12(0.14)	0.13(0.15)	0.14(0.15)		0.15(0.18)
140–160	0.09(0.11)	0.10(0.12)	0.11(0.13)	0.11(0.14)	0.12(0.14)			(0.17)
160–180	0.10(0.11)	0.10(0.12)	0.10(0.12)	0.10(0.12)				
>180	0.09	0.09(0.11)	0.10(0.11)					

Modified from Guntheroth WG: *Pediatric Electrocardiography*. Philadelphia, 1965, WB Saunders.

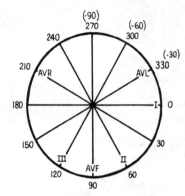

FRONTAL AXIS

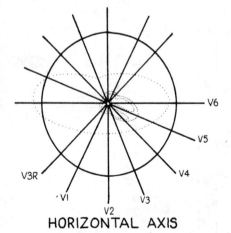

HORIZONTAL AXIS

FIG. 7.5. Frontal and horizontal axes.

TABLE 7.3.

QRS Axis

Age	2%	Mean	98%
<1 day	59	137	−167
1–2 days	64	134	−161
3–6 days	77	132	−167
1–3 wk	65	110	161
1–2 mo	31	74	113
3–5 mo	1	60	104
6–11 mo	1	56	99
1–2 yr	1	55	101
3–4 yr	1	55	104
5–7 yr	1	65	143
8–11 yr	1	61	119
12–15 yr	1	59	130

2. Left atrial enlargement (LAE)
    a. P wave duration >0.10 sec; may have "plateau" or "notched" contour
    b. Terminal and deep inversion of the P wave in V_3R or V_1 (Fig. 7.6)
G. **Ventricular Hypertrophy**
    1. Normal voltage range for R and S waves: Voltages are measured in millimeters, 1 mV = 10 mm paper (Table 7.5.)
    2. Normal R/S ratios (Table 7.5)
    3. Criteria for right ventricular hypertrophy
        a. Primary criteria—at least one of criteria below
            1) R in V_1 above the 98th percentile for age
            2) S in V_6 above the 98th percentile for age

TABLE 7.4.

T Wave Axis

Age	V_1, V_2	aVF	I, V_5, V_6
Birth–1 day	±	+	±
1–4 days	±	+	+
4 days–adolescent	−	+	+
Adolescent–adult	+	+	+

+, T wave positive; −, T wave negative; ±, T wave normally either positive or negative.

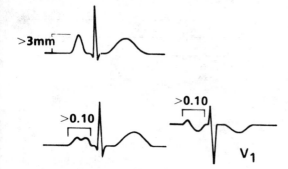

FIG. 7.6. Criteria for atrial enlargement.

3) Upright T wave in V_1 after 3 days of age until adolescence
- T wave up in V_1, with normal R = mild RVH
- T wave up in V_1, with tall R wave = severe RVH
- T wave down in V_1, with tall R wave = RV strain

b. Secondary criteria—may be used in conjunction with primary criteria to support a diagnosis of RVH
1) R/S ratio in V_1 above the 98% for age
2) R/S ratio in V_6 < 1 after one month of age
3) A qR pattern in V_1
4) Normal duration RSR′ in V_{3R} or V_1 with R′ >15 mm if < 1 yr; >10 mm thereafter (suggestive of diastolic volume overload [e.g., ASD])

4. Right ventricular hypertrophy in the newborn—at least one of criteria below
a. Pure R wave in V_1 > 10 mm
b. R in V_1 > 25 mm, or R in a VR > 8 mm
c. Right axis deviation > +180°

5. Criteria for left ventricular hypertrophy
a. Primary criteria—at least one of criteria below
1) R in V_6 above the 98th percentile for age
- Tall R waves in II, III, and aVF reflect pressure overload (aortic stenosis)

TABLE 7.5.

R VOLTAGES ACCORDING TO LEAD AND AGE

Lead	<1 day	1–2 days	3–6 days	1–3 wk	1–2 mo	3–5 mo	6–11 mo	1–2 yr	3–4 yr	5–7 yr	8–11 yr	12–15 yr
2%	5.2	5.3	2.8	3.2	3.3	2.7	1.4	2.6	1.0	0.5	0.0	0.0
V_1 Mean	13.8	14.4	12.9	10.6	9.5	9.8	9.4	8.9	8.1	6.7	5.4	4.1
98%	26.1	26.9	24.2	20.8	18.4	19.8	20.3	17.7	18.2	13.9	12.1	9.9
2%	0.0	0.0	0.3	2.6	5.2	6.4	5.8	5.9	8.1	8.4	9.2	6.5
V_6 Mean	4.2	4.5	5.2	7.6	11.6	13.1	12.6	13.3	14.8	16.3	16.3	14.3
98%	11.1	12.2	12.1	16.4	21.4	22.4	22.7	22.6	24.4	26.5	25.4	23.0

S VOLTAGES ACCORDING TO LEAD AND AGE

Lead	<1 day	1–2 days	3–6 days	1–3 wk	1–2 mo	3–5 mo	6–11 mo	1–2 yr	3–4 yr	5–7 yr	8–11 yr	12–15 yr
2%	0.0	0.0	0.0	0.0	0.0	0.0	0.4	0.7	1.8	2.9	2.7	2.8
V_1 Mean	8.5	9.1	6.6	4.2	5.0	5.7	6.4	8.4	10.2	12.0	11.9	10.8
98%	22.7	20.7	16.8	10.8	12.4	17.1	18.1	21.0	21.4	23.8	25.4	21.2
2%	0.0	0.0	0.0	0.0	0.0	0.0	0.0	0.0	0.0	0.0	0.0	0.0
V_6 Mean	3.2	3.0	3.5	3.4	2.7	2.9	2.1	1.9	1.5	1.2	1.0	0.8
98%	9.6	9.4	9.8	9.8	6.4	9.9	7.2	6.6	5.2	4.0	3.9	3.7

R/S RATIOS ACCORDING TO LEAD AND AGE

Lead	<1 day	1–2 days	3–6 days	1–3 wk	1–2 mo	3–5 mo	6–11 mo	1–2 yr	3–4 yr	5–7 yr	8–11 yr	12–15 yr
2%	0.1	0.1	0.2	1.0	0.3	0.1	0.1	0.05	0.03	0.02	0.0	0.0
V_1 Mean	2.2	2.0	2.7	2.9	2.3	2.3	1.6	1.4	0.9	0.7	0.5	0.5
98%	U	U	U	U	U	U	3.9	4.3	2.8	2.0	1.8	1.7
2%	0.0	0.0	0.1	0.1	0.2	0.2	0.2	0.3	0.6	0.9	1.5	1.4
V_6 Mean	2.0	2.5	2.2	3.3	4.8	6.2	7.6	9.3	10.8	11.5	14.3	14.7
98%	U	U	U	U	U	U	U	U	U	U	U	U

Note: U = undefined (S wave may equal zero)

• Tall R waves in V_5 and V_6 reflect volume overload (PDA)

2) S in V_1 above the 98th percentile for age
3) Inverted T waves in V_6 are always abnormal and suggest LV strain.

b. Secondary criteria—may be used in conjunction with primary criteria to support a diagnosis of LVH
1) R/S ratio in V_1 below the 2nd percentile for age
2) Q wave >4 mm in V_5 or V_6 (suggests volume overload)

6. Precautions
a. In the event of abnormal conduction, abnormal cardiac position, or complex congenital heart disease, these criteria may not be applicable.
b. There is a gradual progression from LV to RV predominance as an infant approaches term. Therefore these conventional electrocardiographic criteria for interpretation of ventricular hypertrophy are not reliable in the premature infant.

H. **Superiorly Oriented Vector**
1. S wave > R wave in aVF
2. aVF is downgoing with a QRS axis between 0° and −90°
3. An abnormally superior vector is associated with endocardial cushion defects (especially with RVH), double outlet right ventricle, transposition with large VSD, hypoplastic right ventricle with tricuspid atresia (especially with LVH), and Noonan syndrome.

From Liebman J, Plonsey R, Gilette P: *Pediatric Electrocardiography,* Baltimore, 1982, Williams & Wilkins.

I. **The ECG and Myocardial Infarction in Children**
1. Predisposing conditions: Myocardial infarction (MI) and ischemia (see below) in children occur infrequently but can be seen in the setting of such diseases as anomalous origin of the coronary artery from the pulmonary artery, myocarditis, Kawasaki disease (with coronary artery aneurysms), asphyxia, cocaine ingestion, and adrenergic drugs (e.g., beta agonists in asthma).
2. ECG criteria for MI have not been well established in children, and adult criteria may not be useful; however, the following criteria have been proposed recently:

        a. New-onset Q waves >35 msec in duration
        b. Increased amplitude/duration (>35 msec) of preexisting Q waves
        c. New-onset Q waves in serial tracings
        d. Notching of Q waves
        e. ST segment elevation (>2 mm) and long QTc (> 440 msec) when associated with any other criterion

Note: These criteria seem to be useful in detecting acute MI but are less useful for diagnosing nonacute MI in children. They may provide a useful adjunct to other tests of myocardial injury, such as creatine phosphokinase (CPK)/MB fraction and lactate dehydrogenase (LDH).

From JA, Bricker TB, Garson A: Electrocardiographic criteria for diagnosis of acute myocardial infarction in childhood, *Am J Cardiol* 69:1545, 1992.

      3. Myocardial ischemia may be subtle to detect. An ECG may exhibit flat or inverted T waves overlying the ischemic area. In the case of subendocardial ischemia, however, peaked and symmetrical T waves overlie the ischemic area.

From Garson A Jr: Electrocardiography. In *The Science and Practice of Pediatric Cardiology,* Philadelphia, 1990, Lea and Febiger.

J.   Conduction and Rhythm Disturbances
      1. Sinus arrhythmia
        a. Definition: Normal respiratory variation of the RR interval without morphologic changes of the P wave or QRS complex
        b. ECG

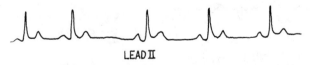

LEAD II

      2. Sinus bradycardia
        a. Definition: Heart rate less than 5th percentile for age with normal sinus rhythm
        b. ECG

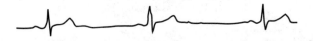

    c. Treatment: Usually indicated only in symptomatic patients

      1) Treatment based on underlying cause such as hypoxemia, hypercapnea, acidosis, increased intracranial pressure

      2) Epinephrine: 0.01 mg/kg bolus IV/IO or 0.1 mg/kg per ETT. May repeat every 3–5 minutes at same dose.

      3) Atropine: 0.02 mg/kg IV bolus (min dose 0.1 mg; max single dose 0.5 mg for child, 1 mg for adolescent)

      4) Isoproterenol drip: 0.1 mcg/kg/min. May increase every 5–10 minutes by 0.1 mcg/kg/min (max dose 2 mcg/kg/min).

3. Sinus tachycardia

    a. Definition: Heart rate greater than 95th percentile for age with normal sinus rhythm. Causes include sepsis, fever, hypovolemia, etc. Rate is usually less than 230/min. Rate may vary with respiration. P waves are same as sinus P waves and are almost always visible. QRS morphology same as slower sinus rhythm.

    b. Treatment: Treat underlying cause.

4. Low right atrial pacemaker (coronary sinus rhythm)

    a. Definition: Shortened to normal PR interval with positive P in I, negative P in II, III, aVF. P wave axis is 180°–360°

    b. ECG

LEAD I   LEAD III   LEAD AVF

5. Left atrial rhythm

    a. Definition: Varying P configurations in limb leads depending on site of origin (high, low, mid); however, frequently negative in I and positive in III. Dome and dart configuration diagnostic of left atrial rhythm with the dome representing the left atrium and the dart the right atrium. Best seen in II and V_1. P wave axis is 90°–270°.

b. ECG

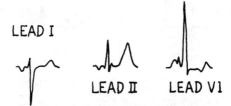

6. Premature atrial contraction (PAC)
   a. Definition: Premature beat with abnormal P wave, normal QRS complexes, and usually not followed by a fully compensatory pause.
   b. ECG

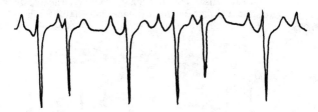

   c. Treatment: Usually stable. No treatment required.
7. PAC with aberrancy
   a. Definition: Similar to PAC, but with wide QRS complex resembling a right bundle branch block (RBBB) or left bundle branch block (LBBB) pattern. The initial vector is often in the same direction as the normal sinus QRS.
   b. ECG

Lead V₁

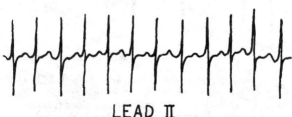

V₁

8. Supraventricular tachycardia (PAT or SVT)
   a. Definition: Normal QRS complexes at a rapid rate
      with or without discernible P waves. After the first
      10–20 beats, the QRS in SVT almost always has
      the same morphology as the QRS in sinus rhythm.
      If after the first 10–20 beats the QRS has a BBB
      pattern, consider ventricular tachycardia (see p.
      152). History usually noncontributory; usually
      rate greater than 230 bpm (infants 260–300); 60% have
      visible P waves; however, the P waves usually do
      not look like the sinus P waves.
   b. ECG

LEAD II

   c. Treatment
      1) Vagal maneuvers (i.e., ice to face, knee to chest,
         valsalva, carotid massage)
      2) Adenosine: 0.1 mg/kg/dose rapid IV push. If no
         effect may double dose and repeat. Max single
         dose 12 mg. (IV should be as close to the heart
         as possible.)
      3) Digoxin (see Formulary)

4) Beta blockade (e.g., esmolol) (see Formulary)
5) Synchronous cardioversion 0.5–1.0 joules/kg (do not delay in unstable patient)
6) Atrial esophageal overdrive pacing
7) Procainamide drip (see Formulary)

9. Wolff-Parkinson-White (WPW)
   a. Definition: Prolonged QRS duration and shortened PR interval secondary to initial slurring of the upstroke of the QRS (delta wave)
   b. ECG

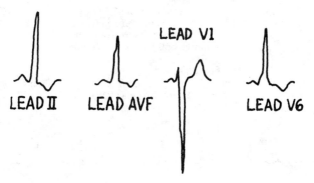

c. Treatment
   1) See treatment of SVT above.
   2) Obliteration of accessory pathway may be required if recurrent SVT.

Note: If a delta wave is present and treating to prevent recurrence of SVT, do not use digoxin or verapamil. Beta blockers are the treatment of choice.

10. Atrial flutter
    a. Definition: Normal QRS complexes, flutter (p) waves between QRS complexes. 92% have abnormal heart. Atrial rate is usually 250–500 bpm. Ventricular 1:1 to 4:1 conduction. May have variable block giving different ventricular rates.
    b. ECG

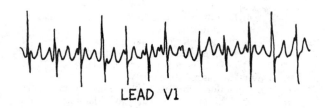

LEAD V1

    c. Treatment
      1) Digoxin (see Formulary)
      2) Synchronous cardioversion 0.5–1.0 joules/kg
      3) Atrial esophageal overdrive pacing
      4) Quinidine orally or procainamide IV (see Formulary)
  11. Atrial fibrillation
    a. Definition: Normal QRS complexes, absent P waves, irregularly irregular RR interval
    b. ECG

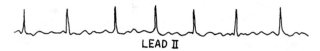

LEAD II

    c. Treatment: Emergency treatment usually not required; however, if acute or if hemodynamic changes occur:
      1) Digoxin to slow ventricular rate
      2) Beta-blockers to slow ventricular rate (e.g., atenolol)
      3) Cardioversion 0.5–1.0 joules/kg; recurrence common

Note: Must anticoagulate before cardioversion.

      4) Quinidine to prevent recurrence
  12. First degree AV block
    a. Definition: PR interval longer than normal for age and rate (see Table 7.2).
    b. ECG

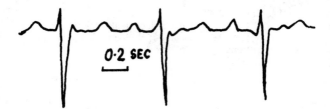

13. Second degree AV block
    a. Definition: Atrial rate greater than ventricular rate with conduction of the atrial impulse at regular intervals (i.e., every other [2:1 block], every third [3:1 block], three atrials for every 2 ventricular [3:2 block]).
    b. Types and ECG
       1) Type I (Wenckebach): Progressive lengthening of the PR interval until an atrial impulse is not conducted and a ventricular contraction does not occur. P-P interval is regular, R-R interval shortens. The pause is less than 2 times the P-P interval. Usually does not progress to complete heart block.

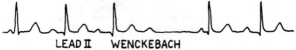

LEAD II   WENCKEBACH

       2) Type II: Paroxysmal skipped ventricular contractions without lengthening of the PR interval. May progress to complete heart block.

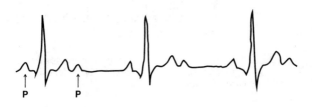

14. Complete AV block
    a. Definition: No conducted atrial impulses (complete AV dissociation), with a slow unrelated junctional or ventricular rhythm
    b. ECG

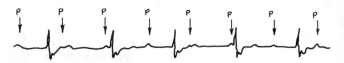

    c. Treatment
        1) Epinephrine: 0.01 mg/kg bolus IV/IO or 0.1 mg/kg per ETT. May repeat every 3–5 minutes at same dose.
        2) Atropine: 0.02 mg/kg IV bolus (min dose 0.1 mg; max single dose 0.5 mg for child; 1 mg for adolescent)
        3) Isoproterenol drip: 0.1 mcg/kg/min. May increase every 5–10 minutes by 0.1 mcg/kg/min (max dose 2 mcg/kg/min)
        4) Pacemaker may be required.
15. AV dissociation with junctional tachycardia
    a. Definition: Failed conduction of atrial impulse through AV node with a faster independent nodal or ventricular rhythm
    b. ECG

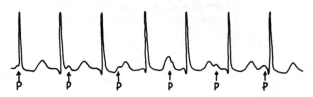

    c. Treatment: Usually seen in postoperative period. Will not respond to vagal maneuvers, adenosine, or cardioversion.

      1) Avoid anything inducing endogenous catecholamines (e.g., fever, agitation, pain). Avoid exogenous catecholamines (e.g., epinephrine).
      2) Digoxin (see Formulary)
      3) Hypothermia
      4) Procainamide drip (see Formulary)
      5) Amiodarone IV (see Formulary)

16. Complete bundle branch block (BBB)
   a. Definition: The normal QRS duration is less than 0.08 seconds for children under 2 years of age, less than 0.09 seconds for 2–8 years, and less than 0.10 seconds over 8 years. BBB is present when QRS is prolonged.
   b. Complete left BBB (LBBB)
     1) Definition: Monophasic R wave in I; absence of Q wave in V_6. (LBBB is rare in children; WPW frequently mimics LBBB.)
     2) ECG

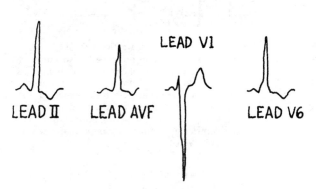

LEAD II   LEAD AVF   LEAD V1   LEAD V6

   c. Complete right BBB (RBBB)
     1) Wide S wave in I, V_6; M-shaped QRS (RSR′ in V_1, right axis deviation [RAD]).
     2) ECG

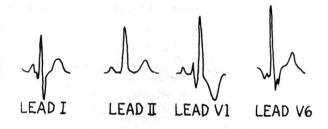

LEAD I   LEAD II   LEAD V1   LEAD V6

17. Left anterior hemiblock
    a. Definition: Normal QRS duration, left axis deviation; qR in I, rS in III.
    b. ECG

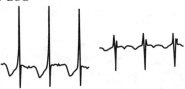

18. Premature ventricular contraction (PVC)
    a. Definition: Unusually prolonged QRS complexes that always differ morphologically from sinus; ST segments slope away from QRS, and T waves are inverted. PVCs occur before the expected atrial beat and are usually followed by a compensatory pause. Bigeminy is alternating normal and abnormal ventricular complexes. Couplets are two consecutive PVCs.
    b. ECG

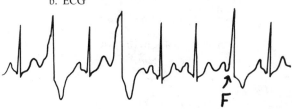

   c. Treatment
     1) Usually indicated only in symptomatic patients
     2) Investigate underlying cause (e.g., drugs, metabolic derangement, myocarditis, etc.).
     3) Lidocaine 1 mg/kg IV bolus, then 20–50 mcg/kg/min
     4) Procainamide or quinidine (see Formulary)
19. Fusion beat
   a. Definition: Characteristics of both a sinus beat and a PVC. It has the same early activation of a sinus beat and late activation of a PVC. (*Arrow* in preceding PVC figure marks fusion beat.)
20. Ventricular tachycardia (VT)
   a. Definition: ≥3 serial PVCs occurring at a rapid rate. P waves, if present, may be dissociated. Usually no Q wave in V_{5-6}. Presence of fusion beats before onset or at termination of VT is usually diagnostic. The QRS in VT is wider than the upper limit of normal for age (see section above under complete heart block for normals for age). If (after 10–20 beats) morphology of the QRS differs from the sinus QRS, the diagnosis is probably VT.

Note: 70% have abnormal heart. Rate is usually less than 250 bpm (infants 250–500). May have sinus P waves that are unrelated to VT (AV dissociation), retrograde P waves, or no visible P waves.

   b. ECG

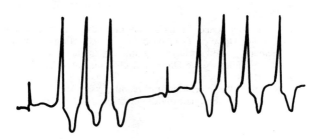

    c. Treatment
      1) Hemodynamically stable
- Lidocaine: 1 mg/kg bolus IV then 20–50 mcg/kg/min
- Bretylium: 5 mg/kg rapid IV infusion

      2) Hemodynamically unstable
- See decision tree back cover.
- Remember to treat underlying illness.

      3) Pulseless V-tach (see decision tree back cover)
21. Ventricular fibrillation
    a. Definition: Rapid irregular ventricular depolarization, low voltage, without identifiable QRS complexes. Rare in children.

Note: Asystole (more common in children) may be mistaken for fine ventricular fibrillation.

    b. ECG

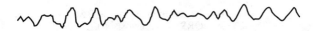

    c. Treatment (See Decision Tree-back inside cover)
K.   **Systemic Effects on Electrocardiogram (Table 7.7)**

IV.   **ECHOCARDIOGRAPHY**
A.   **Techniques for Assessment**
1. 2-D Echo: Provides a 2 dimensional image of the heart
2. M-mode: Used for assessment of cardiac function
3. Color Doppler: Displays blood flow direction and velocity while viewing a 2-D image of the heart
4. Continuous wave Doppler: Useful for measuring high velocity flow
5. Pulsed Doppler: Measures blood flow velocity; however, this technique provides better spatial localization

TABLE 7.7.

Systemic Effects on Electrocardiogram

	Short QT	Long QT-U	Prolonged QRS	ST-T changes	Sinus tach	Sinus brady	AV block	V tach	Miscellaneous
CHEMISTRY									
Hyperkalemia			X	X			X	X	Low voltage Ps; peaked Ts
Hypokalemia		X	X	X					
Hypercalcemia	X								
Hypocalcemia		X					X	X	
Hypermagnesemia					X		X		
Hypomagnesemia		X							
DRUGS									
Digitalis	X			X		T	X	T	
Phenothiazines		T						T	
Phenytoin	X								
Propranolol	X					X	T		
Quinidine		X	X			T	T	X	
Tricyclics		T	T	T	T		T	T	
Verapamil						X	X		
Imipramine							T	T	Atrial flutter

(Continued.)

TABLE 7.7. (cont.)

	Short QT	Long QT-U	Prolonged QRS	ST-T changes	Sinus tach	Sinus brady	AV block	VTach	Miscellaneous
MISCELLANEOUS									
CNS injury		X		X		X	X		
Freidreich's ataxia				X	X				Atrial flutter
Duchenne's disease				X	X				Atrial flutter
Myotonic dystrophy			X	X	X		X		
Collagen disease				X			X	X	
Hypothyroidism						X			Low voltage
Hyperthyroidism				X	X		X		
Other diseases		Romano-Ward	Lyme disease				Holt-Oram, maternal lupus		

X, Present; T, present only with drug toxicity.
From Garson A Jr: *The electrocardiogram in infants and children: a systematic approach,* Philadelphia, 1983, Lea and Febiger; Walsh EP: Electrocardiography and introduction to electrophysiologic techniques. In Fyler DC, editor. Nadas A: *Pediatric cardiology.* Philadelphia, 1992, Hanley and Belfus.

B.   Indications for Echocardiography
1. Defining congenital and aquired structural heart defects using both 2-D echo and Doppler interrogation
2. Detection and quantification of valvular dysfunction using Doppler interrogation (i.e., valve stenosis and regurgitation)
3. Assessment of ventricular function by M-mode analysis: Shortening fraction measures percent change in left ventricular end systolic dimension (LVESD) and left ventricular end diastolic dimension (LVEDD).

$$\text{Shortening fraction} = \frac{(\text{LVEDD} - \text{LVESD})}{\text{LVEDD}} \times 100$$

   Functional parameters are affected by loading conditions (i.e., preload [stretch on fiber before shortening] and afterload [stress fiber must generate in order to shorten]). (Fig 7.7)
4. Assessment of ventricular contractility by M-mode analysis: Intrinsic contractile properties are measured using wall stress analysis, which determines velocity of shortening and afterload.
5. Identification of intracardiac masses
6. Identification of pericardial effusions
7. Estimation of pulmonary artery pressure/right ventricular pressure: When tricuspid regurgitation is present the jet velocity can be measured by Doppler interrogation. This measurement can provide an accurate estimate of pulmonary artery pressure. If there is no pulmonary artery stenosis, right ventricular pressure will closely approximate pulmonary artery pressure.

C.   Special Applications
1. Fetal echocardiography
   a. At 18–20 weeks most major heart defects can be reliably identified.
   b. Indications for fetal echo include a sibling or parent with congenital heart disease, maternal diabetes, chromosomal anomaly, or multiple noncardiac anomalies.
2. Transesophageal echocardiography
   a. The heart is viewed from the stomach and esophagus.

b. Offers superior sensitivity for detection of vegetations.
c. Superior images are obtained when transthoracic windows are limited (i.e., cardiac postoperative patients or the older child with congenital heart disease).

From Sanders SP: Echocardiography. In DC Fyler, editor: *Nadas' pediatric cardiology,* Philadelphia, 1992, Hanley and Belfus.

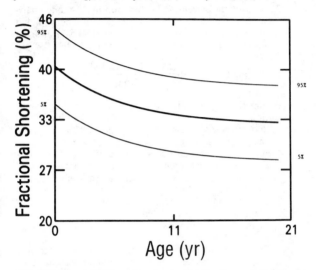

FIG. 7.7. Normal range for shortening fraction related to age. (From Colon S et al: Developmental modulation of myocardial mechanics: age- and growth-related alterations in afterload and contractility, *JACC* 19:619, 1992.)

V. OXYGEN CHALLENGE TEST
A. Technique

Used to evaluate etiology of cyanosis in neonates. Obtain baseline arterial blood gases (ABG) or pulse oximetry saturation at $Fio_2 = 0.21$, then place infant in oxygen hood at $Fio_2 = 1$ for a minimum of 10 minutes, and repeat ABG or pulse oximetry. Pulse oximetry will not be useful for following the change in oxygenation once the saturations reach 100% (approximately $Po_2 \geq 90$).

B.   Interpretation (Table 7.8)

TABLE 7.8.

Interpretation

	F_iO_2 = .21 PaO_2 (% saturation)	F_iO_2 = 1.00 PaO_2 (% saturation)	$PaCO_2$
Normal	70 (95)	>200 (100)	35
Pulmonary disease	50 (85)	>150 (100)	50
Neurologic disease	50 (85)	>150 (100)	50
Methemoglobinemia	70 (95)	>200 (100)	35
Cardiac disease			
Separate circulation*	<40 (<75)	<50 (<85)	35
Restricted PBF†	<40 (<75)	<50 (<85)	35
Complete mixing without restricted PBF‡	50 (85)	<150 (<100)	35
Persistent pulmonary hypertension	Preductal	Postductal	
PFO (no R to L shunt)	70 (95)	<40 (<75)	Variable	35–50
PFO (with R to L shunt)	<40 (<75)	<40 (<75)	Variable	35–50

PBF, Pulmonary blood flow.
*D-Transposition of the great arteries (D-TGA) with intact ventricular septum.
†Tricuspid atresia with pulmonary stenosis or atresia; pulmonary atresia or critical pulmonary stenosis with intact ventricular septum; or tetralogy of Fallot.
‡Truncus, total anomalous pulmonary venous return, single ventricle, hypoplastic left heart, D-TGA with ventricular septal defect, tricuspid atresia without pulmonary stenosis or atresia.
From Lees MH: J *Pediatr* 77:484, 1970; Kitterman JA: *Pediatr Rev* 4:13, 1982; Jones RWA et al: *Arch Dis Child* 51:667, 1976.

VI.   SELECTED CARDIAC PROCEDURES
A.   Cardiac Catheterization Lab Procedures
1. Park: A knife-tipped cardiac catheter enlarges the intraatrial communication at the foramen ovale.
2. Rashkind: A balloon-tipped cardiac catheter is rapidly pulled across the foramen ovale to create a defect in the atrial septum.
3. Interventional devices: Umbrellas, clamshells, and coils are used to close septal defects, PDAs, or collaterals. Stents are used to keep stenotic vessels open.

B.   Closed-heart Procedures
1. Shunts (Fig. 7.8)
   a. Blalock-Taussig (classic): Subclavian artery to pulmonary artery anastomosis

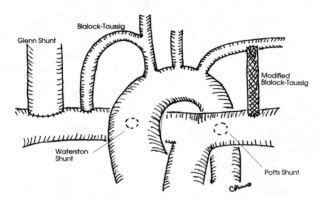

FIG. 7.8. Schematic diagram of cardiac shunts.

      b. Blalock-Taussig (modified): Gore-Tex graft interposed between subclavian artery and pulmonary artery

      c. Glenn: Superior vena cava to right pulmonary artery anastomosis. The original Glenn shunt required ligation of the proximal RPA, while the now more commonly used "bidirectional" Glenn shunt (cavopulmonary anastomosis) allows flow to both the RPA and LPA.

      d. Potts: Descending aorta to left pulmonary artery anastomosis

      e. Waterston: Ascending aorta to right pulmonary artery anastomosis

   2. Heart

      a. Blalock-Hanlon: Closed-heart atrial septectomy

      b. Brock: Closed-heart pulmonary valvulotomy or infundibulotomy

      c. Waldhausen: Use of left subclavian artery as an onlay patch for repair of coarctation of the aorta

C.   **Open-heart Procedures**

   1. Mustard: Intraatrial baffle (usually pericardium) for repair of simple transposition of the great arteries

   2. Senning: Intraatrial baffle constructed using flaps of native atrial septum and atrial wall as repair for transposition of great arteries (TGA)

3. Arterial Switch (of Jatene): Pulmonary artery and aorta transected above valves and switched for repair of TGA. Coronaries moved from old aortic root to new aorta (former pulmonary root).

4. Rastelli
   a. Placement of valved conduit or graft between right ventricle and pulmonary arteries; used for pulmonary atresia and complex TGA
   b. Repair of AV canal by resuspension of mitral and tricuspid valves upon the newly created ventricular septum

5. Fontan: Anastomosis of the right atrium, or the SVC and IVC to the pulmonary artery in order to separate systemic and pulmonary circulations in lesions without two AV valves and two ventricles (e.g., tricuspid atresia, hypoplastic left heart syndrome)

6. Norwood (Palliation for hypoplastic left heart)
   a. Stage 1: Anastomosis of proximal pulmonary artery to aorta, with transection of distal main pulmonary trunk; central shunt between new aorta and distal main pulmonary artery; atrial septectomy
   b. Stage 2: Modified Fontan. More recently, Stage 2 has been subdivided into two stages: a hemi-Fontan (essentially a Glenn shunt) followed later by completion of Fontan in which the IVC is also directly incorporated into the pulmonary circulation.

7. Damus-Kaye-Stansel (for double-outlet right ventricle with subpulmonic VSD): VSD patched to right of PA; anastomosis of PA to aorta; conduit placed between RV and distal main PA

8. Konno: Replacement of aortic valve and patch augmentation of LVOT

9. Ross: Pulmonary autograft replacement of aortic root and homograft conduit from RV to PA

From Arciniegas E: *Pediatric cardiac surgery,* Chicago, 1985, Year Book Medical Publishers; Fyler DC, editor: *Nadas' pediatric cardiology,* Philadelphia, 1992, Hanley and Belfus.

VII. PAROXYSMAL HYPERPNEA—"TETRALOGY SPELLS"

Emergency management of paroxysmal hyperpnea in cyanotic heart disease. Mechanism is usually infundibular spasm and may be incited by anything that distresses the infant. The spasm severely reduces pulmonary blood flow and shunts blood right-to-left across the VSD. As with any emergency, the rule **"do what you can do easily first"** applies: dim the lights; quiet the room; avoid agitating the infant; oxygen; knee-chest position; morphine; correct underlying abnormalities of volume, anemia, hypoglycemia (Table 7.9).

TABLE 7.9.

Treatment	Rationale
Oxygen	Reduces hypoxemia (limited value)
Knee-chest position	Decreases venous return and increases systemic resistance
Propranolol	Negative inotropic effect on infundibular myocardium; may block drop in systemic vascular resistance
Morphine	Decreases venous return, depresses respiratory center, relaxes infundibulum
Phenylephrine HCl	Increases systemic vascular resistance
Methoxamine	Increases systemic vascular resistance
Sodium bicarbonate	Reduces metabolic acidosis
Correct anemia	Increases delivery of oxygen to tissues
Correct pathologic tachyarrhythmias	May abort hypoxic spell
Infuse glucose	Avoids hypoglycemia from increased utilization and depletion of glycogen stores

VIII. NEURALLY-MEDIATED HYPOTENSION

A. Definition

Also known as vasovagal syncope or neurocardiogenic syncope. Presents commonly with lightheadedness or fainting.

Associated with autonomic dysfunction associated with the cardiovascular system resulting in hypotension and bradycardia.

B. Diagnostic Evaluation

1. Thorough history and physical examination. Associated factors are thought to be standing upright for pro-

longed periods, diet, emotional stress, or prolonged heat exposure.
2. Tilt table testing
3. Treatment options
   a. Increase salt and fluids in diet.
   b. Avoid circumstances that induce symptoms.
   c. Drug therapy with florinef, atenolol, norpace, and others.
4. Recent evidence shows that some patients with chronic fatigue syndrome may have symptoms explained by neurally mediated hypotension.

From Bou-Halaigah I et al: The relationship between neurally mediated hypotension and the chronic fatigue syndrome, *JAMA:* 274(12): 961, 1995; Perry J et al: The child with recurrent syncope: autonomic function testing and beta-adrenergic hypersensitivity, *J Am Coll Cardiology* 17:1168, 1991.

IX. KAWASAKI DISEASE
For diagnostic criteria and treatment see Chapter 18.
A. Cardiovascular Complications
1. Leading cause of acquired pediatric heart disease in developed countries
2. If untreated, 15%–25% develop coronary artery dilatation.
   a. Acutely at risk for coronary thrombosis
   b. Long term risk of decreased coronary distensibility and coronary stenosis
B. Cardiovascular Follow Up
1. Obtain echocardiogram early in the acute phase of the illness, 3 weeks after onset, and 8 weeks after onset.
2. See Table 7.10 for follow up based on risk level.
3. If patient develops varicella or influenza, stop aspirin therapy and place on dipyridamole for duration of illness to reduce risk of Reye syndrome.

From *Diagnosis and therapy of Kawasaki disease in children,* American Heart Association Special Report, **Circulation,** Vol 87, No 5, May 1993; **Circulation,** Vol 89, No 2, February 1994

TABLE 7.10.

Risk level	Pharmacologic therapy	Physical activity	Follow-up and diagnostic testing	Invasive testing
I (no coronary artery changes at any stage of illness)	None beyond initial 6–8 weeks	No restrictions beyond initial 6–8 weeks	None beyond first year unless cardiac disease suspected	None recommended
II (transient coronary artery ectasia that disappears during acute illness)	None beyond initial 6–8 weeks	No restrictions beyond initial 6–8 weeks	None beyond first year unless cardiac disease suspected. Physician may choose to see patient at 3- to 5-year intervals	None recommended
III (small to medium solitary coronary artery aneurysm)	3–5 mg/kg aspirin per day, at least until abnormalities resolve	For patients in first decade of life, no restriction beyond initial 6–8 weeks. For patients in second decade, physical activity guided by stress testing every other year. Competitive contact athletics with endurance training discouraged.	Annual follow-up with echocardiogram ± electrocardiogram in first decade of life	Angiography, if stress testing or echocardiography suggests stenosis

IV (one or more giant coronary artery aneurysms or multiple small to medium aneurysms, without obstruction)	Long-term aspirin (3–5 mg/kg per day) ± warfarin	For patients in first decade of life, no restriction beyond initial 6–8 weeks. For patients in second decade, annual stress testing guides recommendations. Strenuous athletics are strongly discouraged. If stress test rules out ischemia, noncontact recreational sports allowed.	Annual follow-up with echocardiogram ± electrocardiogram ± chest x-ray ± additional electrocardiogram at 6-month intervals. For patients in first decade of life, pharmacologic stress testing should be considered.	Angiography, if stress testing or echocardiography suggest stenosis. Elective catheterization may be done in certain circumstances.
V (coronary artery obstruction)	Long-term aspirin (3–5 mg/kg per day) ± warfarin. Use of calcium channel blockers should be considered to reduce myocardial oxygen consumption.	Contact sports, isometrics, and weight training should be avoided. Other physical activity recommendations guided by outcome of stress testing or myocardial perfusion scan.	Echocardiogram and electrocardiogram at 6-month intervals and annual Holter and stress testing	Angiography recommended for some patients to aid in selecting therapeutic options. Repeat angiography with new-onset or worsening ischemia.

± Indicates with or without.

X.   **BACTERIAL ENDOCARDITIS: PROPHYLAXIS**
A.   **Cardiac Conditions**
  1. Endocarditis prophylaxis recommended
     a. Prosthetic cardiac valves, including bioprosthetic and homograft valves
     b. Previous history of bacterial endocarditis
     c. Surgically constructed systemic-pulmonary shunts
     d. Most congenital cardiac malformations (e.g., VSD, ASD)
     e. Rheumatic and other acquired valvular dysfunction
     f. Hypertrophic cardiomyopathy
     g. Mitral valve prolapse with valvular regurgitation
  2. Endocarditis prophylaxis not recommended
     a. Isolated secundum atrial septal defect
     b. Surgical repair without residua beyond 6 months of secundum atrial septal defect, ventricular septal defect, or patent ductus arteriosus
     c. Previous coronary artery bypass graft surgery
     d. Mitral valve prolapse without valvular regurgitation (thickened or redundant leaflets may be at higher risk for SBE)
     e. Physiologic, functional, or innocent heart murmurs
     f. Previous Kawasaki disease without valvular dysfunction
     g. Previous rheumatic fever without valvular dysfunction
     h. Cardiac pacemakers and implanted defibrillators
B.   **Procedures for which Prophylaxis is Recommended**
  1. All **dental procedures** likely to cause gingival bleeding, including routine professional cleaning (not simple adjustment of orthodontic appliances or shedding of deciduous teeth)
  2. Tonsillectomy and/or adenoidectomy
  3. Surgical procedures involving **intestinal or respiratory mucosa**
  4. Bronchoscopy with a **rigid bronchoscope**
  5. Incision and drainage of infected tissue, in addition to proper antibiotics for the tissue infection

6. Specific **genitourinary and gastrointestinal procedures** including cystoscopy, urethral dilatation, urethral catheterization if UTI is present, urinary tract surgery if UTI is present, vaginal hysterectomy, vaginal delivery in presence of infection, dilatation/curettage (D and C) if infection is suspected, esophageal dilatation, and gallbladder surgery. Prophylactic antibiotics are recommended in addition to appropriate antibiotic coverage for other infection(s).

7. In patients with prosthetic heart valves, previous history of endocarditis, or surgically constructed systemic-pulmonary shunts/conduits, physicians may choose to administer prophylaxis even for low risk procedures involving the lower respiratory, GU, or GI tracts.

C. **Procedures for which Prophylaxis is not Recommended**
1. Injection of local intraoral anesthetic (except intraligamentary injections)
2. Tympanostomy tube insertion
3. Endotracheal intubation alone or flexible bronchoscopy (with or without biopsy)
4. Cardiac catheterization
5. Endoscopy (with or without GI biopsy), cesarean section.
6. In the absence of infection: urethral catheterization, D & C, uncomplicated vaginal delivery, therapeutic abortion, sterilization procedures, or insertion and removal of IUDs

D. **Antibiotic Regimen**
1. Dental, oral, or upper respiratory tract procedures
   a. Standard regimen: Amoxicillin 50 mg/kg PO 1 hour before procedure, then half of initial dose 6 hours after initial dose (max 3 g initial dose, 1.5 g follow-up dose)
   b. High-risk regimen (prosthetic heart valves, history of endocarditis, surgically constructed systemic-pulmonary shunts): Ampicillin 50 mg/kg (max 2 g) plus gentamicin 2 mg/kg (adults 1.5 mg/kg; max 80 mg) IV/IM 30 minutes before procedure; followed by amoxicillin 25 mg/kg PO 6 hours after initial dose (max 1.5 g). Alternatively, the parenteral regimen may be repeated 8 hours after the initial dose.

  c. Penicillin-allergic patients: Erythromycin (EES or stearate) 20 mg/kg (max EES 800 mg; stearate 1.0 g) PO 2 hours before procedure; then half of initial dose 6 hours after initial dose, or clindamycin 10 mg/kg (max 300 mg) PO 1 hour before procedure, then half of initial dose 6 hours after initial dose. For high-risk patients: Vancomycin 20 mg/kg (max 1 g) IV over 1 hour, 1 hour before procedure. No repeat dose necessary.

  d. Alternate regimens for patients at risk

   1) Patients unable to take PO meds: Ampicillin 50 mg/kg (max 2 g) 30 minutes before procedure IV/IM, then ampicillin at half initial dose **or** amoxicillin 25 mg/kg PO (max 1.5 g) 6 hours after the initial dose.

   2) Penicillin-allergic patients unable to take PO medications: Clindamycin 10 mg/kg (max 300 mg) IV 30 minutes before the procedure; 5 mg/kg IV/PO (max 150 mg) 6 hours after the initial dose.

 2. Gastrointestinal/genitourinary procedures

  a. Standard regimen: Ampicillin 50 mg/kg (max 2 g) plus gentamicin 2 mg/kg (adults 1.5 mg/kg; max 80 mg) IV/IM 30 minutes before procedure; followed by amoxicillin 25 mg/kg PO 6 hours after initial dose (max 1.5 g). Alternatively, the parenteral regimen may be repeated once 8 hours after the initial dose.

  b. Penicillin-allergic patients: Vancomycin IV 20 mg/kg (max 1 g) over 1 hour plus gentamicin IV/IM 2 mg/kg (adults 1.5 mg/kg, max 80 mg) 1 hour before procedure. May repeat once 8 hours after initial dose.

  c. Alternate low-risk regimen: Amoxicillin 50 mg/kg PO 1 hour before procedure, then half of initial dose 6 hours after initial dose (max 3 g initial dose, 1.5 g follow-up dose).

Note: Children may also be on penicillin prophylaxis (e.g., for sickle cell disease) or amoxicillin prophylaxis (e.g., for recurrent otitis media) for conditions other than rheumatic fever; they too should placed on an alternate regimen as well.

E.   Specific Situations and Circumstances
1. Rheumatic fever: Antibiotic regimens used to prevent recurrence of acute rheumatic fever are inadequate for the prevention of bacterial endocarditis. Individuals on penicillin prophylaxis may have resistant *viridans* streptococci and should be placed on erythromycin or other alternate regimen instead of amoxicillin/penicillin for endocarditis prophylaxis.
2. Patients on anticoagulants: Avoid IM injections.
3. Renal dysfunction: Modify doses in patients with significant renal insufficiency (see Chapter 29).
4. Patients undergoing cardiac surgery: Perioperative antibiotics are recommended for patients with cardiac conditions or in whom "hardware" is to be placed. Prophylaxis should be directed against staphylococci and should be of short duration; modify according to institutional susceptibility patterns.

From Committee on Rheumatic Fever, Endocarditis, and Kawasaki Disease of the Council on Cardiovascular Disease in the Young, the American Heart Association, *JAMA* 264:2919, 1990.

XI.   BLOOD PRESSURE NORMS
A.   Premature and Term Infants (Figs. 7.9 to 7.13)

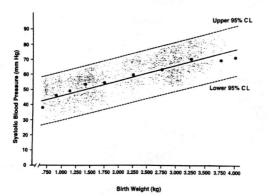

FIG. 7.9. Linear regression of mean SBP on birthweight on day 1 of life. *(From Zubrow AB, Hulman S:* J Perinatol *15: 470, 1995.)*

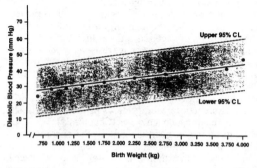

FIG. 7.10. Linear regression of mean DBP on birthweight on day 1 of life. *(From Zubrow AB, Hulman S: J Perinatol 15: 470, 1995.)*

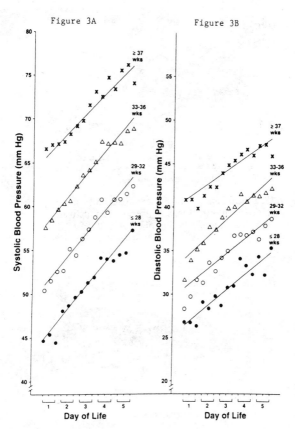

FIG. 7.11. SBP and DBP in the first 5 days of life. *(From Zubrow AB, Hulman S: J Perinatol 15: 470, 1995.)*

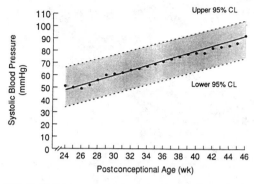

FIG. 7.12. Linear regression of mean SBP on postconceptional age (gestational age in weeks + weeks after delivery). *(From Zubrow AB, Hulman S: J Perinatol 15: 470, 1995.)*

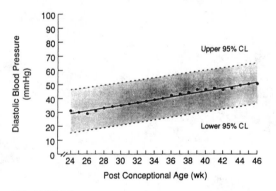

FIG. 7.13. Linear regression of mean DBP on postconceptional age (gestational age in weeks + weeks after delivery). *(From Zubrow AB, Hulman S: J Perinatol 15: 470, 1995.)*

B. **Age birth–12 months (Figs. 7.14 and 7.15)**

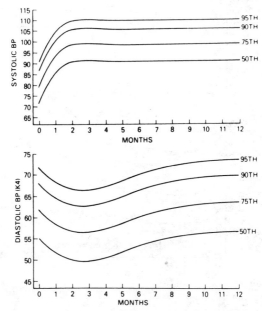

90TH PERCENTILE												
SYSTOLIC BP	87	101	106	106	106	105	105	105	105	105	105	105	105
DIASTOLIC BP	68	65	63	63	63	65	66	67	68	68	69	69	69
HEIGHT CM	51	59	63	66	68	70	72	73	74	76	77	78	80
WEIGHT KG	4	4	5	5	6	7	8	9	9	10	10	11	11

FIG. 7.14. Age-specific percentiles of BP measurements in boys-birth to 12 months of age; Korotkoff phase IV (K4) used for diastolic BP. *(From Horan MJ:* Pediatrics *79: 1, 1987.)*

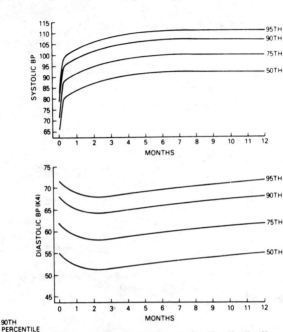

90TH PERCENTILE												
SYSTOLIC BP	76	98	101	104	105	106	106	106	106	106	105	105
DIASTOLIC BP	68	65	64	64	65	66	66	66	67	67	67	67
HEIGHT CM	54	55	56	58	61	63	66	68	70	72	74	75	77
WEIGHT KG	4	4	4	5	5	6	7	8	9	9	10	10	11

FIG. 7.15. Age-specific percentiles of BP measurements in girls from birth to 12 months of age; Korotkoff phase IV (K4) used for diastolic BP. *(From Horan MJ: Pediatrics 79: 1, 1987.)*

C.   Age 1–17 Years (Tables 7.11 and 7.12)

From Update on the Task Force Report (1987) on high blood pressure in children and adolescents: a working group of the National High Blood Pressure Education Program. Tables used with permission of Dr. Edward Rocella, PhD, MPH.

TABLE 7.11.

Blood pressure levels for the 90th and 95th percentiles of blood pressure for boys age 1 to 17 years by perdentiles of height

Age (yr)	Percentiles BP↓	Systolic BP (mm Hg) by percentile of height							Diastolic BP (DBP5) (mm Hg) by percentile of height						
	Height* →	5%	10%	25%	50%	75%	90%	95%	5%	10%	25%	50%	75%	90%	95%
1	90th	94	95	97	98	100	102	102	50	51	52	53	54	54	55
	95th	98	99	101	102	104	106	106	55	55	56	57	58	59	59
2	90th	98	99	100	102	104	105	106	55	55	56	57	58	59	59
	95th	101	102	104	106	108	109	110	59	59	60	61	62	63	63
3	90th	100	101	103	105	107	108	109	59	59	60	61	62	63	63
	95th	104	105	107	109	111	112	113	63	63	64	65	66	67	67
4	90th	102	103	105	107	109	110	111	62	62	63	64	65	66	66
	95th	106	107	109	111	113	114	115	66	67	67	68	69	70	71
5	90th	104	105	106	108	110	112	112	65	65	66	67	68	69	69
	95th	108	109	110	112	114	115	116	69	70	70	71	72	73	74
6	90th	105	106	108	110	111	113	114	67	68	69	70	70	71	72
	95th	109	110	112	114	115	117	117	72	72	73	74	75	76	76
7	90th	106	107	109	111	113	114	115	69	70	71	72	72	73	74
	95th	110	111	113	115	116	118	119	74	74	75	76	77	78	78
8	90th	107	108	110	112	114	115	116	71	71	72	73	74	75	75
	95th	111	112	114	116	118	119	120	75	76	76	77	78	79	80
9	90th	109	110	112	113	115	117	117	72	73	73	74	75	76	76
	95th	113	114	116	117	119	121	121	76	77	78	79	80	80	81
10	90th	110	112	113	115	117	118	119	73	74	74	75	76	77	78
	95th	114	115	117	119	121	122	123	77	78	79	80	80	81	82

(Continued.)

TABLE 7.11. (cont.)

Age (yr)	Height* → BP† ↓	Systolic BP (mm Hg) by percentile of height							Diastolic BP (DBP5) (mm Hg) by percentile of height						
	Percentiles	5%	10%	25%	50%	75%	90%	95%	5%	10%	25%	50%	75%	90%	95%
11	90th	112	113	115	117	119	120	121	74	74	75	76	77	78	78
	95th	116	117	119	121	123	124	125	78	79	79	80	81	82	83
12	90th	115	116	117	119	121	123	123	75	75	76	77	78	78	79
	95th	119	120	121	123	125	126	127	79	79	80	81	82	83	83
13	90th	117	118	120	122	124	125	126	75	76	76	77	78	79	80
	95th	121	122	124	126	128	129	130	79	80	81	82	83	83	84
14	90th	120	121	123	125	126	128	128	76	76	77	78	79	80	80
	95th	124	125	127	128	130	132	132	80	81	81	82	83	84	85
15	90th	123	124	125	127	129	131	131	77	77	78	79	80	81	81
	95th	127	128	129	131	133	134	135	81	82	83	83	84	85	86
16	90th	125	126	128	130	132	133	134	79	79	80	81	82	82	83
	95th	129	130	132	134	136	137	138	83	83	84	85	86	87	87
17	90th	128	129	131	133	134	136	136	81	81	82	83	84	85	85
	95th	132	133	135	136	138	140	140	85	85	86	87	88	89	89

*Height percentile determined by standard growth curves.
†Blood pressure percentile determined by a single measurement.

TABLE 7.12.

Blood pressure levels for the 90th and 95th percentiles of blood pressure for girls age 1 to 17 years by percentiles of height

Age (yr)	Height* → BP† ↓	Systolic BP (mm Hg) by percentile of height							Diastolic BP (DBP5) (mm Hg) by percentile of height						
		5%	10%	25%	50%	75%	90%	95%	5%	10%	25%	50%	75%	90%	95%
1	90th	97	98	99	100	102	103	104	53	53	53	54	55	56	56
	95th	101	102	103	104	105	107	107	57	57	57	58	59	60	60
2	90th	99	99	100	102	103	104	105	57	57	58	58	59	60	61
	95th	102	103	104	105	107	108	109	61	61	61	62	63	64	65
3	90th	100	100	102	103	104	105	106	61	61	61	62	63	63	64
	95th	104	104	105	107	108	109	110	65	65	65	66	67	67	68
4	90th	101	102	103	104	106	107	108	63	63	64	65	65	66	67
	95th	105	106	107	108	109	111	111	67	67	68	69	69	70	71
5	90th	103	103	104	106	107	108	109	65	66	66	67	68	68	69
	95th	107	107	108	110	111	112	113	69	70	70	71	72	72	73
6	90th	104	105	106	107	109	110	111	67	67	68	69	69	70	71
	95th	108	109	110	111	112	114	114	71	71	72	73	73	74	75
7	90th	106	107	108	109	110	112	112	69	69	69	70	71	72	72
	95th	110	110	112	113	114	115	116	73	73	73	74	75	76	76
8	90th	108	109	110	111	112	113	114	70	70	71	71	72	73	74
	95th	112	112	113	115	116	117	118	74	74	75	75	76	77	78
9	90th	110	110	112	113	114	115	116	71	72	72	73	74	74	75
	95th	114	114	115	117	118	119	120	75	76	76	77	78	78	79

(Continued.)

TABLE 7.12. (cont.)

Age (yr)	BP†	Height* →	Systolic BP (mm Hg) by percentile of height							Diastolic BP (DBP5) (mm Hg) by percentile of height						
		Percentiles	5%	10%	25%	50%	75%	90%	95%	5%	10%	25%	50%	75%	90%	95%
10	90th		112	112	114	115	116	117	118	73	73	73	74	75	76	76
	95th		116	116	117	119	120	121	122	77	77	77	78	79	80	80
11	90th		114	114	116	117	118	119	120	74	74	75	75	76	77	77
	95th		118	118	119	121	122	123	124	78	78	79	79	80	81	81
12	90th		116	116	118	119	120	121	122	75	75	76	76	77	78	78
	95th		120	120	121	123	124	125	126	79	79	80	80	81	82	82
13	90th		118	118	119	121	122	123	124	76	76	77	78	78	79	80
	95th		121	122	123	125	126	127	128	80	80	81	82	82	83	84
14	90th		119	120	121	122	124	125	126	77	77	78	79	79	80	81
	95th		123	124	125	126	128	129	130	81	81	82	83	83	84	85
15	90th		121	121	122	124	125	126	127	78	78	79	79	80	81	82
	95th		124	125	126	128	129	130	131	82	82	83	83	84	85	86
16	90th		122	122	123	125	126	127	128	79	79	79	80	81	82	82
	95th		125	126	127	128	130	131	132	83	83	83	84	85	86	86
17	90th		122	123	124	125	126	128	128	79	79	79	80	81	82	82
	95th		126	126	127	129	130	131	132	83	83	83	84	85	86	86

*Height percentile determined by standard growth curves.
†Blood pressure percentile determined by a single reading.

CONVERSION FORMULAS

8

I. TEMPERATURE
A. Calculation
1. To convert degrees Celsius to degrees Fahrenheit: (9/5 × temperature) + 32
2. To convert degrees Fahrenheit to degrees Celsius: (temperature − 32) × 5/9

B. Temperature Equivalents

Centigrade	Fahrenheit	Centigrade	Fahrenheit
34.0	93.2	38.6	101.4
34.2	93.6	38.8	101.8
34.4	93.9	39.0	102.2
34.6	94.3	39.2	102.5
34.8	94.6	39.4	102.9
35.0	95.0	39.6	103.2
35.2	95.4	39.8	103.6
35.4	95.7	40.0	104.0
35.6	96.1	40.2	104.3
35.8	96.4	40.4	104.7
36.0	96.8	40.6	105.1
36.2	97.1	40.8	105.4
36.4	97.5	41.0	105.8
36.6	97.8	41.2	106.1
36.8	98.2	41.4	106.5
37.0	98.6	41.6	106.8
37.2	98.9	41.8	107.2
37.4	99.3	42.0	107.6
37.6	99.6	42.2	108.0
37.8	100.0	42.4	108.3
38.0	100.4	42.6	108.7
38.2	100.7	42.8	109.0
38.4	101.1	43.0	109.4

II. LENGTH AND WEIGHT
A. Length
To convert inches to centimeters, multiply by 2.54.
B. Weight

Ounces	1 lb	2 lb	3 lb	4 lb	5 lb	6 lb	7 lb	8 lb
0	454 g	907	1,361	1,814	2,268	2,722	3,175	3,629
1	482	936	1,389	1,843	2,296	2,750	3,204	3,657
2	510	964	1,418	1,871	2,325	2,778	3,232	3,686
3	539	992	1,446	1,899	2,353	2,807	3,260	3,714
4	567	1,021	1,474	1,928	2,381	2,835	3,289	3,742
5	595	1,049	1,503	1,956	2,410	2,863	3,317	3,771
6	624	1,077	1,531	1,985	2,438	2,892	3,345	3,799
7	652	1,106	1,559	2,013	2,466	2,920	3,374	3,827
8	680	1,134	1,588	2,041	2,495	2,948	3,402	3,856
9	709	1,162	1,616	2,070	2,523	2,977	3,430	3,884
10	737	1,191	1,644	2,098	2,552	3,005	3,459	3,912
11	765	1,219	1,673	2,126	2,580	3,033	3,487	3,941
12	794	1,247	1,701	2,155	2,608	3,062	3,515	3,969
13	822	1,276	1,729	2,183	2,637	3,090	3,544	3,997
14	851	1,304	1,758	2,211	2,665	3,119	3,572	4,026
15	879	1,332	1,786	2,240	2,693	3,147	3,600	4,054

1 lb = 454 g; 1 kg = 2.2 lb. To convert pounds to grams, multiply by 454. To convert kilograms to pounds, multiply by 2.2.

DEVELOPMENT 9

Developmental disabilities are a group of interrelated chronic, nonprogressive neurologic disorders occurring in childhood. This chapter focuses on screening and assessment of neurodevelopment to identify possible developmental disability.

I. KEY CONCEPTS

Since development takes place in an orderly and sequential manner, the phenomena of developmental delay, dissociation, and deviancy are important in the detection of developmental disabilities.

A. Streams of Development: Development can be divided into four major streams or skill areas: gross motor, language, visual-motor/problem solving, and social/adaptive. Assessment of all four streams is a necessary part of ongoing developmental surveillance (Table 9.1).

TABLE 9.1.

Streams of Development

Disorder	Gross motor	Language (CLAMS)	Problem solving (CAT)	Social/adaptive
Cerebral palsy	Decreased	Normal	Normal	Normal to decreased
Mental retardation	Normal	Decreased	Decreased	Decreased
Communication disorder	Normal	Decreased	Normal	Normal to decreased

From Capute AJ et al: *Contemp Pediatr* 4:24, 1987.
CLAMS, Clinical Linguistic and Auditory Milestone Scale; *CAT*, Clinical Adaptive Test.

B. Developmental Quotient (DQ)

1. The **DQ** can be calculated for a given stream or overall.

   DQ = (developmental age/chronological age) × 100

2. The DQ reflects the child's rate of development over time and holds considerable predictive value in children with

delay whose deficits are static. Two separate developmental assessments are more predictive than a single assessment. Testing should be performed in several areas of skill.

   3. Language remains the best predictor of future intellectual endowment. Language development can be divided into two streams, receptive and expressive, each assigned a separate DQ. Language should serve as the common denominator comparing its rate of development with other skill areas.

C. **Delay:** Performance significantly below average in a given area of skill. A developmental quotient below 70 constitutes developmental delay.

D. **Deviancy:** Atypical development within a single stream, such as developmental milestones occurring out of sequence. Examples are the infant who walks before crawling or the early development of hand preference.

E. **Dissociation:** A substantial difference in the rate of development between two streams. Examples include the cognitive-motor differences in some children with mental retardation or cerebral palsy (see Table 9.1).

From Capute AJ et al: *Orthop Clin North Am* 12:3, 1981.

II. DISORDERS

A developmental diagnosis is a functional description and classification that does not specify an etiology or medical diagnosis. The Diagnostic and Statistical Manual-IV (DSM-IV) includes the following classifications: mental retardation, motor skills disorders, communication disorders, learning disorders, pervasive developmental disorders, and attention-deficit and disruptive behavior disorders.

A. **Mental Retardation (MR):** Mental retardation refers to substantial limitations in present functioning. It is characterized by significantly subaverage intellectual functioning (IQ below 70–75), existing concurrently with related limitations in two or more of the following adaptive skill areas: communications, self-care, home living, social skills, community use, self direction, health and safety, functional academics, leisure, and work. Mental retardation manifests itself before age 18 (Table 9.2).

TABLE 9.2.

Mental Retardation

Degree of mental retardation*	Measured intelligence quotient	Expected mental age as an adult (yr)
Low normal	80–90	—
Borderline	70–79	—
Mild (educable)	55–69	9–11
Moderate (trainable)	40–54	5–8
Severe	25–39	3–5
Profound	Below 25	Below 3

*Based on Wechsler scales.

From *Mental retardation: definition, classification, and systems of supports,* ed 9, 1992, American Association on Mental Retardation.

B. **Cerebral palsy (CP):** A disorder of movement and posture resulting from a permanent nonprogressive deficit or lesion of the immature brain. Manifestations, however, may change with brain growth and development. CP may be classified by a description of the motor handicap in terms of physiologic (motor), topographic, etiologic, functional, and therapeutic categories. CP is divided into three main physiologic categories: pyramidal (spastic), extrapyramidal (nonspastic), and mixed types. Extrapyramidal CP includes choreoathetoid, ataxic, rigid, hypotonic, and dystonic types. Spastic CP may be further characterized by topographic classification (Table 9.3).

C. **Communication disorders:** A group of disorders that can be further subdivided into expressive language disorders, mixed receptive-expressive language disorders, phonologic disorders, and stuttering. Developmental language disorders can be characterized by deficits of comprehension, production, and use of language. These deficits can be seen in children with more global disorders such as MR, autism, and pervasive developmental disorder (PDD) or can be seen as a specific language disability. All children suspected of having a communication disorder should undergo a hearing assessment.

TABLE 9.3.

Topographic Classification of Spastic Cerebral Palsy

Type	Pattern of involvement
Hemiplegia	Homolateral arm and leg; arm usually more impaired than leg
Diplegia	All four extremities; legs more involved than arms, which are relatively spared
Quadriplegia	All four extremities; some asymmetry, but all severely impaired with lower extremities more involved than upper
Double hemiplegia	All four extremities; both upper extremities more involved than both lower extremities
Monoplegia	One extremity, usually upper; probably reflects a mild hemiplegia or a birth palsy
Triplegia	One upper extremity and both lower extremities; probably represents a hemiplegia plus diplegia or incomplete quadriplegia
Paraplegia	Involves the legs only with normal upper extremity function (spinal cord injuries)

From Capute AJ, Accardo PJ: Cerebral palsy. In Capute AJ, editor: *Developmental disabilities in infancy and childhood,* Baltimore, 1991, Paul H Brookes.

D. Learning disabilities: A heterogeneous group of disorders that manifest as significant difficulties in one or more of seven areas (as defined by the federal government): basic reading skills, reading comprehension, oral expression, listening comprehension, written expression, mathematical calculation, and mathematical reasoning. Specific learning disabilities are diagnosed when the individual's achievement on standardized tests in a given area is substantially (i.e., 2 standard deviations) below that expected for age, schooling, and level of intelligence.

E. Pervasive developmental disorders: Disorders include autism, Rett syndrome, childhood disintegrative disorder, and Asperger's syndrome. They are characterized by severe and pervasive impairment in several areas of development: reciprocal social interaction skills; communication skills; or the presence of stereotyped behavior, interests, and activities. Autism is characterized by marked deficits in socialization, adaptive behavior, and language. There is a high rate of self-stimulatory, stereotyped behavior and a markedly restricted repertoire of activities and interests.

Development   **181**

F. **Attention-deficit hyperactivity disorder:** A neurobehavioral disorder characterized by inattention, impulsivity, and hyperactivity that is more frequent and severe than is typically observed in individuals of the same developmental age. There is significant inability to sit still, concentrate, and complete tasks. To meet DSM-IV criteria, symptoms must have been present before age 7, impairment must be present in at least two settings, and the disturbance must not be due to another disorder.

From American Psychiatric Association: *Diagnostic and statistical manual of mental disorders,* ed 4, Washington, DC, 1994, American Psychiatric Association.

III. DEVELOPMENTAL SCREENING
A. **Developmental Milestones (Table 9.4)**
B. **Denver Developmental Screening Test (Denver II):**
   (See fold-out following page 192)
C. **CLAMS/CAT**
   1. **CLAMS** (Clinical Linguistic and Auditory Milestone Scale): Developed, standardized, and validated for office assessment of language development from birth to 36 months of age.
   2. **CAT** (Clinical Adaptive Test): Consists of problem-solving items adapted from well-standardized infant psychological tests.
   3. Scoring: A DQ can be derived by assigning an age to the child's best performance and dividing it by chronological age (with age adjustments for prematurity). For example, a 12-month-old performing at a 9-month level has a DQ of 75%. A child with a DQ of less than 80% should have an evaluation to rule out mental retardation or hearing impairment. Dissociation between the CAT/CLAMS components can identify and help differentiate between cerebral palsy, mental retardation, and communication disorders (see Tables 9.1 and 9.5).

TABLE 9.4.

Developmental Milestones

Age	Gross motor	Visual-motor/problem solving	Language	Social/adaptive
1 mo	Raises head slightly from prone, makes crawling movements	Birth: visually fixes 1 mo: has tight grasp, follows to midline	Alerts to sound	Regards face
2 mo	Holds head in midline, lifts chest off table	No longer clenches fist tightly, follows object past midline	Smiles socially (after being stroked or talked to)	Recognizes parent
3 mo	Supports on forearms in prone, holds head up steadily	Holds hands open at rest, follows in circular fashion, responds to visual threat	Coos (produces long vowel sounds in musical fashion)	Reaches for familiar people or objects, anticipates feeding
4 mo	Rolls front to back, supports on wrists and shifts weight	Reaches with arms in unison, brings hands to midline	Laughs, orients to voice	Enjoys looking around environment
5 mo	Rolls back to front, sits supported	Transfers objects	Says "ah-goo," razzes orients to bell (localizes laterally)	
6 mo	Sits unsupported, puts feet in mouth in supine position	Unilateral reach, uses raking grasp	Babbles	Recognizes strangers
7 mo	Creeps	7–8 mo: inspects objects	Orients to bell (localized indirectly)	7–9 mo: fingerfeeds

Age	Gross Motor	Fine Motor	Language	Social/Adaptive
8 mo	Comes to sit, crawls		"Dada" indiscriminately	Starts to explore environment; plays gesture games (e.g., pat-a-cake)
9 mo	Pivots when sitting, pulls to stand, cruises	Uses pincer grasp, probes with forefinger, holds bottle, throws objects	"Mama" indiscriminately, waves bye-bye, gestures, understands "no"; 10 mo: "dada/mama" discriminately; orients to bell (directly); 11 mo: 1 word other than "dada/mama," follows 1-step command with gesture	
12 mo	Walks alone	Uses mature pincer grasp, releases voluntarily, marks paper with pencil	Uses 2 words other than "dada/mama," immature jargoning (runs several unintelligible words together); 13 mo: uses 3 words; 14 mo: follows 1-step command without gesture	Imitates actions, comes when called, cooperates with dressing
15 mo	Creeps up stairs, walks backwards	Scribbles in imitation, builds tower of 2 blocks in imitation	Uses 4–6 words; 17 mo: uses 7–20 words, points to 5 body parts, uses mature jargoning (includes intelligible words in jargoning)	15–18 mo: uses spoon, uses cup independently
18 mo	Runs, throws objects from standing without falling	Scribbles spontaneously, builds tower of 3 blocks, turns 2–3 pages at a time	Uses 2-word combinations; 19 mo: knows 8 body parts	Copies parent in tasks (sweeping, dusting), plays in company of other children
21 mo	Squats in play, goes up steps	Builds tower of 5 blocks	Uses 50 words, 2-word sentences	Asks to have food and to go to toilet

(Continued.)

TABLE 9.4. (cont.)

Age	Gross motor	Visual-motor/ problem solving	Language	Social/adaptive
24 mo	Walks up and down steps without help	Imitates stroke with pencil, builds tower of 7 blocks, turns pages one at a time, removes shoes, pants, etc.	Uses pronouns (I, you, me inappropriately), follows 2-step commands	Parallel play
30 mo	Jumps with both feet off floor, throws ball overhand	Holds pencil in adult fashion, performs horizontal and vertical strokes, unbuttons	Uses pronouns appropriately, understands concept of "1," repeats 2 digits forward	Tells first and last names when asked; gets self drink without help
3 yr	Can alternate feet when going up steps, pedals tricycle	Copies a circle, undresses completely, dresses partially, dries hands if reminded	Uses minimum 250 words, 3-word sentences; uses plurals, past tense; knows all pronouns; understands concept of "2"	Group play, shares toys, takes turns, plays well with others, knows full name, age, sex
4 yr	Hops, skips, alternates feet going down steps	Copies a square, buttons clothing, dresses self completely, catches ball	Knows colors, says song or poem from memory, asks questions	Tells "tall tales," plays cooperatively with a group of children
5 yr	Skips alternating feet, jumps over low obstacles	Copies triangle, ties shoes, spreads with knife	Prints first name, asks what a word means	Plays competitive games, abides by rules, likes to help in household tasks

From Caputo AJ, Biehl RF: *Pediatr Clin North Am* 20:3, 1973; Caputo AJ, Accardo PJ: *Clin Pediatr* 17:847, 1978; Caputo AJ et al: *Am J Dis Child* 140:694, 1986; Rounded norms from Caputo AJ et al: *Devel Med Child Neurol* 28:762, 1986.

TABLE 9.5.

CLAMS/CAT

Age (mo)	CLAMS	Yes	No	CAT	Yes	No
1	1. Alerts to sound (0.5)*	——	——	1. Visually fixates momentarily upon red ring (0.5)	——	——
	2. Soothes when picked up (0.5)			2. Chin off table in prone (0.5)		
2	1. Social smile (1.0)*	——	——	1. Visually follows ring horizontally and vertically (0.5)	——	——
				2. Chest off table prone (0.5)		
3	1. Cooing (1.0)			1. Visually follows ring in circle (0.3)	——	——
				2. Supports on forearms in prone (0.3)		
				3. Visual threat (0.3)	——	——
4	1. Orients to voice (0.5)*	——	——	1. Unfisted (0.3)	——	——
	2. Laughs aloud (0.5)			2. Manipulates fingers (0.3)	——	——
				3. Supports on wrists in prone (0.3)		
5	1. Orients toward bell laterally (0.3)*	——	——	1. Pulls down rings (0.3)		
	2. Ah-goo (0.3)	——	——	2. Transfers (0.3)	——	——
	3. Razzing (0.3)	——	——	3. Regards pellet (0.3)	——	——
6	1. Babbling (1.0)			1. Obtains cube (0.3)	——	——
				2. Lifts cup (0.3)	——	——
				3. Radial rake (0.3)	——	——
7	1. Orients toward bell (1.0) *(upwardly/indirectly 90°)			1. Attempts pellet (0.3)	——	——
				2. Pulls out peg (0.3)	——	——
				3. Inspects ring (0.3)	——	——
8	1. "Dada" inappropriately (0.3)			1. Pulls out ring by string (0.3)	——	——
	2. "Mama" inappropriately (0.5)			2. Secures pellet (0.3)	——	——
				3. Inspects bell (0.3)		
9	1. Orients toward bell (upward directly 180°) (0.5)*	——	——	1. Three finger scissor grasp (0.3)	——	——

(Continued.)

TABLE 9.5. (cont.)

Age (mo)	CLAMS	Yes	No	CAT	Yes	No
	2. Gesture language (0.5)	—	—	2. Rings bell (0.3)	—	—
				3. Over the edge for toy (0.3)	—	—
10	1. Understands "no" (0.3)	—	—	1. Combine cube-cup (0.3)	—	—
	2. Uses "dada" appropriately (0.3)	—	—	2. Uncovers bell (0.3)	—	—
	3. Uses "mama" appropriately (0.3)	—	—	3. Fingers pegboard (0.3)	—	—
11	1. One word (other than "mama" and "dada") (1.0)	—	—	1. Mature overhand pincer movement (0.5)	—	—
				2. Solves cube under cup (0.5)	—	—
12	1. One step command with gesture (0.5)	—	—	1. Release one cube in cup (0.5)	—	—
	2. Two word vocabulary (0.5)	—	—	2. Crayon mark (0.5)	—	—
14	1. Three word vocabulary (1.0)	—	—	1. Solves glass frustration (0.6)	—	—
	2. Immature jargoning (1.0)	—	—	2. Out-in with peg (0.6)	—	—
				3. Solves pellet-bottle with demonstration (0.6)	—	—
16	1. Four-six word vocabulary (1.0)	—	—	1. Solves pellet-bottle spontaneously (0.6)	—	—
	2. One step command without gesture (1.0)	—	—	2. Round block on form board (0.6)	—	—
				3. Scribbles in imitation (0.6)	—	—
18	1. Mature jargoning (0.5)	—	—	1. Ten cubes in cup (0.5)	—	—
	2. 7–10 word vocabulary (0.5)	—	—	2. Solves round hole in form board reversed (0.5)	—	—
	3. Points to one picture (0.5)*	—	—	3. Spontaneous scribbling with crayon (0.5)	—	—
	4. Body parts (0.5)	—	—	4. Pegboard completed spontaneously (0.5)	—	—
21	1. 20 word vocabulary (1.0)	—	—	1. Obtains object with stick (1.0)	—	—
	2. Two word phrases (1.0)	—	—	2. Solves square in form board (1.0)	—	—
	3. Points to two pictures (1.0)*	—	—	3. Tower of three cubes (1.0)	—	—

(Continued.)

TABLE 9.5. (cont.)

Age (mo)	CLAMS	Yes	No	CAT	Yes	No
24	1. 50 word vocabulary (1.0)	___	___	1. Attempts to fold paper (0.7)	___	___
	2. Two-step command (1.0)	___	___	2. Horizontal four cube train (0.7)	___	___
	3. Two word sentences (1.0)	___	___	3. Imitates stroke with pencil (0.7)	___	___
				4. Completes form board (0.7)	___	___
30	1. Uses pronouns appropriately (1.5)	___	___	1. Horizontal-vertical stroke with pencil (1.5)	___	___
	2. Concept of one (1.5)*	___	___	2. Form board reversed (1.5)	___	___
	3. Points to seven pictures (1.5)*	___	___	3. Folds paper with definite crease (1.5)	___	___
	4. Two digits forward (1.5)*	___	___	4. Train with chimney (1.5)	___	___
36	1. 250 word vocabulary (1.5)	___	___	1. 3 cube bridge (1.5)	___	___
	2. Three-word sentence (1.5)	___	___	2. Draws circle (1.5)	___	___
	3. Three digits forward (1.5)*	___	___	3. Names one color (1.5)	___	___
	4. Follows two prepositional commands (1.5)*	___	___	4. Draw-a-person with head plus one other part of body (1.5)	___	___

IV. VISUAL-MOTOR SKILLS/PROBLEM SOLVING

The Goodenough-Harris Draw-a-Person Test, Gesell Figures, and Block Skills are three tests that focus on visual-motor skills and problem solving abilities. For these tests it is important to observe *how* **they are done as well as the final product.**

A. Goodenough-Harris Draw-a-Person Test

1. Procedure: Give the child a pencil (preferably a No. 2 with eraser) and a sheet of blank paper. Instruct child to "Draw a person; draw the best person you can." Supply encouragement if needed (i.e., "Draw a whole person"); however, do not suggest specific supplementation or changes.
2. Scoring: Give the child one point for each detail present using the guide in Table 9.6.
3. Goodenough age **norms** (Table 9.7)

B. Gesell Figures (Fig. 9.1)

TABLE 9.6.

Goodenough scoring

General
   1. Head present
   2. Legs present
   3. Arms present

Trunk
   4. Present
   5. Length greater than breadth
   6. Shoulders

Arms/legs
   7. Attached to trunk
   8. At correct point

Neck
   9. Present
   10. Outline of neck continuous with head, trunk, or both.

Face
   11. Eyes
   12. Nose
   13. Mouth
   14. 12 and 13 in two dimensions
   15. Nostrils

Hair
   16. Present
   17. On more than circumference; nontransparent

Clothing
   18. Present
   19. Two articles; nontransparent
   20. Entire drawing nontransparent (sleeves and trousers)
   21. Four articles
   22. Costume complete

Fingers
   23. Present
   24. Correct number
   25. Two dimension; length, breadth
   26. Thumb opposition
   27. Hand distinct from fingers and arm

Joints
   28. Elbow, shoulder or both
   29. Knee, hip, or both

Proportion
   30. Head: $1/10$ to $1/2$ of trunk area
   31. Arms: Approx. same length as trunk

(Continued.)

TABLE 9.6. (cont.)

32. Legs: 1–2 times trunk length; width less than trunk width
33. Feet: $\frac{1}{10}$ to $\frac{1}{3}$ leg length
34. Arms and legs in two dimensions
35. Heel

Motor Coordination

36. Lines firm and well connected
37. Firmly drawn with correct joining
38. Head outline
39. Trunk outline
40. Outline of arms and legs
41. Features

Ears

42. Present
43. Correct position and proportion
44. Brow or lashes

Eye Detail

45. Pupil
46. Proportion
47. Glance directed front in profile drawing

Chin

48. Present; forehead
49. Projection

Profile

50. Not more than one error
51. Correct

TABLE 9.7.

Goodenough norms

Age (yr)	3	4	5	6	7	8	9	10	11	12	13
Points	2	6	10	14	18	22	26	30	34	38	42

From Taylor E: *Psychological appraisal of children with cerebral defects*, Boston, 1961, Harvard University.

C. **Block Skills:** The structures in Fig. 9.2 should be demonstrated for the child. Figure 9.2 includes the developmental age at which each structure can usually be accomplished.

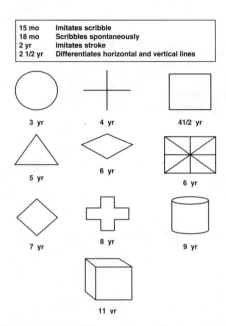

15 mo	Imitates scribble
18 mo	Scribbles spontaneously
2 yr	Imitates stroke
2 1/2 yr	Differentiates horizontal and vertical lines

FIG. 9.1. Gesell Figures *(From Illingsworth RS: The development of the infant and young child, normal and abnormal, ed 5, Baltimore, 1972, Williams and Wilkins;* Bayley Scales of Infant Development, *ed 2, 1993, The Psychological Corporation.)*

V.   PRIMITIVE REFLEXES

Intrauterine/birth reflexes appear late in gestation, are present at birth, and normally disappear by 6 to 9 months. Late infant reflexes appear after suppression of the birth reflexes. These are the postural reactions, which precede voluntary motor function. A primitive reflex profile can be helpful in identifying infants at risk for cerebral palsy or other developmental disability. An infant with an abnormally absent, asymmetric, or obligatory reflex is at high risk (Tables 9.8 and 9.9).

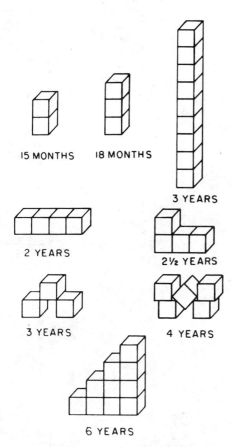

15 MONTHS   18 MONTHS

3 YEARS

2 YEARS

2½ YEARS

3 YEARS

4 YEARS

6 YEARS

FIG. 9.2. Block Skills *(From Capute AJ, Accardo PJ:* The pediatrician and the developmentally disabled child: a clinical textbook on mental retardation, *Baltimore, 1979, University Press.)*

TABLE 9.8.

Primitive Reflexes

Primitive reflexes	Elicitation	Response	Timing
Moro (MR, "embrace" response)	Supine: sudden neck extension; allow head to fall back about 3 cm	Extension, adduction and then abduction of UEs, with semiflexion of fingers, wrists, and elbows	Present at birth disappears by 3–6 mo
Galant reflex (GR)	Prone suspension: stroking paravertebral area from thoracic to sacral region	Produces truncal incurvature with concavity towards stimulated side	Present at birth disappears by 2–6 mo
Asymmetric tonic neck reflex (ATNR, "fencer" response)	Supine: rotate head laterally about 45–90 degrees	Relative extension of limbs on chin side and flexion on occiput side	Present at birth disappears by 4–9 mo
Symmetric tonic neck reflex (STNR, "cat" reflex)	Sitting: head extension/flexion	Extension of UEs and flexion of LEs/flexion of UEs and LE extension	Appears at 5 mo; not present in most normal children disappears by 8–9 mo
Tonic labyrinthine supine (TLS)	Supine: extension of the neck (alters relation of labyrinths)	Tonic extension of trunk and LEs, shoulder retraction and adduction, usually with elbow flexion	Present at birth disappears by 6–9 mo
Tonic labyrinthine prone (TLP)	Prone: flexion of the neck	Active flexion of trunk with protraction of shoulders	Present at birth disappears by 6–9 mo
Positive support reflex (PSR)	Vertical suspension; bouncing hallucal areas on firm surface	**Neonatal:** momentary LE extension followed by flexion **mature:** extension of LEs and support of body weight	Present at birth disappears by 2–4 mo appears by 6 mo

19. Using doll, tell child: Show me the nose, eyes, mouth, hands, feet, tummy, hair. Pass 6 of 8.
20. Using pictures, ask child: Which one flies?... says meow?... talks?... barks?... gallops? Pass 2 of 5, 4 of 5.
21. Ask child: What do you do when you are cold?... tired?... hungry? Pass 2 of 3, 3 of 3.
22. Ask child: What do you do with a cup? What is a chair used for? What is a pencil used for?
    Action words must be included in answers.

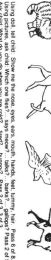

23. Pass: If child correctly places **and** says how many blocks are on paper. (1, 5).
24. Tell child: Put block **on** table, **under** table, **in front** of me, **behind** me. Pass 4 of 4.
    (Do not help child by pointing, moving head or eyes.)
25. Ask child: What is a ball?... lake?... desk?... house?... banana?... curtain?... fence?... ceiling? Pass if defined in terms
    of use, shape, what it is made of, or general category (such as banana is fruit, not just yellow). Pass 5 of 8, 7 of 8.
26. Ask child: If a horse is big, a mouse is ____? If fire is hot, ice is ____? If the sun shines during the day, the moon shines
    during the ____? Pass 2 of 3.
27. Child may use wall or rail only, not person. May not crawl.
28. Child must throw ball overhand 3 feet to within arm's reach of tester.
29. Child must perform standing broad jump over width of test sheet (8 1/2 inches).
30. Tell child to walk forward, heel within 1 inch of toe. Tester may demonstrate.
    Child must walk 4 consecutive steps.
31. In the second year, half of normal children are non-compliant.

OBSERVATIONS:

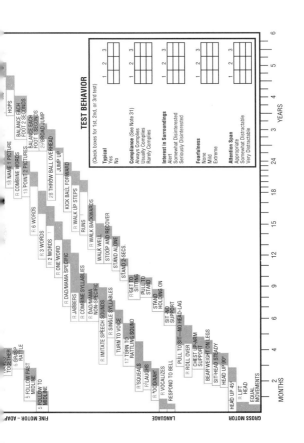

TEST BEHAVIOR

(Check boxes for 1st, 2nd, or 3rd test)

Typical
Yes
No

Compliance (See Note 31)
Always Complies
Usually Complies
Rarely Complies

Interest in Surroundings
Alert
Somewhat Disinterested
Seriously Disinterested

Fearfulness
None
Mild
Extreme

Attention Span
Appropriate
Somewhat Distractable
Very Distractable

MONTHS   YEARS

FINE MOTOR – ADAPTIVE

HANDS
6 TOGETHER
GRASP
RATTLE

5 FOLLOW PAST
MIDLINE

5 FOLLOW TO
MIDLINE

R SQUEALS

R PLAUGHS

R COO/AAH

R VOCALIZES

RESPOND TO BELL

R IMITATE SPEECH SOUNDS

R TURN TO VOICE

1? TURN TO
RATTLING SOUND

R SINGLE SYLLABLES

R DADA/MAMA
NON-SPECIFIC

R COMBINE SYLLABLES

R JABBERS

R DADA/MAMA SPECIFIC

R ONE WORD

R 2 WORDS

R 3 WORDS

R 6 WORDS

1B POINT 2 PICTURES

R COMBINE WORDS

1B NAME 1 PICTURE

LANGUAGE

GROSS MOTOR

EQUAL
MOVEMENTS

R LIFT
HEAD

HEAD UP 45°

HEAD UP 90°

SIT-HEAD STEADY

BEAR WEIGHT ON LEGS

CHEST UP-ARM
SUPPORT

R ROLL OVER

PULL TO SIT—NO HEAD-LAG

SIT-NO
SUPPORT

STAND
HOLDING ON

R PULL TO
STAND

R GET TO
SITTING

STAND 2 SECS.

STAND ALONE

STOOP AND RECOVER

WALK WELL

R WALK BACKWARDS

RUNS †

R WALK UP STEPS

KICK BALL FORWARD

JUMP UP

28 THROW BALL OVERHEAD

29 BROAD JUMP

BALANCE EACH
FOOT 1 SECONDS

BALANCE EACH
FOOT 2 SECONDS

HOPS

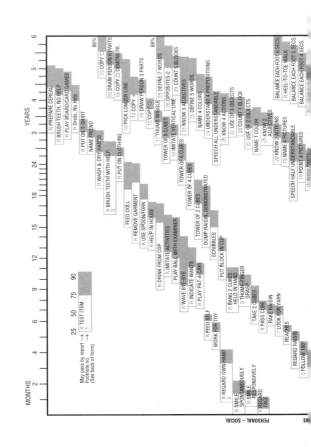

DIRECTIONS FOR ADMINISTRATION

1. Try to get child to smile by smiling, talking or waving. Do not touch him/her.
2. Child must stare at hand several seconds.
3. Parent may help guide toothbrush and put toothpaste on brush.
4. Child does not have to be able to tie shoes or button/zip in the back.
5. Move yarn slowly in an arc from one side to the other, about 8" above child's face.
6. Pass if child grasps rattle when it is touched to the backs or tips of fingers.
7. Pass if child tries to see where yarn went. Yarn should be dropped quickly from sight from tester's hand without arm movement.
8. Child must transfer cube from hand to hand without help of body, mouth, or table.
9. Pass if child picks up raisin with any part of thumb and finger.
10. Line can vary only 30 degrees or less from tester's line.
11. Make a fist with thumb pointing upward and wiggle only the thumb. Pass if child imitates and does not move any fingers other than the thumb.

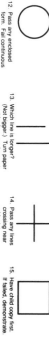

12. Pass any enclosed form. Fail continuous round motions.

13. Which line is longer? (Not bigger.) Turn paper upside down and repeat. (pass 3 of 3 or 5 of 6)

14. Pass any lines crossing near midpoint.

15. Have child copy first. If failed, demonstrate.

When giving items 12, 14, and 15, do not name the forms. Do not demonstrate 12 and 14.

16. When scoring, each pair (2 arms, 2 legs, etc.) counts as one part.
17. Place one cube in cup and shake gently near child's ear, but out of sight. Repeat for other ear.
18. Point to picture and have child name it. (No credit is given for sounds only.)

If less than 4 pictures are named correctly, have child point to picture as each is named by tester.

Reflex	Stimulus	Response	Timing
Stepping reflex (SR, walking reflex)	Vertical suspension; hallucal stimulation	Stepping gait	Present at birth disappears by 2–3 mo
Crossed extension reflex (CER)	Prone; hallucal stimulation of a LE in full extension	Initial flexion, adduction, then extension of contralateral limb	Present at birth disappears by 2–3 mo
Plantar grasp (PG)	Stimulation of hallucal area	Plantar flexion grasp	Present at birth disappears by 9 mo
Palmar grasp	Stimulation of palm	Palmar grasp	Present at birth disappears by 4 mo
Lower extremity placing (LEP)	Vertical suspension; rubbing tibia or dorsum of foot against edge of tabletop	Initial flexion, then extension, the placing of LE on tabletop	Appears at 1 day
Upper extremity placing (UEP)	Rubbing lateral surface of forearm along edge of tabletop from elbow to wrist to dorsum	Flexion, extension, then placing of hand on tabletop	Appears at 3 mo
Downward thrust (DT)	Vertical suspension; thrust LEs downward	Full extension of LEs	Appears at 3 mo

TABLE 9.9.

Postural Reactions

Postural reaction	Age of appearance	Description	Importance
Head righting	6 wk–3 mo	Lifts chin from tabletop in prone position	Necessary for adequate head control and sitting
Landau response	2–3 mo	Extension of head, then trunk and legs when held prone	Early measure of developing trunk control
Derotational righting	4–5 mo	Body follows turning of head in a derotative fashion	Prerequisite to independent rolling
Anterior propping	4–5 mo	Arm extension anteriorly in supported sitting	Necessary for tripod sitting
Lateral propping	6–7 mo	Arm extension laterally in protective response	Allows independent sitting
Posterior propping	8–10 mo	Arm extension posteriorly	Allows pivoting in sitting

From Milani-Comparetti A, Gidoni EA: *Dev Med Child Neurol* 9:631, 1967; Capute AJ: *Pediatr Ann* 15:217, 1986; Capute AJ et al: *Dev Med Child Neurol* 26:375, 1984; Palmer FB, Capute AJ: Developmental disabilities. In Oski FA, editor: *Principles and practice of pediatrics*, Philadelphia, 1994, Lippincott.

ENDOCRINOLOGY *10*

I. NORMAL VALUES

Normal values may differ among laboratories because of variation in technique and in type of radioimmunoassay used. Unless otherwise noted, values that follow come from laboratory standards at the Johns Hopkins Hospital. Ranges include 2 standard deviations (SDs) above and below the mean.

A. Gonadotropins (Table 10.1)

B. Steroid Hormone Pathway (Fig. 10.1)

C. Steroid Hormones

1. Plasma
   a. Testosterone (Table 10.2)
   b. Dihydrotestosterone (DHT), ng/dl (Table 10.2A)
   c. Estradiol, pg/ml (Table 10.3)
   d. Androgens (Table 10.4)
   e. 17, OH-progesterone, ng/dl (increased in most forms of congenital adrenal hyperplasia [CAH]) (Table 10.5)
   f. Cortisol, mcg/dl (Table 10.6)
2. Urine
   a. 17-ketosteroids, mg/24 hr (increased in most forms of CAH and adrenal tumors) (Table 10.7)
   b. Dehydroepiandrosterone (DHEA), mg/24 hr (Table 10.8)

TABLE 10.1.

Gonadotropins

	FSH (mIU/ml)	LH (mIU/ml)
Adult males	1.0–10.3	1.0–10.0
Adult females, follicular phase	1.9–10.2	2.1–15.3
Prepubertal children	0.0–2.0	0.0–1.9

Normal infants have a transient rise in follicle-stimulating hormone (FSH) and luteinizing hormone (LH) to pubertal levels or higher within the first 3 months, which then declines to prepubertal values by the end of the first year. There is no rise with central gonadotropin deficiency.

      c. 17, OH-corticosteroids (increased in Cushing's syndrome; decreased in adrenal insufficiency) (Table 10.9)

      d. Free cortisol, 25–125 mcg/24 hr:

From Migeon CJ. In Rudolf AM, editor: *Pediatrics,* Norwalk, 1987, Appleton & Lange.

D. Catecholamines

    Urinary catecholamines are elevated with neuroblastoma, ganglioneuroma, ganglioblastoma, and pheochromocytoma. Any urinary catecholamine (total catecholamines, homovanillic acid [HVA], vanillylmandelic acid [VMA], metanephrines [and dopamine]) may be elevated with neuroblastoma, ganglioneuroma, or ganglioblastoma; HVA and dopamine are usually not elevated with neuroblastoma. (Table 10.10)

E. Miscellaneous

    1. Insulin-like growth factor 1 (IGF-1) (< 25 ng/ml in most growth hormone deficient subjects; elevated with growth hormone excess) (Table 10.11)

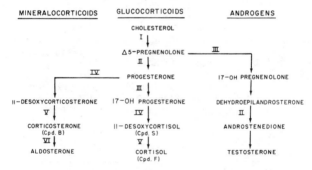

FIG. 10.1. Steroid hormone pathway and the enzymatic deficiencies in congenital adrenal hyperplasia. Enzyme deficiency: I, *cholesterol (20, 22) desmolase;* II, *3-β-ol-dehydrogenase;* III, *17-hydroxylase;* IV, *21-hydroxylase;* V, *11-hydroxylase;* VI, *18-"oxidation" defect;* Cpd, *compound.* (From Bacon GE et al: A practical approach to pediatric endocrinology, ed 3, Chicago, 1990, Yearbook Medical Publishers.)

TABLE 10.2. Testosterone

Age	Testosterone, total (ng/dl)	Testosterone, free (ng/dl)
Adult males	275–285	1.4–5.79
Adult females	23–75	0.2–0.73
	(35–195 during pregnancy)	(0.3–1.2 in 3rd week of cycle)
Prepubertal children	10–20	0.06–0.38

Ref: Endocrine Sciences Laboratory, Calabasas Hills, CA.

Table 10.2A. Dihydrotestosterone (DHT)

Age	Dihydrotestosterone (ng/dl)
Adult males	30–85
Adult females	4–22
Prepubertal children	<3
Male, Tanner stage	
2	3–17
3	8–33
4	22–52

Ref: Endocrine Sciences Laboratory, Calabasas Hills, CA.

TABLE 10.3. Estradiol (pg/ml)

Prepubertal Children	<25
Adult female	
Luteal phase	15–260
Follicular phase	10–200
Midcycle	120–375
Adult male	6–44

Infants: elevated at birth and decrease to prepubertal values during first week, then increase again between 1–2 months, then return to prepubertal levels by 6–12 months.

TABLE 10.4. Androgens

	Androstenedione* (ng/dl)	Dehydroepiandrosterone† (DHEA) (ng/dl)	Dehydroepiandrosterone sulfate † (DHEA-S) (mcg/dl)
Prepubertal children	0–50	0–100	10–60
Adult female	74–230‡	215–855	82–338
Adult male	69–149	195–915	200–335

*Increased in most forms of congenital adrenal hyperplasia (CAH).
†Increased in most forms of adrenal tumors and CAH; DHEA-S is the more steady state compound.
‡Can increase in pregnancy

TABLE 10.5.

17, OH Progesterone	ng/dl
Adult male	36–154
Adult female	
(non-pregnant)	
Follicular	15–102
Luteal	150–386
Prepubertal	
Male	0–81
Female	0–92
CAH (well-controlled)	0–430

CAH, congenital adrenal hyperplasia.

TABLE 10.6.

Cortisol	mcg/dl
Any sex/any age/pre-ACTH, at 8 AM	5.7–16.6
Post-ACTH, 1 hour	16–36

ACTH, Adrenocorticotropic hormone.

TABLE 10.7.

17-Ketosteroids	mg/24hr
Adult male	6–18
Adult female	4–13
Prepubertal	
<1 mo	<2.0
1 mo–5 yr	<0.5
6–8 yr	1.0–2.0
>8 yr	Gradually increases to adult levels

TABLE 10.8.

DHEA
<15% of total 17-ketosteroids (mg/24hr)

TABLE 10.9.

17-OH Corticosteroids	
Adult male	3–9 mg/24 hr
Adult female	2–8 mg/24 hr
Body weight variable	2.5 mg/m^2/24 hr

TABLE 10.10.

Catecholamine's

24-hour Urine

Dopamine	100–440 mcg/24 hr
Epinephrine	<15 mcg/24 hr
Norepinephrine	11–86 mcg/24 hr
Metanephrines	<0.9 mg/24 hr
HVA	1–10 mg/24 hr
VMA	2–10 mg/24 hr

From Smith Klein Beecham Clinical Laboratories
HVA, Homovanillic acid; *VMA,* vanillylmandelic acid.

TABLE 10.11.

Insulin-Like Growth Factor		ng/ml
Age	Males	Females
2 mo–6 yr	17–248	17–248
6 yr–9 yr	88–474	88–474
9 yr–12 yr	110–565	117–771
12 yr–16 yr	202–957	261–1096
16 yr–26 yr	182–780	182–780
>26 yr	123–463	123–463

2. Insulin (fasting), 1.8–24.6 mcU/ml
3. Glycosylated hemoglobin, 5.6%–7.7% (method dependent)
4. C Peptide (Table 10.12)
5. Prolactin <18 ng/ml (may be increased with pituitary and hypothalamic tumors and hypothyroidism)
6. Parathyroid hormone (Table 10.13)
7. 1,25-dihydroxy Vitamin D (pg/ml) (physiologically active form) (Table 10.14)
8. 25-hydroxy Vitamin D (ng/ml) (Table 10.15)
9. Calcitonin (pg/ml) (Table 10.16)

For sections 4, 6–9 above: from Endocrine Sciences Laboratory, Calabasas Hills, CA.

F. Thyroid Function Tests
  1. Routine studies (Table 10.17)

From Fisher DA. In Rudolf AM, editor: *Pediatrics,* Norwalk, 1991, Appleton & Lange.

  2. Thyroid antibodies: High titers are consistent with Hashimoto's thyroiditis (Table 10.18)

TABLE 10.12.

C-Peptide	
8 AM fasting	0.4–2.2 ng/ml
2 hr post prandial (sustacal)	1.2–3.4 ng/ml
2 hr post glucose	2.0–4.5 ng/ml

TABLE 10.13.

Parathyroid Hormone		
Intact	<10–65 pg/ml	(with normal calcium)
C-terminal	50–340 pg/ml	

TABLE 10.14.   1,25-dihydroxy Vitamin D

	pg/ml
Newborns	8–72
Infants and children	15–90
Adults	21–48

TABLE 10.15.   25-hydroxy Vitamin D

	ng/ml
Newborns	5–42
Children and adults	10–55

TABLE 10.16.

Calcitonin	pg/ml
Newborns	70–348
Children	<25–70
Adults	<25–150
Children, after stimulation (short Ca infusion)	25–150

G. Thyroid Function: Premature Infants
   1. Serum T_4 (mcg/dl) (Table 10.19)
   2. Free T_4 (ng/dl) (Table 10.20)

From LaFranchi SH: *Ped Clin North Am* 26:46, 1979; Travert G et al: *Clin Chem* 31:1830, 1985; Migeon CJ. In Rudolf AM, editor: *Pediatrics,* Norwalk, 1987, Appleton & Lange; Cuestas RA: *J Pediatr* 92:963, 1978.

TABLE 10.17.

Routine Studies (Thyroid)

Test	Age	Normal	Comments
T_4RIA (mcg/dl)	Cord	6.6–17.5	Measures total T_4 by radioimmunoassay.
	1–3 days	11.0–21.5	
	1–4 wk	8.2–16.6	
	1–12 mo	7.2–15.6	
	1–5 yr	7.3–15.0	
	6–10 yr	6.4–13.3	
	11–15 yr	5.6–11.7	
	16–20 yr	4.2–11.8	
	21–50 yr	4.3–12.5	
T_3RU		25–35%	Measures thyroid hormone binding, not T_3.
T index		1.25–4.20	T_4RIA X T_3RU
Free T_4 (ng/dl)	1–10 days	0.6–2.0	Metabolically active form.
	>10 days	0.7–1.7	
T_3RIA (ng/dl)	Cord	14–86	Measures triiodothyronine by radioimmunoassay.
	1–3 days	100–380	
	1–4 wk	99–310	
	1–12 mo	102–264	
	1–5 yr	105–269	
	6–10 yr	94–241	
	11–15 yr	83–213	
	16–20 yr	80–210	
	21–50 yr	70–204	
TSH (mIU/ml)	Cord	<2.5–17.4	Best sensitivity for primary hypothyroidism. TSH surge peaks between 80–90 mIU/ml in term newborn by 30 minutes after birth. Values after 1 week are within adult normal range.
	1–3 days	<2.5–13.3	
	1–4 wk	0.6–10.0	
	1–12 mo	0.6–6.3	
	1–15 yr	0.6–6.3	
	16–50 yr	0.2–7.6	
TBG (mg/dl)	Cord	0.7–4.7	With TBG deficiency: 0.1–0.9 mg/dl
	1–3 days	—	
	1–4 wk	0.5–4.5	
	1–12 mo	1.6–3.6	
	1–5 yr	1.3–2.8	
	6–20 yr	1.4–2.6	
	21–50 yr	1.2–2.4	
Reverse T_3 (ng/dl)	Newborns	90–250	Reach adult range by 1 wk.
	Children	10–50	
	Adults	10–50	

TSH, Thyroid stimulating hormone; *TBG,* thyroxine-binding globulin.

TABLE 10.18.

Thyroid Antibodies

Interpretation	Antithyroglobulin	Antimicrosomal
Insignificant	≤1:40	<1:400
Borderline	1:80	1:400
Significant	1:160–1:640	1:1600–1:6400
Very significant	>1:640	>1:6400

II. SEXUAL DEVELOPMENT

A. **Penile Length:** Measured from pubic ramus to tip of glans while traction is applied along length of phallus to point of increased resistance. Penile length >2.5 SD below mean is considered abnormal (Table 10.21).

From Feldman KW, Smith DW: *J Pediatr* 86:395, 1975; Winter JSD, Faiman C: *Ped Res* 6:126, 1972; Lee PA, O'Dea L. In Hung W: *Clinical pediatric endocrinology,* St Louis, 1992, Mosby.

B. **Testicular Size:** Testicular growth is the earliest sign of puberty. Testicular volume of > 4 ml or a long axis > 2.5 cm is evident that pubertal testicular growth has begun (Table 10.22).

From Lee PA, O'Dea L. In Hung W: *Clinical pediatric endocrinology,* St Louis, 1992, Mosby.

C. **Clitoris**
1. Anogenital ratio: Distance between anus and posterior fourchette divided by distance between anus and base of clitoris. It is independent of body size and gestational age. Ratio >0.5 suggests virilization with labioscrotal fusion.

From Callegari C: *J Pediatr* 111:240, 1987.

2. Length: Newborn (mean ± SD) = 4.3 ± 1.1 mm.

From Yoyaka S: Horumon To Rinsho 31:69, 1983.

3. Premature infants: Clitoris normally is more prominent because clitoral size is fully developed by 27 weeks gestation, and there is less fat in labia majora.

TABLE 10.19.

Serum T$_4$ (mcg/dl)

Age	30–31	32–33	34–35	36–37	Term
		Estimated gestational age (wk)			
Cord	4.5–8.5	3.3–11.7	4.3–9.1	1.9–13.1	4.6–11.8
12–72 hr	7.3–15.7	5.9–18.7	6.2–18.6	10.3–20.7	14.8–23.2
3–10 days	4.1–11.3	4.7–12.3	5.2–14.8	7.7–17.7	9.9–21.9
11–20 days	3.9–11.1	5.1–11.5	6.9–14.1	5.4–17.0	8.2–16.2
21–45 days	4.8–10.8	4.6–11.4	6.7–11.9	3.0–19.8	9.1–15.1
46–90 days	6.2–13.0	6.2–13.0	6.2–13.0	6.2–13.0	6.4–14.0

TABLE 10.20.

Free T$_4$ (ng/dl)

GA (wk)	27–28	29–30	31–32	33–34	35–36	37–38
Free T$_4$	0.03–1.3	0.3–1.2	0.2–1.6	0.5–1.4	0.5–1.7	0.6–1.9

GA, Estimated gestational age (wk).

TABLE 10.21.

Mean Stretched Penile Length (cm)

Age	Mean ± SD	−2.5 SD
Birth		
30 wk gestation	2.7 ± 0.5	1.5
34 wk gestation	3.0 ± 0.4	2.0
Full term	3.5 ± 0.4	2.5
0–5 mo	3.8 ± 0.8	1.8
6–12 mo	4.1 ± 0.8	2.1
1–2 yr	4.6 ± 0.8	2.6
2–3 yr	5.0 ± 0.8	3.0
3–4 yr	5.4 ± 1.0	2.9
4–5 yr	5.6 ± 0.7	3.4
5–7 yr	6.0 ± 0.9	3.8
7–9 yr	6.3 ± 1.0	3.8
9–11 yr	6.3 ± 1.0	3.8
11–14 yr	6.3 ± 2.0	5.0
14–16 yr	8.6 ± 2.4	6.0
16–18 yr	9.9 ± 1.7	4.3
18–20 yr	11.0 ± 1.1	2.8
Adult	12.4 ± 1.6	4.0

TABLE 10.22.

Testicular Size

Age (yr)	Length (cm) (mean ± SD)	Corresponding volume (ml) (approximate)	Tanner stage (genital)
<2	1.4 ± 0.4		
2–4	1.2 ± 0.4		
4–6	1.5 ± 0.6	1	
6–8	1.8 ± 0.3		
8–10	2.0 ± 0.5	2	1
10–12	2.7 ± 0.7	5	2
12–14	3.4 ± 0.8	10	3
14–16	4.1 ± 1.0	20	4
16–18	5.0 ± 0.5	29	5
18–20	5.0 ± 0.3	29	

SD, Standard deviation.

D. Secondary Sex Characteristics
(See Chapter 5 for diagramatic representations.)
    1. Tanner stages (mean age ± SD)
        a. Breast development (Table 10.23)
        b. Genital development (male) (Table 10.24)
        c. Pubic hair (male and female) (Table 10.25)
From Oski FA et al: *Principles and practice of pediatrics,* ed 2, Philadelphia, 1994, JB Lippincott as adapted from Marshall WA, Tanner JM: *Archives Dis Childhood* 44:291, 1969 and Marshall WA, Tanner JM: *Archives Dis Childhood* 45:13, 1970.
    2. Pubertal events See Fig. 5.1 for the temporal relation between the biologic, psychologic, and psychosocial events of adolescence.

TABLE 10.23.

Breast Development

Stage I	Preadolescent; elevation of papilla only
Stage II	Breast bud; elevation of breast and papilla as small mound; enlargement of areolar diameter (11.15 ± 1.10)
Stage III	Further enlargement and elevation of breast and areola; no separation of their contours (12.15 ± 1.09)
Stage IV	Projection of areola and papilla to form secondary mound above level of breast (13.11 ± 1.15)
Stage V	Mature stage; projection of papilla only due to recession of areola to general contour of breast (15.33 ± 1.74)

Note: Stages IV and V may not be distinct in some patients.

TABLE 10.24.

Genital Development (Male)

Stage I	Preadolescent; testes, scrotum, and penis about same size and proportion as in early childhood
Stage II	Enlargement of scrotum and testes; skin of scrotum reddens and changes in texture; little or no enlargement of penis (11.64 ± 1.07)
Stage III	Enlargement of penis, first mainly in length; further growth of testes and scrotum (12.85 ± 1.04)
Stage IV	Increased size of penis with growth in breadth and development of glans; further enlargement of testes and scrotum and increased darkening of scrotal skin (13.77 ± 1.02)
Stage V	Genitalia adult in size and shape (14.92 ± 1.10)

TABLE 10.25.

Pubic Hair (Male and Female)

Stage I	Preadolescent; vellus over pubes no further developed than that over abdominal wall (i.e., no pubic hair)
Stage II	Sparse growth of long, slightly pigmented downy hair, straight or only slightly curled, chiefly at base of penis or along labia (Male: 13.44 ± 1.09, Female: 11.69 ± 1.21)
Stage III	Considerably darker, coarser and more curled; hair spreads sparsely over junction of pubes (Male: 13.9 ± 1.04, Female: 12.36 ± 1.10)
Stage IV	Hair resembles adult in type; distribution still considerably smaller than in adult; no spread to medial surface of thighs (Male: 14.36 ± 1.08, Female: 12.95 ± 1.06)
Stage V	Adult in quantity and type with distribution of the horizontal pattern (Male: 15.18 ± 1.07, Female: 14.41 ± 1.12)
Stage VI	Spread up linea alba: "male escutcheon"

III. TESTS AND PROCEDURES
A. Sexual development
1. **Karyotype:** Purpose is to determine chromosomal sex in patients with ambiguous genitalia. Y-chromosome specific markers are available. Further details are in Chapter 13.
2. **Vaginal smear**
   a. Purpose: To test for estrogenization of vaginal mucosa; useful in evaluating precocious puberty
   b. Method: Make a wet mount of internal vaginal secretions with normal saline. Methylene blue may be used

to stain nuclei, but an unstained preparation can also be read. To make a permanent slide for cytopathology, place in 95% ethanol fixative.

c. Interpretation
1) Low estrogen states: Predominance of round or oval parabasal cells with thick cytoplasm and vesicular nuclei displaying chromatin detail
2) High estrogen states: Predominance of polygonal squamous (superficial) cells with small pyknotic nuclei and thin cytoplasm
3) Intermediate cells with squamelike cytoplasm and nuclei with a reticular chromatin pattern may be variably present but will predominate in high cortisol or high progestin states (e.g., the second half of the menstrual cycle)

From Gold JJ, Josimovich JB: *Gynecologic endocrinology,* ed 4, New York, 1987, Plenum Medical Book Co.

3. **Dexamethasone suppression test (DST)**
a. Purpose: To evaluate premature adrenarche or precocious puberty.
b. Interpretation: Increased urinary 17-ketosteroids (17-KS) confirm the diagnosis of CAH. Incomplete suppression of 17-KS suggests that patient has entered puberty. Markedly increased, nonsuppressible 17-KS suggests the presence of an androgen-producing tumor, most likely adrenal in origin.

From Kelch RP. In Rudolf AM, editor: *Pediatrics,* Norwalk, 1987, Appleton & Lange.

4. **Gonadotropin releasing hormone (Gn-RH, or LHRH) stimulation test**
a. Purpose: Measures pituitary luteinizing hormone (LH) and follicle stimulating hormone (FSH) reserve. Helpful in the differential diagnosis of precocious or delayed sexual development.
b. Interpretation: Normal prepubertal children should show no or minimal increase in LH and FSH to an Gn-RH injection. An exaggerated response of a rise of LH into the adult range is obtained in central precocious puberty and in primary gonadal failure (e.g., Turner's syndrome).

From Kelch RP. In Rudolf AM, editor: *Pediatrics,* Norwalk, 1987, Appleton and Lange; Reiter EO et al: *Pediatr Res* 9:111, 1975; Hughes IA: *Handbook of endocrine tests in children,* Bristol, 1986, Wright.

5. **Human chorionic gonadotropin (HCG) stimulation test:** Used to differentiate cryptorchidism (undescended testes) from anorchia (absent testes). In cryptorchidism, after IM HCG testosterone rises to adult levels; in anorchia there is no rise. A 4–6 week course of HCG may be used by some to induce descent of cryptorchid testes; the timing and value of this procedure is controversial.

From Penny R. In Kaplan SA, editor: *Clinical pediatric and adolescent endocrinology,* Philadelphia, 1982, WB Saunders Co; Lee PA et al: *Johns Hopkins Medical Journal* 146:159, 1980; Garagorri et al: *J Pediatr* 101:923, 1982.

B. **Growth**
   1. **Adult height prediction**
      a. Bayley-Pinneau method: Uses Greulich and Pyle bone age (left hand and wrist radiograph) and present stature.
      b. RWT (Roche-Wainer-Thissen) method: Uses Greulich and Pyle bone age, recumbent length, weight, and midparental heights.
      c. Genetic potential formula, using mean parental stature:
         1) Boys: Paternal height + maternal height + 5 in/2
         2) Girls: Paternal height + maternal height − 5 in/2
            Target height is midparental height ± 2 SD, with 1 SD approximately 2 inches.
      d. Growth curves: Available for early, normal, and late maturers. Predict height percentile by plotting patient's height and extrapolating to adult height at the same percentile.

From Roche A: *Pediatrics* 56:1026, 1975; Tanner JM et al: *Assessment of skeletal maturity and prediction of adult height* (TW-2 method), ed 2, New York, 1983, Academic Press; Cohen P. In McAnarney ER et al, editors: *Textbook of adolescent medicine,* Philadelphia, 1992, WB Saunders.

   2. **Growth hormone (GH) detection:** Because GH secretion is pulsatile, a random GH may be low, even undetectible, in normal individuals. Diagnosis of GH deficiency requires two abnormal stimulation tests (not screening tests). A single value of >10 ng/ml on a screening or stimulation test rules out GH deficiency; values must be <3 to rule out excessive GH. Patients must be euthyroid for these tests to be valid.

From Johns Hopkins Laboratory for reference values.

a. Screening tests
   1) Sleep specimen: Draw GH samples from an indwelling catheter 30 and 60 minutes after onset of sleep. Most subjects will have a rise in GH 45–60 minutes after the onset of nocturnal sleep.
   2) Exercise test: After fasting the patient for at least 4 hours, get baseline GH level. Obtain a GH sample immediately after exercising (e.g., steady jogging for 20 minutes); 80% or more of normal persons will release significant amounts of GH after vigorous exercise.
   3) IGF-1 (Somatomedin C): May be drawn at any time during the day. May be useful in detecting patients with quantitative or qualitative deficiencies in GH not picked up by standard provocative tests. A clearly normal IGF-1 level argues against GH deficiency, although in young children there is considerable overlap between normals and those with GH deficiency. (Normal values are in Table 10.11.)

From Eisenstein E et al: *Pediatrics* 62:526, 1978; Reiter E: *Compr Ther* 9(2):45, 1983; Hughes IA: *Handbook of endocrine tests in children,* Bristol, 1986, Wright.

b. Stimulation tests: GH secretion may be stimulated by arginine, insulin-induced hypoglycemia, L-dopa, glucagon, and clonidine. A GH level >10 ng/ml effectively rules out GH deficiency. (Note that some labs use 7 ng/ml as the cut-off for normal vs. abnormal.) Values between 7 and 10 ng/ml are equivocal and may indicate partial deficiency and require further evaluation. Results <7 ng/ml are definitely abnormal.

From Bacon GE et al: *A practical approach to pediatric endocrinology,* ed 3, Chicago, 1990, Year Book Medical Publishers; Hughes IA: *Handbook of endocrine tests in children,* Bristol, 1986, Wright.

C. **Adrenal and Pituitary Function**
   1. **Urinary 17-hydroxycorticosteroids (17-OHCSs)**
      a. Measures approximately one third of the end products of cortisol metabolism.
      b. Method: Collect a 24-hour urine specimen. Refrigerate during collection and process immediately (17-OHCSs are destroyed at room temperature).
      c. Interpretation

1) Decreased in inanition states (anorexia nervosa), pituitary disorders involving ACTH, Addison's disease, administration of synthetic, potent corticosteroids (prednisone, dexamethasone, triamcinolone), 21-hydroxylase deficiency, liver disease, hypothyroidism, newborn period (due to decreased glucuronidation).

2) Increased in Cushing's syndrome; ACTH, cortisone, or cortisol therapy; medical or surgical stress; obesity (occasionally); hyperthyroidism; 11-hydroxylase deficiency.

2. **Urinary 17-ketosteroids**
   a. Measures some end products of androgen metabolism.
   b. Method: Collect and refrigerate 24-hour urine specimen.
   c. Interpretation
      1) Increased in adrenal hyperplasia (in congenital adrenal hyperplasia it may take 1–2 weeks for 17-KS to rise above the normally high newborn levels; other signs of CAH would be hyponatremia, hyperkalemia, high 17-OH progesterone, and high androstenedione). Also increased in virilizing adrenal tumors; Cushing's syndrome; exogenous ACTH, cortisone, or androgen administration (except methyltestosterone); stressful illness (burns, radiation illness, etc.); and androgen-producing gonadal tumors.
      2) Decreased in Addison's disease, anorexia nervosa, panhypopituitarism.

3. **Plasma corticosteroids**
   a. Method: Collect heparinized blood and separate plasma immediately. Measure cortisol (corticosterone and 11-deoxycortisol sometimes may be needed). Because of the diurnal variation in cortisol concentration, 8 AM (the time of peak cortisol level) is the best time to draw plasma cortisol level.
   b. Interpretation: Same as for 17-OHCSs (see Table 10.9); except usually normal in anorexia nervosa, liver disease, hypothyroidism, hyperthyroidism, and obesity. Elevated levels by protein binding assay occur during pregnancy and during estrogen administration.

4. **Plasma 17-OH progesterone (17-OHP)**
   a. Method: Collect heparinized blood and separate plasma immediately.
   b. Interpretation: Measures precursor, which is elevated with 21- and 11-hydroxylase deficiency forms of CAH.
5. **Adrenal capacity test (ACTH stimulation test)**
   a. Purpose: Used to evaluate adrenal insufficiency, either primary (Addison's disease), secondary (ACTH deficiency), or resulting from adrenal suppression after long-term steroid treatment.
   b. Interpretation: With a normal pituitary-adrenal axis there is a rise in serum cortisol after IV ACTH. With ACTH deficiency or prolonged adrenal suppression, there is not a rise in cortisol after a single IV dose, since this does not produce adrenal reactivation. After 3 days of IM ACTH, however, there will be adrenal reactivation with a rise in urinary 17-OHCSs. A lack of response to the IM ACTH stimulation is pathognomonic of Addison's disease; a subnormal response may be seen with adrenal hyperplasia; a normal response is seen with ACTH deficiency.

From Migeon CJ. In Rudolf AM, editor. *Pediatrics,* Norwalk, 1987, Appleton-Lange; Hughes IA: *Handbook of endocrine tests in children,* Bristol, 1986, Wright.

6. **Pituitary ACTH capacity (metyrapone) test:** Metyrapone inhibits 11-hydroxylase in the adrenal and blocks cortisol production. This causes a rise in ACTH, which increases production of cortisol precursors, which accumulate (the measured precursor is 17-deoxycortisol) and are excreted as 17-OHCSs. A failure of 17-deoxycortisol and 17-OHCSs to rise occurs with pituitary ACTH deficiency, hypothalamic tumors, and pharmacologic doses of steroids. An exaggerated response after metyrapone occurs in pituitary-dependent Cushing's syndrome, hypothyroidism, and diabetes mellitus.

Warning: Test can precipitate adrenal crisis.

From Migeon CJ. In Rudolf AM, editor: *Pediatrics,* Norwalk, 1987, Appleton-Lange; Hughes IA: *Handbook of endocrine tests in children,* Bristol, 1986, Wright.

7. **Insulin-induced hypoglycemia:** With insulin-induced (or spontaneous) hypoglycemia, plasma cortisol normally rises by >10 mcg/dl or to a level of >20 mcg/dl.

8. **Dexamethasone suppression test (DST)**
   a. Dexamethasone suppresses secretion of ACTH by the normal pituitary, decreasing endogenous production of cortisol and, hence, the excretion of 17-OHCSs. Dexamethasone is not excreted as 17-OHCSs.
   b. Standard low-dose and high-dose DST
      1) Method: Give dexamethasone PO for 3 days (low dose: 1.25 mg/m^2/day; high dose: 3.75 mg/m^2/day divided Q6 hr) and collect 24-hour urine for 17-OHCS. (If using DST to evaluate premature adrenarche, also measure urinary 17-KS and pregnanetriol.)
      2) Interpretation: Normally, and in obesity, low dose DST causes 17-OHCS to fall to <1 mg/m^2/24 hr. In Cushing's syndrome secondary to adrenal hyperplasia, 17-OHCS levels are not suppressed by the low dose DST, but fall with the high dose DST, unless the hyperplasia is due to ectopic ACTH production (lung, mediastinal tumor, etc.). With Cushing's syndrome caused by adrenocortical carcinoma, and with some hypothalamic tumors, 17-OHCS levels are not suppressed even with the high dose DST.
   c. Overnight screening DST: Give 1 mg dexamethasone at 11 PM. At 8 or 9 AM the following day, draw a fasting serum cortisol level. In normal or obese patients, the serum cortisol should fall below 5 mcg/dl.

From Migeon CJ. In Rudolf AM, editor: *Pediatrics,* Norwalk, 1987, Appleton-Lange; Bongiovanni AM. In Kaplan SA editor: *Clinical pediatric and adolescent endocrinology,* Philadelphia, 1982, WB Saunders.

9. **Water deprivation test**
   a. Used to diagnose diabetes insipidus. Requires careful supervision since dehydration and hypernatremia may occur.
   b. Method: Begin the test in the morning after a 24-hour period of adequate hydration and stable weight. Have the patient empty his or her bladder and obtain a baseline weight. Restrict fluids for 7 hours. Measure

body weight and urinary specific gravity and volume hourly. Check serum sodium and urine and serum osmolality every 2 hours. Hematocrit and blood urea nitrogen (BUN) may also be obtained at these times but are not critical. Monitor carefully to assure that fluids are not ingested during the test. Terminate the test if weight loss approaches 5%.

c. Interpretation

1) Normal individuals who are water deprived will concentrate their urine between 500 and 1400 mOsm/L and plasma osmolality will range between 288 and 291 mOsm/L. In normal children and those with psychogenic diabetes insipidus (DI), urinary specific gravity rises to at least 1.010 and usually greater. The urinary-to-plasma osmolality ratio exceeds 2. Urine volume decreases significantly, and there should be no appreciable weight loss.

2) Specific gravity remains below 1.005 in patients with antidiuretic hormone (ADH)-deficient or nephrogenic DI. Urine osmolality remains below 150 mOsm/L with no significant reduction of urine volume. A weight loss of up to 5% usually occurs. At the end of the test, a serum osmolality >290 mOsm/L, Na >150 mEq/L, and a rise of BUN and hematocrit provide evidence that the patient did not receive water.

10. **Vasopressin test**

a. To test for nephrogenic versus ADH-deficient (central) diabetes insipidus, vasopressin is given subcutaneously, preferably at the end of the water deprivation test. Urine output, urine concentration, and water intake are monitored. Intranasal vasopressin is not recommended for this test.

b. Interpretation: Patients with ADH-deficient DI concentrate their urine (to 1.010 and usually greater) and demonstrate a reduction of urine volume and decreased fluid intake. Patients with nephrogenic DI have no significant change in intake, urine volume, or specific gravity. Constant intake associated with decreased output and increased specific gravity suggests psychogenic DI.

(For sections 7–10 above): From Bacon GE et al: *Pediatric endocrinology,* ed 3, Chicago, 1990, Year Book.

D. Thyroid Function

1. **Thyroid function tests: interpretation** (see Table 10.26)

2. **Thyroid scan:** Used to assess thyroidal clearance, localize ectopic thyroid tissue, and study structure and function of the thyroid. Localizes hyperfunctioning and nonfunctioning thyroid nodules. Uptake is increased in most types of dyshormonogenesis.

3. **Technetium uptake:** Measures uptake of technetium by thyroid gland during the first 20 minutes after administration. Normal: 0.24%–3.4%. Increased in hyperthyroidism. Decreased in TBG deficiency and in hypothyroidism (except dyshormonogenesis, when it may be increased).

4. **Pituitary thyroid-stimulating hormone (TSH) Reserve Test:** Synthetic thyroid-releasing hormone (TRH) can be given IV, which will normally cause a rise in TSH. No rise in TSH in the face of a high T_4 is confirmatory of hyperthyroidism. No rise in TSH in the face of a low T_4 and low TSH suggests pituitary dysfunction. An exaggerated delayed peak TSH response is suggestive of hypothalamic hypothyroidism, but the distinction from normal is not always clear.

From Lee WP. In Kaplan SA, editor: *Clinical pediatric and adolescent endocrinology,* Philadelphia, 1982, WB Saunders.

E. Pancreatic Endocrine Function

1. A **random plasma glucose** of >200 mg/dl in the presence of classic symptoms of diabetes (polyuria, polydipsia, ketonuria, and weight loss) is diagnostic of diabetes mellitus.

2. **Oral glucose tolerance test (OGTT)**

   a. Pretest preparation: Calorically adequate diet required for 3 days before the test, with 50% of total calories as carbohydrate.

   b. Delay test 2 weeks after period of illness. Discontinue all hyperglycemic or hypoglycemic agents (salicylates, diuretics, oral contraceptives, phenytoin, etc.).

TABLE 10.26.

Thyroid Function Tests: Interpretation

	T$_4$RIA	T$_3$RU	T index	Free T$_4$	TSH
1st-degree hypothyroidism	L	L	L	L	H
2nd-degree hypothyroidism	L	L	L	L	N or L
TBG deficiency	L	H	N	N	N
Hyperthyroidism	H	H	H	H	L

L, Low; H, high; N, normal; *TBG,* thyroxine-binding globulin.

> c. Method: Give 1.75 g/kg (**max** 100 g) of glucose orally after a 12 hour fast allowing up to 5 minutes for ingestion. Mix glucose with water and lemon juice as a 20% dilution. Quiet activity is permissible during the OGTT. Draw blood samples at 0, 30, 60, 120, 180, and 240 minutes.
> d. Interpretation (venous plasma using autoanalyzer ferricyanide method): In asymptomatic individuals, diabetes mellitus is diagnosed if the fasting venous plasma glucose is >140 mg/dl and two OGTTs are abnormal. The OGTT is abnormal if the 2-hour sample and one other sample show plasma venous glucose >200 mg/dl.

From American Diabetes Association, 1989.

3. **Estimated insulin requirements:** approximately 1 U/kg/day

2/3 in AM:	2/3 of AM dose as NPH
	1/3 of AM dose as regular
1/3 in PM:	1/2 of PM dose as NPH
	1/2 of PM dose as regular

Note: For management of diabetic ketoacidosis and adrenal crisis, see Chapter 1; for stress dosing of steroids and relative potencies, see Chapter 28.

FLUIDS & ELECTROLYTES

11

I. MAINTENANCE REQUIREMENTS

A. **Caloric Expenditure Method:** This method is based on the understanding that water and electrolyte requirements parallel caloric expenditure but not body weight. It is effective for all ages, shapes, and clinical states.

1. Determine the child's standard basal caloric expenditure (SBC) (Table 11.1).

TABLE 11.1.

Age	Weight (kg)	Caloric expenditure (cal/kg/24 hr)
Newborn	2.5–4	50
1 wk–6 mo	3–8	65–70
6–12 mo	8–12	50–60
1–2 yr	10–15	45–50
2–5 yr	15–20	45
5–10 yr	20–35	40–45
10–16 yr	35–60	25–40
Adult	70	15–20

2. Add 12% of SBC for each degree that the patient's rectal temperature is above 37.8° C.
3. Add 0–30% of SBC to account for activity level; e.g., coma (add nothing) or thrashing/tachypnea (add 30%).
4. For each 100 calories metabolized in 24 hours, the average patient will need 100–120 ml H_2O, 2–4 mEq Na^+, and 2–3 mEq K^+, as derived from Table 11.2.

Average water (ml) and electrolyte (mEq) requirements for different clinical states per 100 calories per 24 hours (Table 11.2).

TABLE 11.2.

Clinical state	H$_2$O	Na	K
Average patient receiving parenteral fluids*	100–120	2–4	2–3
Anuria	45	0	0
Acute CNS infections and inflammation	80–90	2–4	2–3
Diabetes insipidus	Up to 400	Var	Var
Hyperventilation	120–210	2–4	2–3
Heat stress	120–240	Var	Var
High humidity environment	80–100	2–4	2–3

*Adequate maintenance solution: dextrose 5%–10% (as needed) in 0.2% NaCl + 20 mEq/L of KCl.
Var, Variable requirement.

Average water (ml) and electrolyte (mEq) expenditures per 100 calories metabolized over 24 hours (Table 11.3).

TABLE 11.3.

	Usual			Range*		
Route	H$_2$O	Na$^+$	K$^+$	H$_2$O	Na$^+$	K$^+$
Lungs	15	0	0	10–60	0	0
Skin	30	0.1	0.2	20–100	0.1–3.0	0.2–1.5
Stool	5	0.1	0.2	0–50	0.1–4.0	0.2–3.0
Urine	65	3.0	2.0	0–400	0.2–30	0.4–30
Total	115†	3.2	2.4	30–610	0.4–37	0.8–34.5

*High values represent abnormal losses resulting from environmental variation or pathologic states.
†Maintenance H$_2$O requirements are less than estimated total expenditure, because 5–15 ml H$_2$O is produced endogenously during oxidation of carbohydrate, fat and protein.
From Hellerstein, *Pediatr Rev,* 14:109, 1993.

B.   Holiday-Segar Method: This is a quick, simple formula that estimates caloric expenditure from weight alone; it assumes that for each 100 calories metabolized, 100ml of H$_2$O will be required. This method is not suitable for neonates < 14 days old (generally overestimates fluid needs in neonates compared with the caloric expenditure method) and does not account for abnormal losses (Table 11.4).

TABLE 11.4.

Holiday-Segar Method

Body Weight	Water		Electrolytes (mEq per 100ml H_2O)
	ml/kg/day	ml/kg/hr	
First 10 kg	100	$\div$ 24 hr/day $\approx$ 4	Na^+ 3
Second 10 kg	50	$\div$ 24 hr/day $\approx$ 2	Cl^- 2
Each additional kg	20	$\div$ 24 hr/day $\approx$ 1	K^+ 2

EXAMPLE: 8-YEAR-OLD WEIGHING 25 KG

ml/kg/day	ml/kg/hr
100 (for 1st 10 kg) $\times$ 10 kg = 1000 ml/day	4 (for 1st 10 kg) $\times$ 10 kg = 40 ml/hr
50 (for 2nd 10 kg) $\times$ 10 kg = 500 ml/day	2 (for 2nd 10 kg) $\times$ 10 kg = 20 ml/hr
20 (for each add'l kg) $\times$ 5 kg = 100 ml/day	1 (for each add'l kg) $\times$ 5 kg = 5 ml/hr
1600 ml/day	65 ml/hr

C. **Body Surface Area Method:** This method is based on the assumption that caloric expenditure is proportional to surface area. It should not be used for children < 10 kg. It provides no convenient method of taking into account changes in metabolic rate. See Chapter 14 for body surface area nomogram and conversion formula (Table 11.5).

TABLE 11.5.

H_2O	1500 ml/m²/24 hr
Na	30–50 mEq/m²/24 hr
K	20–40 mEq/m²/24 hr

From Finberg et al: *Water and electrolytes in pediatrics,* Philadelphia, 1982, WB Saunders; Behrman et al: *Nelson textbook of pediatrics,* ed 13, Philadelphia, 1987, WB Saunders; Hellerstein: Fluids and electrolytes: clinical aspects, *Pediatr Rev* 14:103, 1993.

II. DEFICIT THERAPY

The most precise method of assessing fluid deficit is based on pre-illness weight, calculated as follows:

$$\% \text{ Dehydration} = \frac{\text{Preillness weight} - \text{illness weight}}{\text{Preillness weight}} \times 100\%$$

If this is not available, then clinical observation may be used, as described below.

A. **Clinical Assessment**
   1. Clinical observation (Table 11.6)

TABLE 11.6.

% Dehydration (ml/kg) Infants	Children	Clinical Observation
5% (50ml/kg)	3% (30ml/kg)	HR (10–15% above baseline)
		Slightly dry mucous membranes
		Concentration of the urine
		Poor tear production*
		Sunken eyeballs
10% (100ml/kg)	6% (60ml/kg)	Increased severity of the above
		Decreased skin turgor
		Oliguria
		Sunken anterior fontanelle
15% (150ml/kg)	9% (90ml/kg)	Decreased blood pressure
		Delayed capillary refill
		Kussmaul breathing
		Obtundation

*This sign may be a less sensitive indicator of dehydration.
From Oski, FA: *Principles and practice of pediatrics*, 1994, Lippincott; Feld, Koskel, Schoeneman: *Adv Pediatr*, 35:507, 1988.

   2. In hypotonic (hyponatremic) dehydration ($Na^+ < 130$), manifestations appear with less fluid deficit. In hypertonic (hypernatremic) dehydration ($Na^+ > 150$), the circulating volume is relatively preserved at the expense of intracellular water, so that circulatory disturbance is not seen until a greater degree of dehydration occurs.
B. **General Guidelines of Deficit Calculation for IV Hydration**
   For all types of dehydration, if dehydration occurs for < 3 days, then 80% of losses are from ECF and 20% from ICF. If ≥ 3 days, then 60% of losses are from ECF and 40% from ICF.

1. Intracellular and extracellular fluid composition (Table 11.7)

TABLE 11.7.

	Intracellular (mEq/L)	Extracellular (mEq/L)
Na^+	20	145
K^+	150	3–5
Cl^-	—	110
HCO_3^-	10	20–25
PO_4^-	110–115	5
Protein	75	10

2. Electrolyte deficits
   a. Formula

mEq required = (CD − CA) × fD × Wt
CD = concentration desired (mEq/L)
CA = concentration present (mEq/L)
fD = distribution factor as fraction of body weight
Wt = baseline weight before illness (kg)

   b. Apparent distribution factor (fD)

Electrolyte	fD
HCO_3	0.4–0.5
Cl^-	0.2–0.3
Na^{+*}	0.6–0.7

*See p. 222 on hyponatremia for further calculations

3. Free water (FW) deficit in hypernatremic dehydration: Calculated based upon the ml/kg of FW required to decrease the serum sodium by 1 mEq/L and is based on the patient's actual serum sodium. The general calculation is as follows:

Example:

If serum Na^+ = 145 mEq/L (normal), then

$$\frac{145 - 144 \text{ mEq/L}}{145 \text{ mEq/L}} \times 1000ml \times (0.6^* \times \text{body wt in kg}) =$$

$$\frac{600}{[Na]_s^\dagger} = \frac{600}{145} = 4 \text{ ml/kg}$$

*This assumes that the FW deficit is distributed throughout the total body water (TBW) and TBW is approximately 60% of body weight.
†[Na]$_s$ Actual serum Na^+.

Using the above formula, one can estimate the following:

Actual serum sodium (mEq/L)	ml/kg FW required to drop serum Na^+ by 1mEq/L
145–170	4
> 170	3

To calculate the liters of FW given in IVF:

$$1.0 - \frac{\text{concentration } Na^+ \text{ in IVF}}{\text{serum } Na^+ \text{ concentration}} \times \text{L IVF given} = \text{L FW given}$$

From Molteni KH: *Clin Pediatr,* 33:738, 1994.

C. **Overview of Parenteral Rehydration**
  1. Phase I (Emergency) Management: If the patient is hemodynamically unstable, this should be carried out regardless of the type of dehydration (isotonic, hypotonic, or hypertonic) suspected.
     a. Symptomatic dehydration or shock requires one to two 20 ml/kg boluses of isotonic fluid (i.e., lactated Ringer's or 0.9% [normal] NaCl) in the first 30 minutes.
     b. Consider blood or plasma (10 ml/kg) if there is no response after 2 boluses of isotonic fluid or if there is acute blood loss.

    c. For seizures caused by hyponatremia, give 10–12
ml/kg of 3% saline over 60 minutes, or to calculate the
number of ml needed of 3% NaCl to raise the serum
Na by 10 mEq/L:

[amount of 3% NaCl (ml)] = 10 mEq/L × body weight (kg) × 0.6

From Fleisher G, Ludwig S: *Textbook of pediatric emergency medicine,* Baltimore, 1993, Williams and Wilkins.

    2. Phase II (Maintenance, Deficit, and Ongoing Losses)
Management: Calculate the fluid and electrolyte requirements for the next 24 hours.
      a. Maintenance: Use methods described on p. 215 to
calculate maintenance requirements.
      b. Deficits
        1) Isonatremic dehydration (Na^+ = 130–150 mEq/L)

*Example: 5-month-old, 6.3 kg illness weight with 10% deficit,
losses over 4 days and serum Na^+ = 137 mEq/L*

        a) Calculate total fluid deficit based on section II
A. If no preillness weight is available, estimate
% deficit based on clinical exam.

          10% deficit = 0.7L

        b) Calculate estimates of ECF and ICF electrolyte
deficits using formula A × B × C where A =
total fluid deficit (liters), B = ECF or ICF
concentration of electrolyte, C = % loss from
ECF or ICF compartment.

Sample calculations:

$[Na]_{ECF}$ = 0.7L × 145 mEq/L × 0.6 = 61 mEq ECF Na^+ deficit

$[Na]_{ICF}$ = 0.7L × 20 mEq/L × 0.4 = 5.6 mEq ICF Na^+ deficit

$[K]_{ECF}$ = 0.7L × 5 mEq/L × 0.6 = 2.1 mEq ECF K+ deficit

$[K]_{ICF}$ = 0.7L × 150 mEq/L × 0.4 = 42 mEq ICF K+ deficit

Total Na^+ deficit = 61 + 5.6 = 66.6 mEq Na^+

Total K^+ deficit = 2.1 + 42 = 44.1 mEq K^+

    Total volume required over 24 hours =
        0.7L deficit + 0.7L maintenance = 1.4L

   c) Add 24 hour maintenance requirements, total fluid deficit, and electrolyte deficits, and replace 50% of this over the first 8 hours and the remainder over the subsequent 16 hours. *Remember to subtract boluses.*

   2) Hyponatremic dehydration (Na^+ < 130 mEq/L)
      a) Calculate fluid and electrolyte deficits as previously described for isonatremic dehydration.
      b) Calculate the additional ECF Na^+ deficit in hyponatremia using the method described on p. 219.
      c) Give 1/2 the total fluid and electrolyte requirements over the first 8 hours and the remainder over the subsequent 16 hours. If Phase I fluids are given, subtract this from the fluids and electrolytes to be given in the first 8 hours.

Note: In the adult it has been reported that very rapid correction of hyponatremia (i.e., an increase in serum Na^+ >2 mEq/L/hr, up to 10–12 mEq/kg/day) may be dangerous and can produce potentially crippling or even fatal osmotic demyelination syndrome.

From Fleisher G, Ludwig S: *Textbook of pediatric emergency medicine,* 1993, Williams and Wilkins.

   3) Hypernatremic dehydration (Na^+ > 150 mEq/L)
      a) Calculate total fluid deficit.
      b) Calculate FW deficit (see p. 219).
      c) Calculate isonatremic fluid losses from total fluid deficit and FW deficit.
      d) Calculate electrolyte deficits based on the isonatremic fluid deficit.
      e) Replace deficits over 48 hours. Include daily maintenance requirements. If patient is anuric, consider only insensible losses when calculating maintenance fluids.

Note: Avoid dropping the serum Na^+ > 15 mEq/L/24 hr to minimize cerebral edema.

4) Probable Deficits of Water and Electrolytes in Severe Dehydration (Table 11.8)

TABLE 11.8.

Condition*	H₂O (ml/kg)	Sodium	Potassium (mEq/kg)	Chloride
DIARRHEAL DEHYDRATION				
Hypotonic [Na] < 130 mEq/L	20–100	10–15	8–15	10–12
Isotonic [Na] = 130–150 mEq/L	100–120	8–10	8–10	8–10
Hypertonic [Na]> 150 mEq/L	100–120	2–4	0–6	0–3
PYLORIC STENOSIS	100–120	8–10	10–12	10–12
DIABETIC KETOACIDOSIS	100	8	6–10	6

*[Na] refers to the serum or plasma sodium concentration
From Hellerstein: *Pediatr Rev* 14:109, 1993.

c. Ongoing losses
  1) Use Table 11.9 to estimate ongoing electrolyte losses for various body fluids.
  2) Losses should be determined and replaced Q6–8 hr. Because of the wide range of normal values, specific analyses are suggested in individual cases.

TABLE 11.9.

Fluid	Na (mEq/L)	K (mEq/L)	Cl (mEq/L)	Protein (g/dl)
Gastric	20–80	5–20	100–150	—
Pancreatic	120–140	5–15	40–80	—
Small bowel	100–140	5–15	90–130	—
Bile	120–140	5–15	80–120	—
Ileostomy	45–135	3–15	20–115	—
Diarrhea	10–90	10–80	10–110	—
Burns	140	5	110	3–5

D. Oral Rehydration Therapy
   1. Indications: This method of rehydration is effective for treating patients with mild to moderate dehydration. It may be contraindicated in patients with shock, severe dehydration, intractable vomiting, >10 ml/kg/hr losses, coma, or severe gastric distention. In patients with severe dehydration, IV therapy should be used initially until pulse, blood pressure, and level of consciousness return to normal. At that time, oral hydration can be safely instituted.
   2. Technique
      a. Give 5–10 ml of fluid (using a syringe or teaspoon) every 5–10 minutes, and gradually increase amount as tolerated (Table 11.10). Monitor this phase of rehydration.
      b. **STOP** if severe vomiting occurs; small amounts of vomiting should not warrant abandoning this mode of rehydration.
   3. Deficit replacement
      a. Mild dehydration: 50 ml/kg over 4 hours
      b. Moderate dehydration: 100 ml/kg over 4 hours
   From Duggan C et al: *MMWR* 41:14, 1992.
   4. Oral rehydration solutions (ORS) (Table 11.10)

TABLE 11.10.

	CHO (g/dl)	mEq/L				mOsm/kg H_2O
		Na+	K+	Cl*	Base	
Infalyte (formerly Ricelyte)	3.0	50	25	45	30	200
Naturalyte	2.5	45	20	35	48	265
Pedialyte	2.5	45	20	35	30	250
Rehydralyte	2.5	75	20	65	30	310
WHO / UNICEF ORS*	2.0	90	20	80	30	310

CHO, Carbohydrate.
*Available from Jaianas Bros. Packaging Co., 2533 SW Boulevard, Kansas City, MO 64108
From Snyder J: *Semin Pediatr Infect Dis* 5:231, 1994.

5. Approximate electrolyte composition of fluids commonly consumed* (Table 11.11)

TABLE 11.11.

	CHO (g/dl)	mEq/L				mOsm/kg H$_2$O
		Na$^+$	K$^+$	Cl$^-$	HCO$_3^-$	
Apple Juice	11.9	0.4	26	—	—	700
Coca-Cola	10.9	4.3	0.1	—	13.4	656
Gatorade	5.9	21	2.5	17	—	377
Ginger Ale	9.0	3.5	0.1	—	3.6	565
Milk	4.9	22	36	28	30	260
Orange Juice	10.4	0.2	49	—	50	654

CHO, Carbohydrate.
*Values vary slightly depending on source
From Behrman: *Nelson textbook of pediatrics,* ed 15, Philadelphia, 1996, WB Saunders.

6. Maintenance replacement
   a. For breastfed infants, give 100 ml/kg of rehydration solution in addition to breast milk ad lib.
   b. For formula fed infants in the outpatient setting, give lactose free formula or half-strength lactose-containing formula at 100–150 ml/kg/24 hr, alternating with an equal volume of rehydration solution. In the inpatient setting, stool output should be monitored and ongoing losses should be replaced in addition to providing maintenance fluid.
   c. For children on a regular diet, give 100 ml/kg of rehydration solution, and continue the regular diet. However, avoid products high in simple carbohydrate content.
      1) Foods to encourage
         • Starchy foods (rice, baked potatoes, noodles, crackers, toast, cereals that are not sugar coated)
         • Soups (clear broths with rice, noodles, or vegetables)
         • Yogurt, vegetables (without butter), fresh fruits (not canned in syrup)

    2) Foods to minimize
- Foods which are high in fat or simple sugars (fried foods, juices, sodas or jello-water)
- Plain water

7. Replacement of ongoing losses: Regardless of the degree of dehydration, give 10ml/kg of rehydration solution for each diarrheal stool.

III. SERUM ELECTROLYTE DISTURBANCES
A. Potassium
    1. Hypokalemia
       a. Etiologies and laboratory data (Table 11.12)
       b. Other labs (dependent upon clinical scenario)
          1) Blood: Electrolytes with BUN/CR, CPK, glucose, renin, ABG, cortisol
          2) Urine: Urinalysis, K^+, Na^+, Cl^-, osmolality, 17-ketosteroids
          3) Other: ECG

TABLE 11.12.

	Decreased Stores		
	Normal BP		
Hypertension	Renal	Extrarenal	Normal stores
CAUSES			
Renovascular disease	RTA	Skin losses	Alkalosis
Excess renin	Fanconi syndrome	GI losses	↑ insulin
Congenital adrenal hyperplasia*	Bartter syndrome	High CHO diet	Leukemia
Excess mineralocorticoid	DKA	Enema abuse	B_2 Catecholamines
	Antibiotics	Laxative abuse	Familial hypokalemic periodic paralysis
Cushing's syndrome	Diuretics	Anorexia nerovsa	
LABS			
↑ Urine potassium	↑ Urine potassium	↓ Urine potassium	↑ Urine potassium

*May also be normotensive.
RTA, Renal tubular acidosis; *DKA,* diabetic ketoacidosis; *GI,* gastrointestinal; *BP,* blood pressure.

    c. Management: Rapidity of treatment should be proportional to severity of symptoms.
      1) Acute: Calculate electrolyte deficit and replace with Potassium acetate or Potassium chloride*
      2) Chronic: Calculate daily requirements and replace with Potassium chloride or Potassium gluconate*

*Consult formulary for dosing

  2. Hyperkalemia
    a. Etiologies (Table 11.13)

TABLE 11.13.

Increased stores		Normal stores
Increased urine Potassium	Decreased urine Potassium	Normal stores
Cell breakdown	Renal failure	Leukocytosis
Transfusion with aged blood	Hypoaldosteronism	Thrombocytosis >750K /mm³
NaCl substitutes	Aldosterone insensitivity	Metabolic acidosis*
Spitzer syndrome	↓ Insulin	Blood drawing
	K-sparing diuretics	

*For every 0.1 unit reduction in arterial pH there is an approximately 0.2–0.4 mEq/L increase in plasma potassium.

    b. Management (see Chapter 1)
B. Sodium
  1. Hyponatremia
    a. Etiologies (Table 11.14)
    b. Factitious etiologies
      1) Hyperlipidemia: Na^+ ↓ by $0.002 \times$ lipid (mg/dl)
      2) Hyperproteinemia: Na^+ ↓ by $0.25 \times$ [protein (g/dl) − 8]
      3) Hyperglycemia: Na^+ ↓ 1.6 mEq/L for each 100 mg/dl rise in glucose (Table 11.14)
  2. Hypernatremia (Table 11.15)

TABLE 11.14.

Decreased weight		Increased or normal weight
Renal losses	Extrarenal losses	
CAUSE		
Na losing nephropathy	GI losses	Nephrotic syndrome
Diuretics	Skin losses	Congestive heart failure
Adrenal insufficiency	Third Space	SIADH
Hyperglycemia		Acute renal failure
		Water intoxication
LAB DATA		Cirrhosis
↑ Urine Na⁺	↓ Urine Na⁺	↓ Urine Na⁺*
↑ Urine volume	↓ Urine volume	↓ Urine volume
↓ Specific gravity	↑ Specific gravity	↑ Specific gravity
↓ Urine osmolality	↑ Urine osmolality	↑ Urine osmolality
MANAGEMENT		
Replace losses	Replace losses	Restrict fluids
Treat cause	Treat cause	Treat cause

*Urine Na⁺ may be appropriate for level of Na⁺ intake in patients with SIADH and water intoxication.
GI, Gastrointestinal; *SIADH,* syndrome of inappropriate antidiuretic hormone.

TABLE 11.15.

Decreased weight		Increased weight
Renal losses	Extrarenal losses	
CAUSE		
Nephropathy	GI losses	Exogenous Na⁺
Diuretic use	Respiratory*	Mineralocorticoid excess
Diabetes insipidus	Skin/other sites	Hyperaldosteronism
LAB DATA		
↑ Urine volume	↓ Urine volume	Relative ↓ urine volume
↑ Urine Na⁺	↓ Urine Na⁺	Relative ↓ urine Na⁺
↓ Specific gravity	↑ Specific gravity	Relative ↑ specific gravity
MANAGEMENT		

Replace losses based on calculations on p. 222 and treat cause. Consider a natriuretic agent if there is increased weight.

*These causes of hypernatremia are usually secondary to free water loss so that fractional excretion of sodium may be decreased or normal.

C. **Calcium**
   1. Hypocalcemia
      a. Laboratory data*
         1) Blood: Calcium (total and ionized), phosphate, alkaline phosphatase, Mg, total protein, albumin, BUN, creatinine, PTH, pH
         2) Urine: Calcium, phosphate, creatinine
         3) Other: ECG, skull and/or chest films

*Labs that need to be followed will depend on clinical situation.

From Fleisher, Ludwig: *Textbook of pediatric emergency medicine,* Baltimore, 1993, Williams and Wilkins.

      b. Management
         1) Chronic: Consider use of PO supplements of calcium carbonate, calcium gluconate, calcium glubionate, or calcium lactate.[†]
         2) Acute symptomatic: Consider use of IV forms such as calcium gluconate, calcium gluceptate, or calcium chloride (cardiac arrest dose).[†]

Significant hyperphosphatemia should be corrected before correction of hypocalcemia, since soft tissue calcification may occur if total [Ca] × [Phos] > 80 mg/dl.

Hypomagnesemia should be considered if a patient's symptoms of hypocalcemia are refractory to Ca^{++} supplementation, and Mg^{++} should be given before Ca^{++} supplements.

[†]Consult Formulary.

   2. HYPERCALCEMIA
      a. Laboratory Data[‡]
         1) Blood: Calcium (total and ionized), phosphate, alkaline phosphatase, total protein, albumin, BUN, creatinine, PTH, vitamin D
         2) Urine: Calcium, phosphate, creatinine
         3) Other: ECG, skull and abdominal films, skeletal survey, IVP

[‡]Labs that need to be followed will depend on clinical situation.

From Fleisher, Ludwig, *Textbook of pediatric emergency medicine,* Baltimore, 1993, Williams and Wilkins.

      b. Management
         1) Treat the underlying disease, since this is often the etiology.
         2) Hydrate to increase urine output and Ca^{++} excretion. If GFR and BP are stable, may give NS + K^+

supplement at 2–3 times maintenance till $[Ca]_i$ is in normal range.
3) Diurese with furosemide.
4) Consider hemodialysis.
5) Steroids (for malignancy, granulomatous disease and vitamin D toxicity) to decrease vitamin D and Ca^{++} absorption. Hydrocortisone or prednisone may be given.*
6) Severe or persistently elevated calcium
   a) Give calcitonin (calcitonin salmon)
   b) 4 units/kg SC / IM Q12 hr, may increase up to 8 units/kg Q12 hr if no improvement after 1–2 days (max 8 units/kg Q6 hr). Skin testing before administration of calcitonin salmon should be considered.†
   c) Mithramycin (if malignancy suspected)†
7) Other options
   a) Elemental phosphate (can cause soft tissue calcification)*
   b) Biphosphonate drugs
D. Magnesium
   1. Hypomagnesemia
      a. Laboratory Data: Mg^{++} and ionized calcium
      b. Management
         1) Acute: Give magnesium sulfate*
         2) Chronic: Magnesium oxide, magnesium gluconate, magnesium sulfate*

From Fleisher, Ludwig: *Textbook of pediatric emergency medicine,* Baltimore, 1993, Williams and Wilkins.

   2. Hypermagnesemia
      a. Laboratory data: Mg^{++}
      b. Management
         1) Stop supplemental Mg^{++}
         2) Diurese
         3) Give calcium supplements†
            a) Calcium chloride (use cardiac arrest doses)
            b) Calcium gluceptate
            c) Calcium gluconate

*Consult Formulary for dosing
†From *American hospital formulary service drug information,* 1995, p. 2195.

　　　　4) Dialysis if life threatening levels are present

From Fonser L: *Pediatric Annals,* 24:44, 1995.

E. Phosphate
　　1. Hypophosphatemia
　　　　a. Laboratory Data
　　　　　　1) Blood: Phosphate, calcium (total and ionized), electrolytes including BUN/creatinine (follow for low K^+, Mg^{++}, Na^+), vitamin D, PTH
　　　　　　2) Urine: Calcium, phosphate, creatinine, pH
　　　　b. Management
　　　　　　1) Insidious onset of symptoms: Give KPhos or NaPhos PO.
　　　　　　2) Acute onset of symptoms: Give KPhos or Na Phos IV.
　　2. Hyperphosphatemia
　　　　a. Laboratory data
　　　　　　1) Blood: Phosphate, calcium (ionized and total), electrolytes including BUN/creatinine CBC, vitamin D, PTH, ABG
　　　　　　2) Urine: Calcium, phosphate, Creatinine, urinalysis
　　　　b. Management
　　　　　　1) Restrict dietary phosphate
　　　　　　2) Give phosphate binders (calcium carbonate, aluminum hydroxide; use with caution in renal failure).*
　　　　　　3) For cell lysis (with normal renal function), NS bolus and IV mannitol*
　　　　　　4) If poor renal function, may consider dialysis

From *Pediatr Ann* 24:43, 1995.

*Consult Formulary for dosing

IV. ANION GAP
A. Definition

The anion gap represents the difference between unmeasured cations (UC) and unmeasured anions (UA). Clinically it is measured by:

$$AG = UC - UA = Na + K - (Cl + HCO_3)$$
$$(\text{Normal: } 12 \text{ mEq/L} \pm 2 \text{ mEq/L})$$

B. Increased Anion Gap: Causes
1. Decreased unmeasured cation: Hypokalemia, hypocalcemia, hypomagnesemia
2. Increased unmeasured anion
   a. Organic anions: Lactate, ketones
   b. Inorganic anions: Phosphate, sulfate
   c. Proteins: Hyperalbuminemia (transient)
   d. Exogenous anions: Salicylate, formate, nitrate, penicillin, carbenicillin, etc
   e. Incompletely identified anions: Anions accumulating with paraldehyde, ethylene glycol, methanol and salicylate poisoning, uremia, hyperosmolar hyperglycemic nonketotic coma
3. Laboratory error
   a. Falsely increased serum sodium
   b. Falsely decreased serum chloride or bicarbonate

C. Decreased Anion Gap: Causes
1. Increased unmeasured cation
2. Increased normally present cation: Hyperkalemia, hypercalcemia, hypermagnesemia
3. Retention of abnormal cation: IgG globulin, tromethamine (TRIS buffer), lithium
4. Decreased unmeasured anion: Hypoalbuminemia
5. Laboratory error
   a. Systematic error: Hyponatremia caused by viscous serum, hyperchloremia in bromide intoxication
   b. Random error: Falsely decreased serum sodium, falsely increased serum chloride or bicarbonate

From Emmett M, Narins R: *Medicine* 56:38, 1977; Oh MS, Carroll HJ: *N Engl J Med* 297:814, 1977.

V. MISCELLANEOUS
A. Conversion Formula of mg to mEq/L

$$\frac{mEq}{L} = \frac{mg/L}{equivalent\ wt} \qquad equivalent\ wt = \frac{atomic\ wt}{valence\ of\ element}$$

From Behrman: *Nelson textbook of pediatrics,* ed 15, Philadelphia, 1996, WB Saunders.

TABLE 11.16.

Atomic Weights

Aluminum (Al)	26.97	Lead (Pb)	207.21
Calcium (Ca)	40.08	Magnesium (Mg)	24.32
Carbon (C)	12.01	Manganese (Mn)	54.93
Chlorine (Cl)	35.46	Nitrogen (N)	14.01
Copper (Cu)	63.57	Oxygen (O)	16.00
Fluorine (F)	19.00	Phosphorus (P)	30.98
Gold (Au)	197.20	Potassium (K)	39.10
Hydrogen (H)	1.01	Sodium (Na)	23.00
Iodine (I)	126.92	Sulfur (S)	32.06
Iron (Fe)	55.85		

TABLE 11.17.

Factors for Conversion of Concentration Expressed in mEq/L to mg/dl (100 ml) and Vice Versa.

Element or Radical	mEq/L to mg/dL		mg/dL to mEq/L	
Sodium	1	2.30	1	0.4348
Potassium	1	3.91	1	0.2558
Calcium	1	2.005	1	0.4988
Magnesium	1	1.215	1	0.8230
Chloride	1	3.55	1	0.2817
Bicarbonate (HCO_3)	1	6.1	1	0.1639
Phosphorus valence 1	1	3.10	1	0.3226
Phosphorus valence 1.8	1	1.72	1	0.5814

Ref: *Nelson's textbook of pediatrics,* ed 15, Philadelphia, WB Saunders.

B. Serum Osmolality
1. Defined as the number of particles per liter. May be approximated by:

$$2 \, (Na) + \frac{glucose \ (mg/dl)}{18} + \frac{BUN \ (mg/dl)}{2.8}$$

2. Normal range: 285–295 mOsm/L.

VI. PARENTERAL FLUID COMPOSITION (Table 11.18)

TABLE 11.18.

Composition of Frequently Used Parenteral Fluids

Liquid	CHO protein (g/100 ml)	Cal/L	Na	K	Cl	HCO3†	Ca	P‡
				(mEq/L)				(mg/dl)
D$_5$W	5	170	—	—	—	—	—	—
D$_{10}$W	10	340	—	—	—	—	—	—
Normal saline (0.9% NaCl)	—	—	154	—	154	—	—	—
1/2 Normal saline (0.45% NaCl)	—	—	77	—	77	—	—	—
D$_5$ (0.2% NaCl)	5	170	34	—	34	—	—	—
3% Saline	—	—	513	—	513	—	—	—
8.4% Sodium bicarbonate (1 mEq/ml)	—	—	1000	—	—	1000	—	—
Ringer's	0–10	0–340	147	4	155.5	—	4.5	—
Ringer's lactate	0–10	0–340	130	4	109	28	3	—
Amino acid 8.5% (Travasol)	8.5	340	3	—	34	52	—	—
Plasmanate	5	200	110	2	50	29	—	—
Albumin 25% (salt poor)	25	1000	100–160	—	<120	—	—	—
Intralipid (Cutter)§	2.25	1100	2.5	0.5	4.0	—	—	08

*Protein or amino acid equivalent.

†Bicarbonate or equivalent (citrate, acetate, lactate).

‡Approximate values: actual values may vary somewhat in various localities depending on electrolyte composition of water supply used to reconstitute solution.

§Values are approximate—may vary from lot to lot.

GASTROENTEROLOGY *12*

"Burn'd on the water, the poop was beaten gold."
William Shakespeare,
Antony and Cleopatra

I. TESTS FOR CARBOHYDRATE MALABSORPTION
A. Fecal pH
1. Purpose: To screen for carbohydrate malabsorption
2. Method: Dip a portion of nitrazine pH paper into the liquid portion of a fresh stool specimen and compare with the color chart provided.
3. Interpretation: pH <5.5 suggests carbohydrate malabsorption.

B. Stool Reducing Substances
1. Purpose: To screen for carbohydrate malabsorption by measuring reducing substances (lactose, maltose, fructose, galactose) in stool
2. Method: Place a small amount of fresh liquid stool in a test tube and dilute with twice its volume of water. Centrifuge and place 15 drops of the supernatant in a second test tube containing a Clinitest tablet. Compare the resulting color with the chart provided for urine testing. To screen for malabsorption of sucrose (not a reducing substance) use 1N HCl instead of water and boil for 30 seconds before centrifuging.
3. Interpretation
   a. >0.5% suggests carbohydrate malabsorption.
   b. 0.25% to 0.5% is indeterminate.
   c. <0.25% is normal.

C. Breath Hydrogen Test
1. Purpose: To diagnose malabsorption of a specific carbohydrate by measuring hydrogen gas in expired air after an oral load of the carbohydrate in question
2. Method: Have infants fast for 4–6 hours, older children for 12 hours. Give a 2 g/kg (max 50 g) oral load of the desired carbohydrate as a 20% solution (10% in infants

<6 months of age). Place nasal prongs or an air-tight face mask attached to a 20 ml syringe with stop-cock on the child, and aspirate 5 ml of end-expiratory air for 4 consecutive breaths before the carbohydrate load and every 30 minutes for 3 hours thereafter. Inject samples into red-topped glass tubes and send for measurement of H_2 by gas chromatography.

Note: Do not give antibiotics for 1 week before test.

3. Interpretation: H_2 is produced by bacterial fermentation of undigested carbohydrate in the bowel, diffuses into the blood, and is expelled in expired air. A rise in H_2 >20 ppm above the lowest test value obtained suggests malabsorption of the test carbohydrate. An elevated baseline or a rise in H_2 >20 ppm above baseline within 30 minutes suggests small bowel bacterial overgrowth.

From Montes R, Perman JA: *Semin Pediatr Gastroenterology and Nutrition,* 2:2, 1991.

D. **Monosaccharide and Disaccharide Absorption**
    1. Purpose: To diagnose malabsorption of a specific carbohydrate (glucose [a monosaccharide] or lactose, maltose, fructose, galactose or sucrose [disaccharides]) by measuring the change in blood glucose after an oral load of the carbohydrate in question. Most useful when gas chromatography is not available.
    2. Method: Have patient fast for 4–6 hours before test. Give a 2 g/kg (max 50 g) oral load of the desired carbohydrate as a 10% solution. For maltose give 1 g/kg. Measure serum glucose before carbohydrate dose and 30, 60, 90, and 120 minutes after the dose. Test all stools passed during and for 8 hours after the test for pH and reducing substances.
    3. Interpretation
        a. Rise in blood glucose <20 mg/dl over the baseline suggests malabsorption of the test carbohydrate.
        b. Malabsorption is also suggested if during or within 8 hours of the test the patient develops diarrhea, stool pH <5.5, or >0.5% stool reducing substances.

From Silverman A, Roy CC: *Pediatric clinical gastroenterology,* St Louis, 1983, Mosby.

E. **D-Xylose Test**
 1. Purpose: To screen for duodenojejunal malabsorption by measuring the amount of D-xylose absorbed after an oral load. Unreliable in patients with edema, renal disease, delayed gastric emptying, severe diarrhea, rapid transit time, or small bowel bacterial overgrowth.
 2. Method: Have infants fast for 4–6 hours, older children for 8 hours. Give a 14.5 g/m^2 (max 25 g) oral load of D-xylose as a 10% water solution. Ensure adequate urine output using supplementary oral or IV fluid, collect all urine for 5 hours, and send for quantitation. Alternatively, send serum specimens for D-xylose concentration before the load and 30, 60, 90, and 120 minutes after the load.
 3. Interpretation (urine)
    a. Children >6 months old:
       1) 5 hours urinary excretion of <15% of the oral load suggests malabsorption.
       2) 15%–24% is indeterminate.
       3) ≥ 25% is normal.
    b. Infants <6 months old: 5 hours urinary excretion <10% suggests malabsorption.
 4. Interpretation (serum): Failure of the serum level to exceed 25 mg/dl in any of the postabsorptive specimens suggests malabsorption.

From Anderson CM, Burke A: *Pediatric gastroenterology,* St Louis, 1975, Mosby; Silverman A, Roy CC: *Pediatric clinical gastroenterology,* St Louis, 1983, Mosby.

II. **TESTS FOR FAT MALABSORPTION: QUANTITATIVE FECAL FAT**
A. **Purpose**
 To screen for fat malabsorption by quantitating fecal fat excretion
B. **Method**
 Patient should be on a normal diet (≥35% fat) with the amount of calories and fat ingested recorded for 2 days before the test and during the test itself. Collect and freeze all stools passed within 72 hours, and send to the laboratory for determination of total fecal fatty acid content.
C. **Interpretation**
 1. Total fecal fatty acid excretion of >5 g fat/24 hr may suggest malabsorption.

Note: Results will vary with amount of fat ingested and normal values have not been established for children <2 years old.

   2. The coefficient of absorption (CA) is a more accurate indicator of malabsorption that does not vary with fat intake.

$$CA = \frac{\text{g fat ingested} - \text{g fat excreted}}{\text{g fat ingested}} \times 100$$

Malabsorption is suggested by the following:

Premature infants	CA <60%–75%
Fullterm infants	CA <80%–85%
10 mo–3 yr old	CA <85%–95%
>3 yr old	CA <95%

Note: Quantitative fecal fat is recommended over qualitative methods (e.g., staining with Sudan III), which depend on spot checks and are thus unreliable for diagnosing fat malabsorption.

III. MISCELLANEOUS TESTS
A. Occult Blood
   1. Purpose: To screen for the presence of heme in stool
   2. Method: Smear a small amount of stool on the test areas of an occult blood test card (such as Hemoccult) and allow to air dry. Apply developer as directed.
   3. Interpretation: A blue color resembling that of the control indicates the presence of heme. Brisk transit of ingested red meat and inorganic iron may yield a false positive result.

Note: Low pH diminishes the sensitivity of a Hemoccult card. Use a Gastroccult or similar card when testing gastric contents for the presence of heme.

B. Fetal Hemoglobin (Apt Test)
   1. Purpose: To differentiate fetal blood from swallowed maternal blood
   2. Method: Mix specimen with an equal quantity of tapwater and centrifuge or filter. Add 1 part of 0.25 N (1%) NaOH to 5 parts of supernatant.

Note: Specimen must be bloody, and supernatant must be pink for proper interpretation.

3. Interpretation: A pink color persisting over 2 minutes indicates fetal hemoglobin. Transition from pink to yellow within 2 minutes indicates adult hemoglobin.

C. Fecal Leukocytes
1. Purpose: To aid in the diagnosis of diarrhea by noting the presence or absence of leukocytes in the stool
2. Method: Place a small amount of stool or mucus (ideally from a rectal swab) on a glass slide. Mix thoroughly with 2 drops of 0.5% methylene blue (Wright or Gram stain can also be used). Wait 2–3 minutes, cover with a coverslip, and examine under low power.
3. Interpretation: Sheets of polymorphonuclear cells suggest an inflammatory enterocolitis, such as that seen with *Shigella, Salmonella, Yersinia, Campylobacter,* invasive *E. coli, C. difficile,* ulcerative colitis, and Crohn's disease.

D. Stool Electrolytes and Osmotic Gap
1. Purpose: To aid in the diagnosis of diarrhea by determining stool electrolytes and osmotic gap
2. Method: Send stool specimen to lab for electrolytes.

Note: Specimen must be liquid to perform analysis.

Stool osmotic gap (mOsm/L) = 290 − 2 (stool Na + stool K)

3. Interpretation
   a. Stool Na >70 mEq/L and osmotic gap <100 mOsm/L suggests a secretory diarrhea.
   b. Stool Na <50 mEq/L and osmotic gap >100 mOsm/L suggests malabsorption or a viral etiology.

From Walker WA et al: *Pediatric gastrointestinal disease,* Philadelphia, 1991, BC Decker.

E. Parasites
1. Direct smear: Place a small amount of stool in a drop of saline on a glass slide, mix, remove particulate matter, and cover with a coverslip. Add iodine stain for identification of protozoan cysts.
2. Lab identification: Specimen must be fresh. If delay is expected, preserve with a commercially available kit.
3. *Giardia lamblia:* In addition to stool examination for cysts, a string test collection system (e.g., Entero/Test)

can assist in identification. An antigen detection test is also now widely available.

4. Pinworms: Obtain specimen in the morning before the child has had a bath. Apply sticky side of cellophane tape to the perianal area, transfer tape to a glass slide sticky side down, and examine for ova.

F. *Helicobacter pylori*

A variety of different tests are available for diagnosing *H. pylori* infection, including the following:

1. Histologic examination of biopsy specimens obtained by endoscopy

2. pH-sensitive dye tests for urease (e.g., CLO-test) performed on biopsy specimens (*H. pylori* produces urease, which hydrolyzes urea to ammonia [a base] and CO_2).

3. Breath urea tests that measure labeled CO_2 in expired air after oral administration of radiolabeled urea (after being formed, CO_2 diffuses into the bloodstream and is expired).

4. Serologic tests for antibody against *H. pylori*

IV. GASTROINTESTINAL HEMORRHAGE

A. **Evaluation**

1. Verify presence of blood with occult blood test card (such as Hemoccult), and rule out nasal, oral, and genitourinary sources of blood by careful examination.

2. Initial laboratory studies: Complete blood count (CBC), chemistry panel, prothrombin time (PT), partial thromboplastin time (PTT), type and cross

3. Gastric lavage: Differentiate upper from lower GI bleeding by placing a nasogastric or orogastric tube and lavaging with 10 ml/kg of room-temperature normal saline.

B. **Upper GI Bleeding**

1. Neonatal period: Swallowed maternal blood, hemorrhagic disease of the newborn, esophagitis, gastritis, peptic ulcer, vascular malformation, intestinal duplication

2. Infancy: Peptic ulcer, esophagitis, gastritis, Mallory-Weiss tear, vascular malformation, intestinal duplication

3. Preschool: Peptic ulcer, gastritis, Mallory-Weiss tear, esophageal varices, esophagitis, foreign body, vascular malformation

    4. School age/adolescence: Peptic ulcer, gastritis, Mallory-Weiss tear, esophageal varices, esophagitis, Crohn's disease, vascular malformation

C. Lower GI Bleeding

    1. Neonatal period: Anal fissure, infectious colitis, milk protein allergy, midgut volvulus, necrotizing enterocolitis, intestinal duplication

    2. Infancy: Anal fissure, infectious colitis, milk protein allergy, intussusception, Meckel's diverticulum, inflammatory bowel disease, polyps, intestinal duplication, pseudomembranous colitis

    3. Preschool: Infectious colitis, polyps, anal fissure, Meckel's diverticulum, intussusception, Henoch-Schonlein purpura, inflammatory bowel disease, pseudomembranous colitis, vascular malformation

    4. School age/adolescence: Infectious colitis, polyps, hemorrhoids, inflammatory bowel disease, pseudomembranous colitis, vascular malformation

V. JAUNDICE

A. Indirect Hyperbilirubinemia

    1. Transient neonatal jaundice: Physiologic jaundice, breastfeeding jaundice, breast milk jaundice, Lucey-Driscoll syndrome, resorption of extravascular blood, polycythemia

    2. Hemolytic disorders

      a. ABO and Rh incompatibility

      b. Hemoglobinopathies: Sickle cell anemia, thalassemia major

      c. Red cell membrane disorders: Spherocytosis, elliptocytosis

      d. Microangiopathies: Hemolytic uremic syndrome, hemangioma

      e. Red cell enzyme deficiencies: Glucose-6-phosphate dehydrogenase, fructokinase, pyruvate kinase, glutathione peroxidase

      f. Autoimmune disease: Viral infection, systemic lupus erythematosus

    3. Enterohepatic recirculation: Hirschprung disease, cystic fibrosis, ileal atresia, pyloric stenosis

4. Disorders of bilirubin metabolism: Crigler-Najjar syndrome, Gilbert syndrome, hypothyroidism, hypoxia, acidosis
5. Miscellaneous: Sepsis, dehydration, hypoalbuminemia, drugs

B. Direct Hyperbilirubinemia

1. Biliary obstruction: Biliary atresia, paucity of intrahepatic bile ducts, Alagille syndrome, choledochal cyst, inspissated bile syndrome, fibrosing pancreatitis, primary sclerosing cholangitis, gallstones, neoplasm, Caroli disease
2. Infection: Sepsis, urinary tract infection, cholangitis, liver abscess, viral hepatitis, other viral infections (Coxsackie, herpes simplex, varicella, echovirus, reovirus, parvovirus), syphilis, toxoplasmosis, tuberculosis, histoplasmosis, visceral larva migrans
3. Metabolic disorders: Alpha 1-antitrypsin deficiency, cystic fibrosis, galactosemia, galactokinase deficiency, Wilson disease, hereditary tyrosinemia, hereditary fructose intolerance, Niemann-Pick disease, Wolman disease, glycogen storage disease, Zellweger syndrome, Gaucher disease, Dubin-Johnson syndrome, Rotor syndrome, other disorders of bilirubin metabolism
5. Chromosomal abnormalities: Turner syndrome, trisomy 18, trisomy 21
6. Drugs: Aspirin, acetaminophen, iron, isoniazid, vitamin A, erythromycin, sulfonamides, oxacillin, rifampin, ethanol, steroids, tetracycline, methotrexate
7. Miscellaneous: Neonatal hepatitis syndrome, hyperalimentation, Reye's syndrome, Langerhans' cell histiocytosis, neonatal lupus erythematosus

VI. GASTROSTOMY DEVICES

A. Placement

Gastrostomy tubes can be placed in one of two ways.

1. Operative gastrostomy: A tube is placed in the stomach through an incision in the abdominal wall, a purse-string suture of the stomach wall is placed around the tube, and the stomach is sutured to the peritoneum (the Stamm procedure).

2. Percutaneous endoscopic gastrostomy (PEG): A gastrostomy tube is pulled through the mouth, down the esophagus, and out through the stomach and abdominal walls through an opening placed percutaneously with the assistance of an endoscope. The stomach is not sutured to the peritoneum but is held in place by the tube itself until fibrosis occurs.

B. Types

Gastrostomy devices come in several different forms.

1. External appearance: A gastrostomy tube is used for initial placement (regardless of the method) and may later be replaced by a low-profile or skin-level device (a gastrostomy "button"). Buttons have an improved appearance, are sometimes easier to manage, and may decrease formation of granulation tissue.

2. Internal bolsters: Tubes and buttons are prevented from coming out by internal bolsters. These devices come in a variety of shapes, including mushroom, disk, bar, and balloon. Only the latter can be identified externally by the presence of a separate port for inflation and deflation of the balloon.

C. Replacement

Only a gastrostomy device having a balloon as an internal bolster can be safely removed by untrained personnel. If the device has come out on its own, it can be replaced with a balloon device or simply a foley catheter with a bottle nipple placed over it to act as an external bolster. If the gastrostomy site appears to have been injured during the removal, a contrast study should be performed before use to confirm placement.

GENETICS   *13*

The purpose of this chapter is to aid the pediatrician in evaluating an acutely ill child with known or suspected metabolic disease, a dysmorphic infant, or an infant with abnormal growth and development. An attempt is also made to describe immediate diagnostic and therapeutic measures that should be instituted by the general pediatrician while awaiting input from a geneticist with expertise in the diagnosis and management of these diseases.

I. **INBORN ERRORS OF METABOLISM**
A. **Metabolic diseases:** Metabolic diseases may present at any time from the neonatal period to adolescence. Although these are often thought of as rare when considered collectively, they represent significant treatable causes of morbidity and mortality. The purpose of the following section is *not* to provide a comprehensive list of diseases but rather to provide a format for evaluating and diagnosing metabolic disease.
B. **Neonatal Onset**
   1. A previously healthy normal full-term infant presents at 24–48 hours of age with anorexia, lethargy, and/or vomiting. In this situation, metabolic disease is nearly as common as sepsis and must be considered when evaluating these infants.
   2. History
      In many cases, a thorough history and family history can aid in diagnosis and raise the level of suspicion.
      a. Family history of neonatal or childhood death, consanguinity, ethnicity, mental retardation or developmental delay, known genetic disorders
      b. In addition, a three generation pedigree can be helpful including the above plus: age, gender, and medical status of each individual; cause of death if deceased; and any history of infertility, miscarriage, stillbirth, birth defects, or seizure disorder.
   3. Initial lab tests
      a. Blood
         1) Complete blood count (CBC)

2) Electrolyte panel (calculate anion gap), liver function tests (T Bili, D Bili, AST, ALT)
3) Arterial blood gases (ABG)
4) Plasma ammonia
5) Serum lactate
b. Urine
1) Dip for pH, ketones, glucose, protein, bilirubin
2) Unusual urine odor (Table 13.1)

TABLE 13.1.

	Odor
ACUTE DISEASE	
Maple syrup urine disease	Maple syrup, burned sugar
Isovaleric acidemia	Cheesy or sweaty feet
Multiple carboxylase deficiency	Cat's urine
3-OH, 3-methyl glutaryl-CoA, lyase deficiency	Cat's urine
NONACUTE DISEASE	
Phenylketonuria	Musty
Hypermethioninemia	Rancid butter, rotten cabbage
Trimethylaminuria	Fishy

3) Ferric chloride ($FeCl_3$) reaction
   a) Ferric iron forms colored derivatives when combined with many organic compounds. Results depend on methodology.
   b) Place 2 drops of 10% $FeCl_3$ in 1 ml of fresh urine; mix and observe color immediately and upon standing.
   c) The test is relatively insensitive and usually requires high concentrations of the reacting metabolite. Salicylate is an exception. Phosphate ions yield cloudy precipitates, which may mask positive results. A negative test does not rule out the disease.
   d) Interpretation (Table 13.2)

Note: The workup of jaundice in a neonate should include urine for reducing substances to r/o galactosemia.

TABLE 13.2.

Color	Interpretation
Green	PKU, tyrosinemia, direct hyperbilirubinemia, L-dopa.
Blue-green	Histidinemia, pheochromocytoma.
Gray-green	MSUD, formiminotransferase deficiency.
Purple	Salicylates, methionine malabsorption.
Blue-purple	Phenothiazines.

From Buist NRM: *Brit Med J* 2:745, 1968; Thomas GH, Howell RR: *Selected screening tests for genetic metabolic disease,* Chicago, 1973, Year Book. *PKU,* Phenylketonuria; *MSUD,* maple syrup urine disease.

4) Urine reducing substances: For method see Chapter 21. Metabolic disorders associated with a positive test include the following:
   a) Galactose: Galactosemia, galactokinase deficiency, severe liver disease
   b) Fructose: Hereditary fructose intolerance, essential fructosuria (see note)
   c) Glucose: Diabetes mellitus, renal glycosuria, Fanconi's type
   d) p-Hydroxyphenyl pyruvic acid: Tyrosinemia
   e) Xylulose: Pentosuria

From Burton BK, Nadler HL: *Pediatrics* 61:398, 1978; Aleck KA, Shapiro LJ: *Pediatr Clin North Am* 25:431, 1978.

4. Further lab evaluation: If any of the above are abnormal, continue the workup with the following and call for genetic consultation. *Early identification and institution of appropriate therapy are essential to prevent irreversible brain damage and death* (Table 13.3).
   a. Blood
      1) Plasma amino acids
      2) Plasma carnitine
      3) Pyruvate
   b. Urine
      1) Urine metabolic screen
      2) Urine organic acids
      3) Urine amino acids (rarely useful)
5. Newborn algorithm-hyperammonemia (Figure 13.1)

TABLE 13.3.

Sample Collection

Specimen	ml	Tube	Handling
Plasma ammonia	1–3	Green top	On ice. Levels rise rapidly on standing. Run to lab and hand to technician.
Plasma amino acids	1–3	Green top	On ice. If must store, spin sample, separate plasma, and freeze. Obtain after 3 hr fast.*
Plasma carnitine	1–3	Green top	On ice
Karyotype	3	Green top	Room temperature
Very-long chain fatty acids	3	Purple top	Room temperature
WBC for enzymes	3	Purple top	Room temperature
Urine organic acids	5–10		Deliver immediately or freeze*
Urine metabolic screen	5–10		Deliver immediately or freeze*
Urine amino acids	5–10		Deliver immediately or freeze*
Skin biopsy		Tissue culture media OR pt.'s plasma	Refrigerate Do not freeze

*Acute samples are the most informative.

      6. Treatment: See section below on acute management.
      7. For further details on specific metabolic diseases of the newborn see Seidel et al: *Primary care of the newborn,* St Louis, 1993, Mosby.

C. Late Onset
    1. Symptoms are usually brought on by intercurrent illness, prolonged fast, dietary indiscretion, or any process causing increased catabolism. They typically present with fever, vomiting, respiratory distress, changes in mental status including confusion, lethargy, irritability, aggressive behavior, hallucinations, or even coma. A history of unusual dietary preferences can often be elicited (e.g., children who refuse proteins such as milk, cheese, and meats and eat only salads).
    2. Examples
       a. Medium chain acyl CoA dehydrogenase deficiency (MCAD)
         1) Present after a prolonged fast or increased caloric need with change in mental status, seizures, hepatomegaly.

a) Most common age of onset 12 to 24 months but may present earlier or later.
b) Some sudden infant death syndrome (SIDS) cases thought to be due to MCAD.

2) Lab results: Hypoglycemia with lack of appropriate degree of ketosis, metabolic acidosis, hyperammonemia, abnormal liver function tests, and urine organic acids are diagnostic.

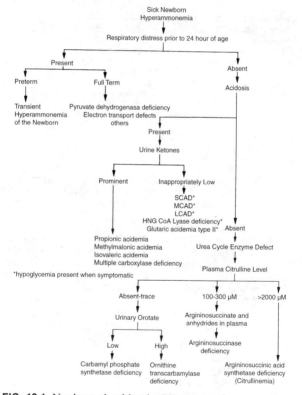

FIG. 13.1. Newborn algorithm-hyperammonemia.

3) Complications: Increased intracranial pressure (ICP), hepatic encephalopathy, cardiomyopathy
4) Treatment
   a) Acute management: See below.
   b) Long-term treatment is to avoid prolonged fast and to provide adequate glucose intake during times of increased need such as intercurrent illness. Also, L-carnitine 100 mg/kg/day is prescribed to prevent secondary carnitine deficiency.

b. Symptomatic ornithine transcarbamylase (Urea cycle) heterozygote
   1) Females who present with vomiting and change in mental status
   2) Lab results: Elevated ammonia, respiratory alkalosis, plasma amino acids, and urine orotic acid are diagnostic.
   3) Treatment
      a) Acute management: See below.
      b) Long-term treatment: Protein restriction, arginine supplementation, sodium (Na) phenylbutyrate (experimental) or Ucephan (Na benzoate and Na phenylacetate) orally

D. Acute Management
1. Stop protein.
2. D_{10} at 1.5–2 × maintenance (this delivers 10–15 mg/kg/min of glucose and stops catabolism).
3. Add Na/K based on degree of dehydration and electrolyte results.
4. In cases of severe dehydration, bolus with NS. Piggyback in D_{10} to provide 1.5–2 × maintenance (this delivers approximately 10–15 mg/kg/min glucose).
5. HCO_3 replacement for severe acidosis (pH<7.1) only

E. Acute Management of Hyperammonemia
1. See above.
2. Na benzoate 250 mg/kg (5.5 g/m^2) and Na phenylacetate 250 mg/kg (5.5 g/m^2) IV, Arginine HCl (10% solution) 2 ml/kg (4.0 g/m^2)
   a. The above amounts are given as a bolus over 90 minutes.
   b. The same amount is then given over a 24-hour period as a maintenance dose.

      c. Zofran (odansetran) may be used to decrease nausea and vomiting associated with these drugs.

Note: These are experimental drugs and should only be used in consultation with a geneticist. Overdose may cause death.

   3. If unresponsive to the above medical management, hemodialysis should be instituted.

      a. Hemodialysis will probably be required in neonates because of the inherently catabolic state.

      b. Hemodialysis is 10 times as efficient as peritoneal dialysis.

      c. Exchange transfusion should NOT be used.

TABLE 13.4.

Algorithm for Considering Metabolic Diseases

Defect	Amino acid metabolism (MSUD)	Fatty acid oxidation (MCAD)	Carbohydrate metabolism (galactosemia)	Urea cycle (OTC)
pH	Acid	+/− Acid	Acid	Alkaline
Ketones	Increased	Decreased	Increased	
Glucose	Increased, decreased, or normal	Decreased	Decreased	Decreased
NH_4	+/−	Increased	Increased	Increased
FTT	Present		Present	Present
DevDelay	Present		Present	Present
△MS	Lethargy to coma	Hepatic encephalopathy	Hypoglycemic seizures	Irritable, combative, confused, lethargy coma

II. NEWBORN METABOLIC SCREEN

It is essential to realize in this day of early postpartum discharge that a formula fed infant is unlikely to have a diagnostic abnormality before 36 hours of age; breastfed infants may not have diagnostic abnormalities until 48 to 72 hours of age. Therefore infants tested before the first 36 to 48 hours of life must have a repeat screen done by the primary care giver in the first week of life (Table 13.5).

Note: All states screen for phenylketonuria (PKU) and hypothyroidism. Thirty-five states screen for only these two disorders.

TABLE 13.5.

Maryland Newborn Metabolic Screen

Disease	Newborn screening level	Diagnostic test	Immediate clinical response
Phenylketonuria	Phe (4–6 mg/dl) Phe (6–12 mg/dl) Phe (>12 mg/dl)	Plasma amino acids (Phe, Tyr); urine phenyl acids; genotyping	1. For mild elevation: Evaluate nutritional developmental, neurological status, hepatic, and renal function. Repeat screening test. 2. For moderate elevation: Consult referral center, and send frozen urine and plasma. 3. For high levels: Arrange for hospitalization and diagnostic evaluation.
Maple syrup urine disease	Leu (4 mg/dl) Leu (4–8 mg/dl) Leu (>8 mg/dl)	Plasma amino acids (Val, Leu, Ileu)	
Homocystinuria	Meth (2–6 mg/dl) Meth (>6 mg/dl)	Plasma amino acids (homocystine, Met)	
Tyrosinemia	Tyr (6–12 mg/dl) Tyr (12–20 mg/dl) Tyr (>20 mg/dl)	Plasma amino acids (Tyr, Phe); blood spot for succinylacetone	
Galactosemia	Beutler test: positive; *E. coli* phage test negative. Beutler test: positive; *E. coli* phage test positive.	Galactose-1-P uridyl transferase; galactokinase; UPD-gal-4-epimerase galactose; galactose-1-P	Evaluate for jaundice, liver dysfunction, sepsis, cataracts, urine reducing substances. Send blood for enzyme analysis. Remove from diet.
Hypothyroidism	RIA (T$_4$ = 5–7.6 mcg/dl) (TSH <25 mcIU/ml) RIA (T$_4$ <5 mcg/dl) (TSH >25 mcIU/ml)	T$_4$ T$_3$, TSH, TBG, thyroid antibodies, bone age	Evaluate for hypothermia, hypoactivity, poor feeding, jaundice, constipation.

From Maryland State Department of Health and Hygiene Laboratories Administration
RIA, Radioimmunoassay; *TSH,* thyroid-stimulating hormone; *TBG,* thyroxine-binding globulin.

III.   CHROMOSOMAL DEFECTS

Some dysmorphic neonates have a poor prognosis because of chromosomal abnormalities. Recognition of the syndrome, with prompt confirmation by karyotype, allows parents and medical personnel to decide the appropriateness of medical intervention for each child.

A.   **Trisomy 21 (Down Syndrome)**
1. Incidence: 1:660 overall, making it the most common malformation.
2. Features: There are ten cardinal features in the neonate: hypotonia, poor Moro, hyperreflexibility, excess skin on back of neck, flat facies, slanted palpebral fissures, ear anomalies, pelvic dysplasia, dysplasia of the midphalanx of fifth finger, and single transverse palmar (simian) creases. Presence of 6 out of 10 of these is highly suggestive.
3. Recommended testing: Echocardiogram, yearly TFTs, LFTs and CBC, x-ray exam of atlantooccipital junction at 2 years of age, and audiologic evaluation
4. Natural History
   a. Cardiac defects (50%)
   b. Leukemia (1%)
   c. Thyroid disease

B.   **Trisomy 13**
1. Incidence: 1:5000
2. Features: Holoprosecephaly, polydactyly, scalp skin defects, seizures, deafness, microcephaly, sloping forehead, cleft lip, cleft palate, retinal anomalies, abnormal ears, single umbilical artery, inguinal hernia, omphalocele, cardiac defects
3. Karyotype using specific probe by fluorescent in-situ hybridization (FISH) analysis; results available as rapidly as 24–48 hours
4. Natural history
   a. 44% die within 1 month.
   b. Less than 18% survive past 1 year.
   c. Profound mental retardation occurs in survivors.

C.   **Trisomy 18**
1. Incidence: 1:3000 with 3:1 female to male predominance

2. Features: Clenched hand with index finger overlapping third or third overlapping fourth, short stature, decreased fetal activity, low arch dermal ridge pattern, inguinal or umbilical hernia, cardiac defects, prominent occiput, low set ears, micrognathia, rocker bottom feet
3. Karyotype/FISH results available in 24–48 hours.
4. Natural history
   a. Many have apnea
   b. Severe FTT
   c. 30% die within 1 month, 50% by 2 months, 90% by 1 year
   d. 10% survive past 1 year
   e. Profound mental retardation in survivors

D. 45, X (Turner syndrome)
1. Incidence: 1:5000
2. Features: Short female with broad chest, wide spaced nipples, webbed neck, and congenital lymphedema (feet most prominent). May have renal anomalies such as horseshoe kidney. Cardiac defects present in greater than 20%, most commonly coarctation of the aorta.
3. Chromosomal analysis of blood or skin diagnostic
4. Natural history
   a. No known shortening of life span
   b. Normal intelligence
   c. Infertility

IV. NORMAL MORPHOLOGY
A. Many syndromes and some chromosomal abnormalities have minor anomalies such as hypotelorism or hypertelorism, epicanthal folds, long, short, or flat philtrum, ear pits or tags, low set or posteriorly rotated ears, micrognathia, retrognathia, asymmetric short stature, long bone overgrowth, abnormal hand creases, and other hand or foot anomalies, such as fifth finger clinodactyly, syndactyly, polydactyly, and many others. The most frequent of these are referenced in the Figures 13.2–13.5. For more complete tables, see the Smith or Hall references. (Hall JG et al: *Handbook of normal physical measurements,* 1989; Oxford Medical Publications. Jones K: *Smith's recognizable patterns of human malformation,* ed 4, Philadelphia, 1988, WB Saunders)

B. **Diagnostic Tests Useful in Workup**
   1. Magnetic resonance image (MRI) of brain for structural defects
   2. Ophthalmologic exam for optic atrophy or coloboma, cataracts, and retinal abnormalities
   3. Echocardiogram for structural defects
   4. Abdominal ultrasound for polysplenia/asplenia, absent or horseshoe kidney, ureteral or bladder defects, and abdominal situs
   5. Skeletal survey

C. **Skeletal dysplasia**
   Examine length of bones by clinical exam and x-ray exam to decide type of shortening
   1. Rhizomelic shortening (i.e., shortening of proximal segment of bones) is typical of conditions such as achondroplasia.
   2. Proportionate dwarfism is characteristic of growth hormone deficiency.
   3. Multiple fractures suggest osteogenesis imperfecta (or abuse).

D. **Upper:Lower Segment Ratio**
   When considering syndromes involving long bone overgrowth, upper:lower segment ratio (see below) measurement is an important key. In addition, arm span should be measured since normally arm span is equal to height. Other features to note are arachnodactyly, scoliosis, and loose jointedness (Fig. 13.2).

E. **Outer Canthal Distance (Fig. 13.3)**
F. **Inner Canthal Distance (Fig. 13.4)**
G. **Palpebral Fissure Length (Fig. 13.5)**

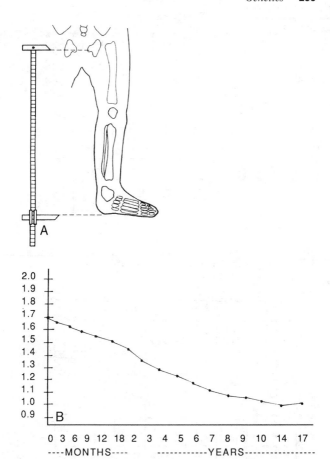

FIG. 13.2 A, To calculate upper: lower segment ratios:

$$\frac{\text{upper segment}}{\text{lower segment}} = \frac{\text{height} - \text{lower segment}}{\text{lower segment}}$$

B, Upper: lower segment ratios.

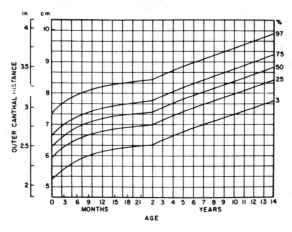

FIG. 13.3. Outer canthal distance. *(From Feingold M, Bossert WH: Birth defects: original article series, 10(13): 8, 1974.)*

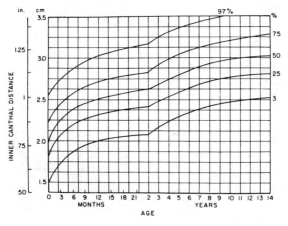

FIG. 13.4. Inner canthal distance.

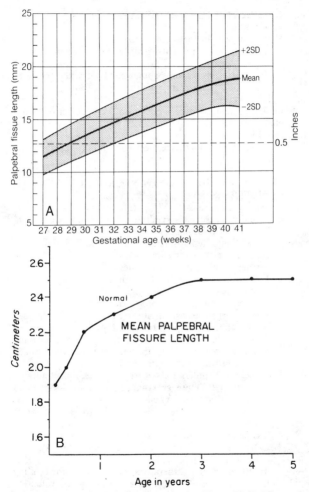

FIG. 13.5. Palpebral fissure length. **A,** (From Hall JG et al: *Handbook of normal physical measurements,* Oxford, 1989, Oxford). **B,** (from Jones KL: *Smith's recognizable patterns of human malformation,* Philadelphia, 1988, WB Saunders).

V. **GLYCOGEN STORAGE DISEASES**
A. **Presentation**
    Hepatomegaly, hypoglycemic seizures
    1. Type I typically presents early, usually as an infant with hepatomegaly.
    2. Type III often presents somewhat later when trying to get a child to sleep through the night.
B. **Lab Workup**
    Glucose, lactate, venons blood gases (VBG), electrolyte and chemistry panels
C. **Lab Findings**
    Increased LFT, cholesterol, uric acid (in I only), hypoglycemia, metabolic acidosis, increased lactate

VI. **LOSS OF MILESTONES/NEURODEGENERATIVE CONDITIONS**
A. **Mucopolysaccharidoses (MPS) (Hurler's syndrome, Hunter's syndrome, Scheie's syndrome, Sly's syndrome [due to deficiencies of lysosomal enzymes])**
    1. Present with hepatosplenomegaly, corneal clouding (except Hunter's syndrome), dysostosis multiplex, coarse features, and neurologic degeneration
    2. Lab workup: CBC with smear for inclusion bodies, MPS spot (urine), eye exam, skeletal survey
    3. Treatment: No pharmacologic therapy currently exists. Bone marrow transplantation cannot reverse damage but is effective if performed before loss of cognitive function. Partial liver transplants may correct enzyme deficiency outside the CNS, but the newly synthesized enzyme fails to cross the blood-brain barrier.
B. **Peroxisomal Disorders Refsum syndrome, X-linked adrenoleukodystrophy, Zellweger syndrome (due to disorders of peroxisome structure or function)**
    1. Present with seizures, loss of milestones and white matter, changes on MRI. Neurodegeneration is relentless leading eventually to death.
    2. Lab workup: Very-long-chain fatty acids (VLCFA), pipecolic acid, phytanic acid
    3. Treatment: Current therapy approaches include treating the adrenal insufficiency. Research protocols evaluating the efficacy of reduction of VLCFA and bone marrow transplant are under investigation.

VII. GENETIC CONSULTATION

In general, dysmorphic children and their families need referral. Other indications for referral are as follows:

A. Indications for Referral to a Genetics Center

1. Known or suspected hereditary disorder
2. Major physical anomalies, unusual body proportions, short stature
3. Major organ malformation
4. Developmental delay, mental retardation, or learning disability in females who have brothers with mental retardation
5. Complete or partial blindness or hearing loss
6. Loss or deterioration of motor or speech abilities in a child who was previously thriving
7. Evidence of maternal exposure to drugs, alcohol, or radiologic agents during pregnancy

B. Indications for Prenatal Counseling

1. Genetic disorder or birth defect in one partner
2. Previous child with a known or suspected genetic disorder
3. Maternal age of >35 yr
4. Family history of known or suspected chromosome error(s)
5. Multiple early miscarriages or stillbirths
6. Membership in an ethnic group known to have a higher incidence of a specific genetic disorder than the general population
7. Known carrier of a gene for a genetic disorder

C. Indications for Karyotype

1. Two major or one major and two minor malformations (small for gestational age and mental retardation are considered major malformations for this purpose)
2. Features of specific chromosomal syndrome
3. At risk for a familial chromosomal aberration
4. Ambiguous genitalia
5. Malignancies
6. Recurrent spontaneous abortions (more than 2) or history of infertility (karyotype both father and mother)

D. DNA testing

Many monogenic disorders now have DNA testing available. The list is too exhaustive to include in this text. For information on those tests available in your area, contact your local genetics department or DNA diagnostic laboratory.

Editor's note: Growth charts for specific disease syndromes:

Down Syndrome:
Piro E et al: *Amer Jour Med Genet:* 7:66, 1990.
Cronk C et al: *Pediatrics* 81:102, 1988.

Turner Syndrome:
Lyon AH et al: *Am J Dis Child* 60:932, 1985.
Sickle Cell Anemia: Platt OS: *NEJM* 311:7, 1984.
Cystic Fibrosis: Cystic Fibrosis Foundation, 1985.

I.   PREMATURE INFANTS (Fig. 14.1)

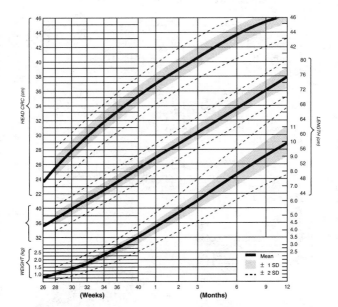

FIG. 14.1. Length, weight, and head circumference for premature infants. *(From Babson SG, Benda GI: Growth graphs for the clinical assessment of infants of varying gestational age,* J Pediatr *89:815, 1976.)*

II. GIRLS: BIRTH TO 36 MONTHS
A. Length and Weight (Fig. 14.2)

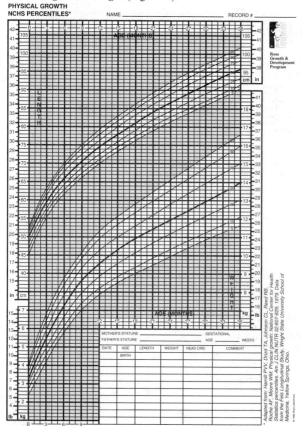

FIG. 14.2. Length and weight for girls, birth to 36 months. *From Hamill PV et al: Physical growth: national center for health statistics percentiles.* Am J Clin Nutr *32:607, 1979; Data from the Fels Longitudinal Study, Wright State Univ School of Medicine, Yellow Springs, Ohio. Copyright Ross Laboratories 1982.*

B. **Head Circumference and Length-Weight Ratio** (Fig. 14.3)

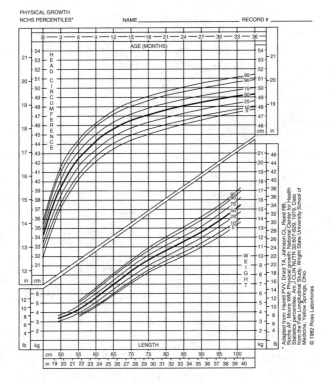

FIG. 14.3. Head circumference and length-weight ratio for girls, birth to 36 months. *From Hamill PV et al: Physical growth: national center for health statistics percentiles,* Am J Clin Nutr 32:607, 1979; *Data from the Fels Longitudinal Study, Wright State Univ School of Medicine, Yellow Springs, Ohio. Copyright Ross Laboratories 1982.*

III.   BOYS: BIRTH TO 36 MONTHS
A.   Length and Weight (Fig. 14.4)

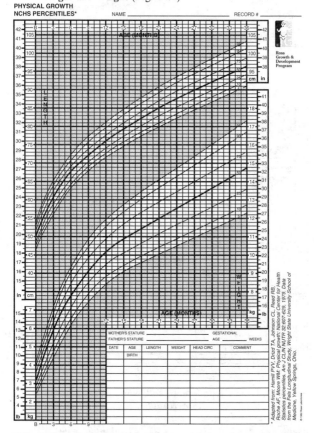

FIG. 14.4. Length and weight for boys, birth to 36 months. *From Hamill PV et al: Physical growth: national center for health statistics percentiles.* Am J Clin Nutr *32:607, 1979; Data from the Fels Longitudinal Study, Wright State Univ School of Medicine, Yellow Springs, Ohio. Copyright Ross Laboratories 1982.*

B.   Head Circumference and Length-Weight Ratio (Fig. 14.5)

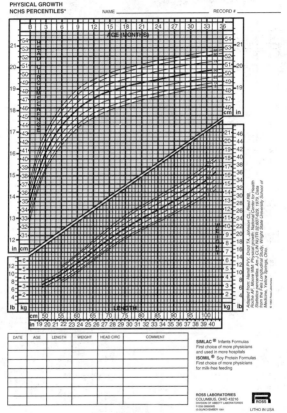

FIG. 14.5. Head circumference and length-weight ratio for boys, birth to 36 months. *From Hamill PV et al: Physical growth: national center for health statistics percentiles.* Am J Clin Nutr *32:607, 1979; Data from the Fels Longitudinal Study, Wright State Univ School of Medicine, Yellow Springs, Ohio. Copyright Ross Laboratories 1982.*

IV. GIRLS: 2 TO 18 YEARS
A. Stature and Weight (Fig. 14.6)

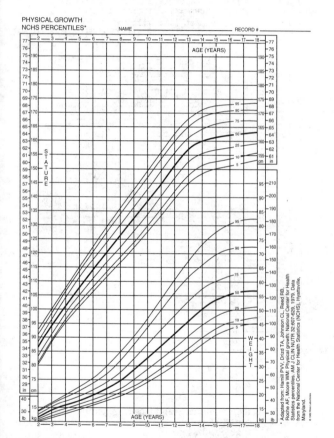

FIG. 14.6. Stature and weight for girls, 2 to 18 years.

B.   Stature-Weight Ratio (Fig. 14.7)

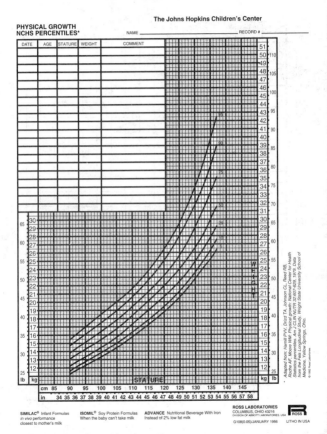

FIG. 14.7. Stature-weight ratio for girls, 2 to 18 years.

C. **Height Velocity** (Fig. 14.8)

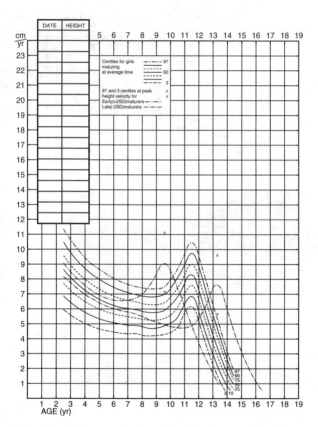

FIG. 14.8. Height velocity for girls, 2 to 18 years. *From Tanner JM, Davis PSW:* J Pediatrics *107:317, 1985; Copyright Castlemead Publications, 1985. Distributed by Sereno Laboratories.*

V. BOYS: 2 TO 18 YEARS
A. Stature and Weight (Fig. 14.9)

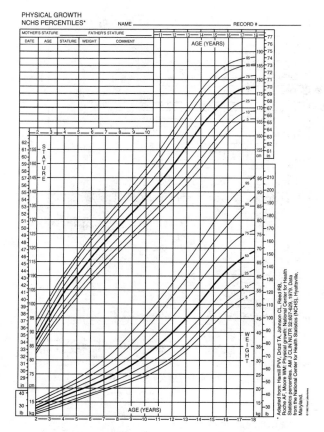

FIG. 14.9. Stature and weight for boys, 2 to 18 years.

B.   **Stature-Weight Ratio** (Fig. 14.10)

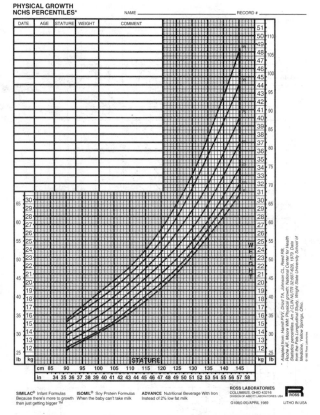

FIG. 14.10. Stature-weight ratio for boys, 2 to 18 years.

C. Height Velocity (Fig. 14.11)

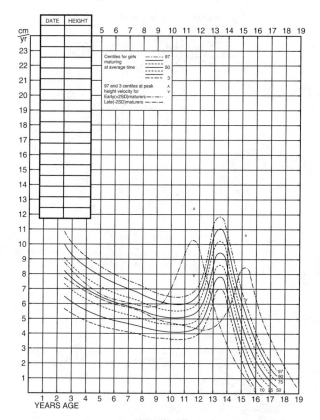

FIG. 14.11. Height velocity for boys, 2 to 18 years. *From Tanner JM, Davis PSW: J Pediatr 107:317, 1985; Copyright Castlemead Publications, 1985. Distributed by Sereno Laboratories.*

VI. HEAD CIRCUMFERENCE: GIRLS AND BOYS 2 TO 18 YEARS (Fig. 14.12)

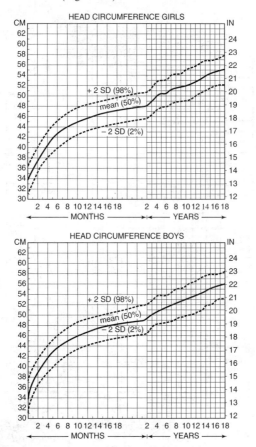

FIG. 14.12. Head circumference for boys and girls, 2 to 18 years. *From Nelhaus G: J Pediatr 41:106, 1968.*

VII. BODY SURFACE AREA NOMOGRAM AND EQUATION (Fig. 14.13)

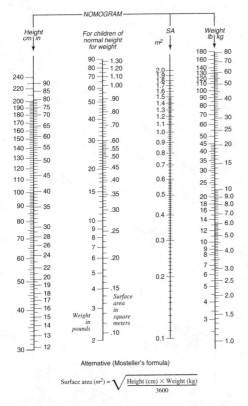

FIG. 14.13. Body surface area nomogram and equation. Ref: *Arch Dis Child,* 70:246, 1994.

Alternative (Mosteller's formula)

$$\text{Surface area }(m^2) = \sqrt{\frac{\text{Height (cm)} \times \text{Weight (kg)}}{3600}}$$

VIII. DENTAL DEVELOPMENT. (Table 14.1)

TABLE 14.1.

Chronology of Human Dentition of Primary or Deciduous and Secondary or Permanent Teeth*

	Age at Eruption		Age at Shedding	
PRIMARY TEETH	Maxillary	Mandibular	Maxillary	Mandibular
Central incisors	6–8 mo	5–7 mo	7–8 yr	6–7 yr
Lateral incisors	8–11 mo	7–10 mo	8–9 yr	7–8 yr
Cuspids (canines)	16–20 mo	16–20 mo	11–12 yr	9–11 yr
First molars	10–16 mo	10–16 mo	10–11 yr	10–12 yr
Second molars	20–30 mo	20–30 mo	10–12 yr	11–13 yr
SECONDARY TEETH				
Central incisors	7–8 yr	6–7 yr		
Lateral incisors	8–9 yr	7–8 yr		
Cuspids (canines)	11–12 yr	9–11 yr		
First premolars (bicuspids)	10–11 yr	10–12 yr		
Second premolars (bicuspids)	10–12 yr	11–13 yr		
First molars	6–7 yr	6–7 yr		
Second molars	12–13 yr	12–13 yr		
Third molars	17–22 yr	17–22 yr		

Max, Maxillary; *Mand*, mandibular.
From Behrman RE, Kliegman RM, Arvin AM: Nelson textbook of pediatrics, ed 15, Philadelphia, 1996, WB Saunders.

HEMATOLOGY   *15*

I. **ROUTINE HEMATOLOGY**
    Methods adapted from Beutler EB et al, editors: *Hematology,* New York, 1995, McGraw-Hill; Wallach J: *Interpretation of diagnostic tests,* Boston, 1992, Little, Brown and Co. For normal values, see section IX.

A. **Microhematocrit**
    1. Because of the risk of exposure to blood borne pathogens, the benefits of a manual hematocrit must be weighed against potential risks to health care personnel. As always when handling blood, universal precautions are recommended.
    2. Fill standard microhematocrit tube with blood, and seal one end with clay. Centrifuge (12,000 g) for 5 minutes.
    3. Falsely high hematocrits caused by increased plasma trapping occur with short centrifugation time and in disorders with decreased red cell deformability (e.g., iron deficiency).

B. **Wright's Staining Technique**
    1. Place air-dried blood smears, film side up, on staining rack.
    2. Cover smear with undiluted Wright's stain and leave for 2 to 3 minutes.
    3. Add equal volume of distilled water, and blow gently on the surface until a greenish metallic sheen appears. Leave diluted stain on smear for 2 to 6 minutes.
    4. Without disturbing the slide, flood with water and wash until stained smear is pinkish red. Blot dry.

C. **Hematologic Indices**
    1. Mean Corpuscular Volume (MCV): Average red blood cell (RBC) volume. Usually measured directly by electronic counters. Expressed in femtoliters (fl, 10^{-15} L). Useful in determining category of anemia.
    2. Mean Corpuscular Hemoglobin (MCH): Average quantity of Hb per red cell expressed in picograms (pg, 10^{-12} g).

3. Mean Corpuscular Hemoglobin Concentration (MCHC): Grams of Hb per 100 ml packed cells. High in congenital spherocytic hemolytic anemia and normal newborns; may be high in Hgb SC disease; low in microcytic anemia, including iron deficiency.

$$MCHC = \frac{Hb \ (g\%) \times 100}{Hct \ (\%)}$$

4. Red Cell Distribution Width (RDW): Statistical description of heterogeneity of red cell size. Increased in anisocytosis, reticulocytosis, iron deficiency, newborns, and hemolysis. Often normal in thalassemia minor.

D. Reticulocyte Count
1. Mix equal amounts of new methylene blue or brilliant cresyl blue with whole blood. After 10–20 minutes, prepare thin smears.
2. Count the number of reticulocytes (cells containing reticulum or blue granules) per 100 red cells and report as % of RBCs.
3. Increases with effective RBC production. Inappropriately low in hypoplastic states and nutritional deficiencies.

E. Platelet Estimation
Use Wright's stained blood smear to approximate platelet count. Always examine periphery of smear or coverslip since platelet clumps may be deposited there. For rough approximation, 1 platelet/oil immersion field corresponds to 10,000–15,000 platelets/mm^3. Platelet clumps usually indicate >100,000 platelets/mm^3.

II. HEMATOLOGIC INDICATORS OF SYSTEMIC DISEASE
A. Erythrocyte Sedimentation Rate (ESR)
ESR should be determined within 1 hour after obtaining blood.
1. Collect venous blood in EDTA or oxalate-containing tube.
2. Place 1 ml in a Wintrobe tube, using a long Pasteur pipette. Fill carefully from the bottom of the tube; do

not shake tube or allow air bubbles to form in the column of blood. Place the tube vertically.

3. Read depth of fall of RBC column at the end of 60 minutes.

4. Tilting of column, warming, or shaking may artificially increase the ESR. Other conditions associated with an increase include anemia, hypercholesterolemia, female sex, pregnancy, and inflammatory disease. Elevated in newborns with infections or with ABO hemolysis. Conditions associated with a decrease in the ESR include sickle cell disease, anisocytosis, spherocytosis, acanthocytosis, polycythemia, extreme leukocytosis, high doses of adrenal steroids, old or cold blood, clotted blood, hypofibrinoginemia or afibrinoginemia, microcytosis, congestive heart failure, trichinosis, pertussis, and cachexia. Body temperature, aspirin, and nonsteroidal antiinflammatory drugs (NSAIDs) exert no effect on the ESR.

From Sox HC, Liang MH: *Ann Intern Med* 104:515, 1986.

B. Cold Agglutinins

Rapid Screening Test

1. Collect 4–5 drops of blood in 60×7 mm Wasserman tube containing about 0.2 ml of 3.8 NaEDTA.

2. Cap tube and place in ice water bath for 30–60 seconds.

3. Tilt tube and observe blood as it runs down wall of tube.

4. Definite floccular agglutination (seen with unaided eye), which disappears upon warming to 37° C is considered a positive (3–4+) test. A control sample is useful for interpretation.

5. Positive test frequently correlates with cold agglutinin titer of >1:64. 75%–85% of patients with atypical pneumonia and a positive test will develop serologic evidence of mycoplasma pneumonia infection.

From Griffin JP: *Ann Intern Med* 70:701, 1969.

III. ANEMIA: EVALUATION

A. General Studies

Anemia is defined by age-specific norms. Common evaluations include the following:

1. Complete history, specifically regarding symptoms or history of anemia, blood loss, pica, medication expo-

sure, and family history of anemia, splenectomy, or cholecystectomy

2. Careful physical exam, particularly any evidence of tachypnea, tachycardia, cardiac murmurs, pallor, jaundice, hepatosplenomegaly, glossitis, or additional signs of systemic illness

3. Complete blood count (CBC) with differential and reticulocyte count

4. Blood smear to examine morphology of cells

5. Urinalysis for bilirubin, blood, protein, glucose. Also perform microscopic exam.

6. Stool for occult blood

7. Serum bilirubin, blood urea nitrogen (BUN), creatinine

B. **Specific Tests**

1. Tests to diagnose sickle hemoglobin: Any substance that reduces O_2 tension will cause red cells containing Hb S to sickle. A positive "sickle prep" is found in the sickle hemoglobinopathies (SS, SC, S thal, and others), as well as in sickle trait; 8% of African-American children in the United States will have a positive sickle prep. All positive tests should be confirmed with cellulose acetate electrophoresis.

   a. Sulfite solution—"sickle prep": Mix one or two drops of 2% sodium metabisulfite or sodium hyposulfite on a slide with one drop of blood; apply coverslip. Read preparation at 30 minutes and again at 3 hours. Positive test: presence of sickled cells.

   b. Sickledex: A solubility test using dithionate reduction of Hb S. Solution is turbid in the presence of Hb S, otherwise clear. Widely used. Hgb S gives a positive result, whereas Hgb C and others do not.

   c. Note that false negatives may be obtained with either the sickle prep or sickledex in neonates and in other patients with a high Hgb F percentage.

2. Hemoglobin electrophoresis: Cellulose acetate electrophoresis: separation of hemoglobin variants based on molecular charge. Hemoglobins found are reported in order of relative abundances in the sample (e.g., sickle cell trait is ASA_2, sickle cell disease is SFA_2).

3. Coombs test: Detects immunoproteins, IgG, or complement adsorbed on RBCs

4. Iron trial: Adequate iron therapy (3–6 mg/kg/24 hr divided TID of elemental iron) should result in reticulocytosis peaking 7–10 days into therapy. A significant increase in Hb concentration should be evident after 3–4 weeks of therapy.

5. Ferritin: Serum ferritin is an accurate reflection of total body iron stores after 6 months of age. Ferritin may be falsely elevated with infection or inflammation.

6. Glucose-6-phosphate dehydrogenase (G6PD) assay, pyruvate kinase assay

7. Bone marrow aspiration

From Siimes MA et al: *Blood* 43:581, 1974.

8. Specific indicators of hemolysis
   a. Haptoglobin: Binds free hemoglobin. Decreased with intravascular and extravascular hemolysis and hepatocellular disease. Falsely normal or increased levels may occur with inflammation, infection, or malignancy.
   b. Hemopexin: Binds free heme groups. Decreased with intravascular hemolysis, renal disease, and hepatocellular disease. Hemopexin usually not increased with inflammation, infection, or malignancy.

9. Free erythrocyte protoporphyrin (FEP): Accumulates when the conversion of protoporphyrin to heme is blocked. Elevated in iron deficiency, plumbism, and erythropoietic protoporphyria. Levels >300 mcg/dl packed RBC generally found only with lead intoxication.

IV. ANEMIA: DIAGNOSIS

A. Diagnostic Categories
Please refer to age-related normal values of MCV in Tables 15.1 and 15.10.

B. Distinguishing Common Causes of Anemia (Table 15.2)

C. Interpretation of Hemoglobin Patterns in Newborns (Table 15.3)

V. COAGULATION

Normal clotting depends on adequate platelet number and function as well as intact coagulation cascade (Figure 15.1).

TABLE 15.1.

Evaluation of Anemia

Reticulocyte count	Microcytic anemia*	Normocytic anemia	Macrocytic anemia
Low	Iron deficiency[†] Lead poisoning Chronic disease Aluminum toxicity Copper deficiency	Chronic disease Red cell aplasia (TEC, infection, drug induced) Splenomegaly Malignancy Endocrinopathies Renal failure	Folate deficiency Vitamin B_{12} deficiency Aplastic anemia Congenital bone marrow dysfunction (Diamond-Blackfan or Fanconi's)
Normal	Thalassemia trait Sideroblastic anemia	Acute bleeding Dyserythropoietic anemia II	Drug-induced
High	Thalassemia syndromes Hb C disorders	Antibody-mediated hemolysis Fragmentation (HUS, TTP, DIC, Kassaback-Merritt) Membrane abnormalities (spherocytosis, elliptocytosis) Enzyme disorders (G6PD, pyruvate kinase, hemoglobinopathies)	Dyserythropoetic anemia I, III Active hemolysis

*As a rule of thumb, the lowest limit of normal for MCV is age + 70 (refer to Section IX for specific values)

†An easy way to differentiate iron deficiency from thalassemia minor is to calculate the discriminate index: MCV/RBC > 13.5 suggests iron deficiency; <11.5 is suggestive of thal minor.

From F. Oski: Personal communication, 1993.

TABLE 15.2.

	Iron deficiency	β-Thalassemia trait	Chronic inflammation	Lead poisoning
Reticulocyte count	Low	Low	Normal	Low
RDW	↑	↓	Normal	↓
Ferritin	↓	Normal to ↑	Normal to ↑	↓ to normal
FEP	↑	Normal	↑	↑
Iron	↓	Normal	↓	↓ to normal
TIBC	↑	Normal	↓	
Electrophoresis	Normal	↑ HbA$_2$ or F	Normal	Normal
ESR	Normal	Normal	↑	Normal
Smear	Hypochromic, target cells, microcytic	Normochromic, microcytic	Varies	Basophilic stippling

ESR, Erythrocyte sedimentation rate; *FEP* free erythrocyte protoporphyrin; *RDW,* red cell distribution width; *TIBC,* total iron binding capacity.

A. **Platelet Function**

Adequacy of platelet function and number can be measured by bleeding time, for example by the Ivy technique:

1. Place blood pressure cuff on upper arm and inflate to 40 mm Hg. Clean forearm with alcohol and allow to dry.
2. Make a standardized incision with a nonheparinized long point disposable lancet (3 mm deep) or with a commercially available template. Avoid lancing a superficial vein.
3. Gently absorb the blood onto filter paper every 30 seconds without disturbing the wound. Bleeding time equals time required for bleeding to cease. A prolonged bleeding time in a nonhemophiliac patient with normal platelet count indicates von Willebrand's disease, acquired or congenital platelet dysfunction, or NSAID ingestion within the past week.

B. **Activated Partial Thromboplastin Time (APTT)**

Measures intrinsic system; requires factors XII, XI, IX, VIII, V, II, I. May be prolonged with polycythemia, inadequate sample volume, blood drawn from heparin-containing catheter. Useful for monitoring heparin therapy (see Figure 15.1).

TABLE 15.3.

FA	Designation for adult normal Hgb with fetal Hgb, which is the normal pattern for a newborn.
FAV	Indicates the presence of both Hgb A and F as would be expected in the newborn. However, an anomalous band (V) is present, which does not appear to be any of the common Hgb variants.
FAS	Indicates the presence of adult normal Hgb and Hgb S. This preliminary finding is consistent with the benign sickle cell *trait*.
FS	Designates the presence of sickle Hgb without detectable adult normal Hgb A. This is consistent with homozygous sickle Hgb genotype (S/S) and could lead to manifestations of sickle cell anemia during infancy.
FC*	Designates the presence of Hgb C without adult normal Hgb A. This finding is consistent with the clinically significant monozygous Hgb genotype (C/C) and could result in a hematologic disorder during childhood.
FSC	Indicates the presence of both Hgbs S and C. This heterozygous condition could lead to manifestations of sickle cell disease during childhood.
FAC	Indicates the presence of both Hgb C and adult normal Hgb A. This finding is consistent with the benign Hgb C *trait*.
FSAA₂	Designates heterozygous S Beta thalassemia, which is a clinically significant sickling disorder.
FAA₂	Designates heterozygous Hgb A thalassemia, which is a clinically significant hematologic disorder.
F*	Designates the presence of fetal Hgb F without adult normal Hgb A. Although this may indicate a delayed appearance of Hgb A, it may also represent a potential hereditary persistence of fetal Hgb. It is not possible to interpret this finding without further laboratory studies.
FV*	Indicates the presence of fetal Hgb F and an anomalous Hgb variant (V). The potential clinical significance can only be ascertained after laboratory studies.
AF	If this is the case, another filter paper blood specimen must be submitted when the infant is about 4 months of age, at which time the transfused blood cells should have been cleared.

* Repeat blood specimen should be submitted to confirm the original interpretation.

C. Prothrombin Time (PT)

Measures extrinsic pathway; requires factors VII, X, V, II, I. May be prolonged with decreased liver synthetic capacity, decreased vitamin K absorption, warfarin therapy, inadequate sample volume and drawing from heparin-containing catheter. Useful for monitoring warfarin thera-

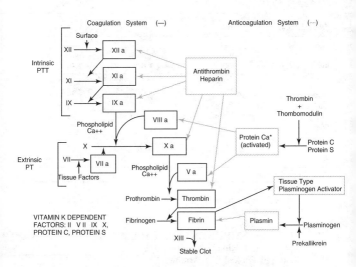

FIG. 15.1. Coagulation cascade *(Modified from Rosenberg RD, Bauer KA: Hosp Pract, 1986.)*
*Also promotes fibrinolysis.

py; systemic heparin has little effect at usual therapeutic doses.

D.   Disseminated Intravascular Coagulation
Usually associated with fragmented RBCs, low or decreasing platelet count, hemoglobinemia (pink plasma), prolonged PT and APTT, and low or decreasing fibrinogen. Confirm by measuring fibrin split products (present) and factors V and VIII (decreased).

E.   Differentiating Etiologies of Coagulopathy (Table 15.4)

F.   Hypercoaguable States
May be documented by decreased levels of protein C, protein S, antithrombin III, or resistance to activated protein C. An increased risk of spontaneous thrombotic events including deep venous thrombosis is incurred. When patients with protein C or S deficiency are treated with warfarin, skin necrosis is an additional risk. Thrombosis may also occur in the presence of antiphospholipid antibodies, lupus anticoagulant, paroxysmal nocturnal,

TABLE 15.4.

Lab test	Vitamin K deficiency	Liver disease	Disseminated intravascular coagulation
PT	↑	↑	↑
Platelets	nl	↓ to nl	↓
Fibrinogen	nl	↓	↓
Factor VIII	nl	nl to ↑	↓
Fibrinogen Degradation Products	nl	nl to ↑	↑
Factor VII	↓	↓	↓ to nl

PT, Prothrombin time.

hemoglobinuria, pregnancy, malignancies, and other clinical syndromes.

VI. **BLOOD COMPONENT REPLACEMENT**
A. **Approximate Blood Volume** (Table 15.5)
B. **Required Packed Cell Volume**
Infuse no faster than 2–3 ml/kg/hr or in 10 ml/kg aliquots over several hours. In cases of severe chronic anemia, reduce replacement to 1 ml/kg/hr to avoid congestive heart failure.

$$\text{Vol of cells (ml)} = \frac{\text{Est blood vol (ml)} \times \text{desired Hct change}}{\text{Hct of PRBC}}$$

Note: The usual Hct of PRBC is 65%.

TABLE 15.5.

Approximate Blood Volume

Age	Total blood volume (ml/kg)
Premature Infants	90–105
Term Newborns	78–86
1 to 12 months	73–78
1 to 3 years	74–82
4 to 6 years	80–86
7 to 18 years	83–90
Adults	68–88

From Nathan DG, Oski FA: *Hematology of infancy and childhood,* Philadelphia, 1993, WB Saunders.

C. **Partial Exchange Transfusion** (Table 15.6)
   (See Chapter 20 for technique in newborns.)
D. **Platelet Transfusions**
   Usually give 4 units/m². Hemorrhagic complications are rare with platelet counts >20,000/mm³. Platelet counts >50,000/mm³ advisable for lumbar puncture. One unit of platelets/m² raises platelet count 10,000/mm³ in the absence of platelet destruction or antiplatelet antibodies.

$$\text{Platelet increment/mm}^3 = \frac{30,000 \times (\text{number of units})}{\text{Est blood vol (L)}}$$

TABLE 15.6.

Diagnosis		Volume of exchange (ml)
Symptomatic polycythemia	Use fresh frozen plasma or 5% albumin solution or normal saline	$\dfrac{\text{Est blood vol (ml)} \times \text{desired Hct change}}{\text{Starting Hct}}$
Severe anemia: rapid correction	Use PRBC (about 22 g/dl)	$\dfrac{\text{Blood vol (ml)} \times \text{desired Hb rise}}{22 \text{ gm/dl} - \text{HbR}}$ $\text{HbR} = \dfrac{\text{Hb (initial)} + \text{Hb (desired)}}{2}$
Sickle cell crisis: double red blood cell volume exchange	Usually reduces sickle cells to <40%; follow Hct during transfusion; use Sickledex negative PRBC.	$\dfrac{\text{Est blood vol (ml)} \times \text{patient's Hct (\%)} \times 2}{\text{Hct of PRBC (\%)}}$
N.B.*		

*N.B.: Do *NOT* exceed Hct of 35%
PRBC, Packed red blood cells.
From Nieburg PI et al: *Am J Dis Child* 131:60, 1977; Zinkham WH: Personal communication, 1989.

E.   **Coagulation Factor Replacement**
   1. Background
      a. 1 unit Factor activity = activity in 1 ml normal plasma.
      b. 1 unit Factor VIII/kg raises VIII levels 2%.
      c. 1 unit Factor IX/kg raises IX levels 1%.
   2. Desired factor level (Table 15.7)
F.   **Blood Products**
   1. Whole blood: Use emergently for hypovolemia due to blood loss. Alternatively, may use PRBCs and fresh frozen plasma (FFP).
   2. PRBC: Contains WBC but few platelets. Usual choice for RBC transfusion.
   3. Leukocyte-poor PRBC: Use if history of nonhemolytic transfusion reaction or in immunocompromised patients or neonates.
      a. Washed: >92%–95% of WBCs and >99% plasma removed
      b. Leukofiltered or frozen deglycerolized: >99% WBCs removed
   4. Platelets
      a. Use in very severe or symptomatic thrombocytopenia.
      b. Pooled-concentrates: From multiple donors.
      c. Single donor product: From hemapheresis. Use in patients with antibodies from multiple transfusions.
      d. Leukocyte-poor: Use if history of significant platelet transfusion reactions.

TABLE 15.7.

Bleeding site	Desired level
Joint or simple hematoma	20%–40%
Simple dental extraction*	50%
Major soft tissue bleed	80%–100%
Serious oral bleeding*	80%–100%
Head injury	100+%
Major surgery (dental, orthopedic, other)	100+%

*Aminocaproic acid, 100 mg/kg IV or PO Q6 hr (up to 24 g/day); may be useful for treatment of oral bleeds and prophylaxis for dental extractions.

5. Granulocytes: Use only in selected patients with very low WBC count and documented severe infection, which is not responsive to antibiotics.
6. Fresh frozen plasma: Contains all clotting factors, except platelets. Indications include acute disseminated intravascular coagulation (DIC), thrombotic thrombocytopenic purpura (TTP), reversal of effect of warfarin, protein C or S deficiency, or in an unknown type of coagulopathy.
7. Cryoprecipitate: Contains factor VIII (5–10 U/cc), Von Willebrand factor (VWF), fibrinogen. Do not use in factor IX deficiency.
8. Monoclonal factor VIII: Relatively purified factor VIII. Use in factor VIII deficiency. Most preparations not effective in Von Willebrand's disease.
9. Recombinant factor VIII: Highly purified factor VIII. Risk of inhibitor formation, which may not exceed that of other products.
10. Activated prothrombin complex concentrates (FEIBA, Autoplex): Contain above factors with some activated IX and X (and VII in some). Consider in factor VIII deficiency with high titer inhibitors.

G. **Irradiated Blood Products**
1. Principle: Many blood products (PRBC, platelet preparations, leukocytes, FFP, and others) contain viable lymphocytes capable of sustained survival in recipient. Irradiation with 1500 rad before transfusion may prevent graft-versus-host disease in immunocompromised patients but does not prevent antibody formation against donor WBCs.
2. Indications: Intensive chemotherapy, leukemia, lymphoma, bone marrow transplantation, solid organ transplantation, known or suspected immune deficiencies, intrauterine transfusions for erythroblastosis fetalis, and transfusions in neonates.

From Von Fliedner V et al: *Am J Med* 72:951, 1982.

H. **Cytomegalovirus (CMV) Negative Blood**
Desirable in neonates and other immunocompromised patients who are CMV-antibody negative, including those undergoing intensive chemotherapy or transplantation.

From Yeager A et al: *J Pediatr* 98:281, 1981.

I. **Complications of Transfusions**
    1. Acute hemolytic reaction: Most often due to blood group incompatibility. Symptoms includes fever, chills, tachycardia, hypotension, shock. Lab findings include disseminated intravascular coagulation (DIC), hemoglobinuria, positive Coombs test. Treatment includes immediate cessation of blood infusion and institution of supportive measures.
    2. Febrile nonhemolytic reaction: Usually due to host antibody response to donor antigens. Seen in previously transfused patients. Symptoms include fever, chills, diaphoresis. Prevention includes premedication with antipyretics, antihistamines, and steroids.
    3. Urticarial reaction: Unknown etiology. Treat with antihistamines. Use washed or frozen RBCs with next transfusion.
    4. Delayed transfusion reaction: Minor blood group antigen incompatibility. Occurs 3–10 days after transfusion. Symptoms include anemia and bilirubinuria. Lab findings are a positive Coombs test and new RBC antibodies.
    5. Transfusion-transmitted disease: Lower incidence at present with increased vigilance in blood product screening. Most common infections include hepatitis B, C, and delta, HIV, HTLV-1, and CMV. Sepsis secondary to bacterial infection may occur, especially with platelet transfusions.

Adapted from Nathan DG Oski FA: *Hematology of infants and children,* Philadelphia, 1993, WB Saunders.

VII. **SCREENING FOR LEAD TOXICITY**
A. **Sources of Lead**
    Lead-based paint, leaded gasoline, soil, air, and dust; drinking water from lead-soldiered pipes; food stored in leaded cans or pottery
B. **Effect of Lead**
    Inhibits enzyme heme synthetase, which prevents incorporation of iron into protoporphyrin III to produce heme, resulting in anemia. May cause encephalopathy, behavior disorders, motor defects, and renal dysfunction.

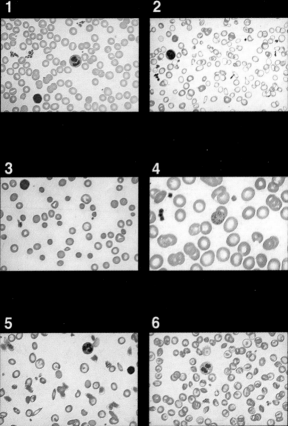

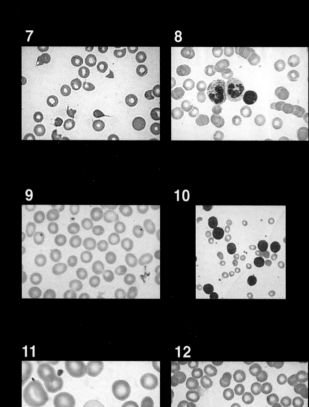

C. **Minimal Screening**
   (Age 6–36 mo) (Table 15.8)
   1. Follow-up of children with Pb >15 mcg/dl:
      a. >15–19 mcg/dl: Screen every 3–4 months; family education and nutrition counseling; identify source of exposure. When Pb is 15–19 in 2 consecutive tests, 3–4 months apart, investigate environment and consider abatement.
      b. >20 mcg/dl: Confirm with venous blood. If still > 20 mcg/dl, refer for medical evaluation.
      c. >45 mcg/dl: Confirm with venous blood. If still >45 mcg/dl, urgent medical and environmental intervention is needed.
      d. >70 mcg/dl: Immediate inpatient chelation therapy

From Centers for Disease Control: Preventing lead poisoning in young children, U.S. Department of Health and Human Services Public Health Service, Oct. 1991. (At the time of this publication, these guidelines are currently being rewritten.)

TABLE 15.8.

Risk groups	Blood Pb level (mcg/dL)	Treatment plan
Low risk: Initial test at 12 months	<10	Retest at 24 mo
	10–14	Retest every 3–4 mo; once 2 consecutive tests are <10 mcg/dL, or 3 are <15 mcg/dL, test once a year.
	≥15	See next section, below.
High risk: Initial test at 6 months	<10	Retest every 6 mo; once two consecutive tests are <10 mcg/dL, or 3 are <15 mcg/dL, test once a year.
	10–14	Retest every 3–4 mo; once two consecutive tests are <10 mcg/dL, or 3 are <15 mcg/dL, test once a year.
	≥15	See above.

VIII. ONCOLOGY
A. **Epidemiology**
   1. There are 6550 new childhood cancer diagnoses in the United States each year, and deaths from malignancy account for 10% of childhood deaths.

2. The most common types of cancer are leukemia, CNS tumors, lymphoma, neuroblastoma, soft tissue sarcoma, Wilm's tumor, bone tumor, and retinoblastoma.
3. Risk factors include radiation exposure, medications, family history, and genetic syndromes.

B. **Diagnosis of Acute Lymphocytic Leukemia (ALL)**
   1. Signs and symptoms include lethargy, fever, infection, respiratory difficulties, extremity/joint pain, bleeding, anorexia, and abdominal pain.
   2. Physical findings include pallor, hepatosplenomegaly, ecchymoses, and lymphadenopathy.
   3. Lab findings include anemia, variable platelet count, and variable WBC count with blasts.

C. **Initial Workup of ALL**
   1. Thoughtful history and physical
   2. Peripheral smear
   3. Additional labs: CBC with differential, electrolytes, and a chemistry panel, amylase, LDH, immunoglobulins, varicella and CMV titers, PT, PTT, fibrinogen and FDP, type and cross, blood culture, and HIV titers
   4. Urinalysis
   5. Chest x-ray exam
   6. Lumbar puncture: If platelets number > 50,000, obtain informed consent. Send cerebrospinal fluid (CSF) for cell count and differential, glucose and protein, culture and cytopathology.
   7. Bone marrow: Obtain informed consent. Send for cell morphology, special stains, immunophenotyping, DNA ploidy, and cytogenetics.
   8. Obtain blood, urine, and throat cultures, if febrile

D. **Initial Management**
   1. Monitor for tumor lysis syndrome (see Chapter 1).
   2. RBC and platelet transfusions as needed with irradiated and leukocyte-poor products.
   3. Hyperleukocytosis: Give hydration and specific chemotherapy. Consider exchange transfusion.
   4. Infection: Broad spectrum antibiotics
   5. Plan for central line placement.

IX. **NORMAL VALUES**
  The following normal values are compiled from published literature and The Johns Hopkins Hospital Department of Laboratory Medicine. Values may vary depending upon analytic technique used. International System (SI) values are in parentheses.
A. **Blood Levels** (Table 15.9)
B. **Age-Specific Indices** (Table 15.10)
C. **Hemoglobin and MCV Percentiles** (Figure 15.2)
D. **Age-Specific White Cell Differential**
  Number of leukocytes are in thousands per mm³; ranges are estimates of 95% confidence limits, and percentages refer to differential counts (Table 15.11).

TABLE 15.9.

Antithrombin III	
Preterm	0.38 (0.14–0.62) units/ml
Term	0.63 (0.39–0.87) units/ml
Child/Adult	1.05 (0.79–1.31) units/ml
Bilirubin	See Chapter 6
Bleeding time	2.5–10 min
D-Dimer	Any positive test is significant
Erythrocyte sedimentation rate (ESR)	
Newborn (0–48 hr)	0–4 mm/hr
Child	4–20 mm/hr
Adult male	0–10 mm/hr
Adult female	0–20 mm/hr
Ferritin	
Child	7–144 mcg/L
Adult male	30–265 mcg/L
Adult female	10–110 mcg/L
Fibrin degradation products (FDPs)	
Titer of 1:25	Borderline positive
Titer of 1:50	Positive
Fibrinogen	
Preterm	2.56 (1.69–5.50) g/L
Term	2.83 (1.67–3.99) g/L
Child/Adult	2.78 (1.56–4.00) g/L

(Continued.)

TABLE 15.9. (cont.)

Folate (RBC)	
Infants (<1 yr)	74–995 mcg/ml
Children 1–11 yr	96–364 mcg/ml
Adults	160–640 mcg/ml
Folate (serum)	
Children 1–10 yr	6.5–16.5 ng/ml
Adults	6.0–18.6 ng/ml
Free erythrocyte protoporphyrin (FEP)	<3 mcg/g Hb <50 mcg/dl whole blood <130 mcg/dl PRBC
Haptoglobin	40–180 mg/dl
Hemoglobin A_1C (glycosylated Hgb)	3.9%–7.7% of total Hb
Hemopexin	
Premature	2–26 mg/dl
Newborn	8–42 mg/dl
1–12 yr	40–70 mg/dl
>12 yr	50–100 mg/dl
Immunoglobulins	See Immunology
Iron	
Newborn	63–201 mcg/dl
2–12 mo	15–164 mcg/dl
Adult	70–190 mcg/dl
Lead	See Section VII
Methemoglobin	
Preterm	0.52 (0.02–0.83) g/dl
Term	0.22 (0.00–0.58) g/dl
1 mo–78 yr	0.11 (0.00–0.33) g/dl
Partial thromboplastin time, activated (APTT)	
Preterm	108 (80–168) sec
Term	42.9 (31.3–54.3) sec
Child/Adult	33.5 (26.6–40.3) sec
Protein C	
Preterm	0.28 (0.12–0.44) units/ml
Term	0.35 (0.17–0.53) units/ml
Infant	0.59 (0.37–0.81) units/ml
Adult	0.96 (0.64–1.28) units/ml

(Continued.)

TABLE 15.9. (cont.)

Protein S	
Preterm	0.26 (0.14–0.38) units/ml
Term	0.36 (0.12–0.69) units/ml
Infant	0.87 (0.55–1.19) units/ml
Adult	0.92 (0.60–1.24) units/ml
Prothrombin time (PT)	
Preterm	15.4 (14.6–16.9) sec
Term	13.0 (10.1–15.9) sec
Child/Adult	12.4 (10.8–13.9) sec
Red cell distribution width (RDW)	
Adults	11.5%–14.5%
Thrombin time	
Preterm	14 (11–17) sec
Term	12 (10–16) sec
Adult	10 sec
Total iron binding capacity (TIBC)	
Newborn	150–240 mcg/dl
2–12 months	200–400 mcg/dl
Adult	250–400 mcg/dl
Transferrin	
Newborn	130–275 mg/dl
Adult	220–400 mg/dl
Vitamin B$_{12}$	30–785 pg/ml

TABLE 15.10.

Age Specific Indices

Age	Hgb (g%), Mean (-2 SD)	Hct (%), Mean (-2 SD)	MCV (fl), Mean (-2 SD)	MCHC (g/% RBC), Mean (-2 SD)	Retic (%)	WBC/mm³ × 1000, Mean (+2 SD)	Platelets (10³/mm³), Mean (+2 SD)
26–30 wk gestation*	13.4 (11)	41.5 (34.9)	118.2 (106.7)	37.9 (30.6)	—	4.4 (2.7)	254 (180–327)
28 wk	14.5	45	120	31.0	(5–10)	—	275
32 wk	15.0	47	118	32.0	(3–10)	—	290
Term† (cord)	16.5 (13.5)	51 (42)	108 (98)	33.0 (30.0)	(3–7)	18.1 (9–30)‡	290
1–3 days	18.5 (14.5)	56 (45)	108 (95)	33.0 (29.0)	(1.8–4.6)	18.9 (9.4–34)	192
2 wk	16.6 (13.4)	53 (41)	105 (88)	31.4 (28.1)	(0.1–1.7)	11.4 (5–20)	252
1 mo	13.9 (10.7)	44 (33)	101 (91)	31.8 (28.1)	(0.1–1.7)	10.8 (4–19.5)	
2 mo	11.2 (9.4)	35 (28)	95 (84)	31.8 (28.3)			
6 mo	12.6 (11.1)	36 (31)	76 (68)	35.0 (32.7)	(0.7–2.3)	11.9 (6–17.5)	
6 mo–2 yr	12.0 (10.5)	36 (33)	78 (70)	33.0 (30.0)		10.6 (6–17)	(150–350)
2–6 yr	12.5 (11.5)	37 (34)	81 (75)	34.0 (31.0)	(0.5–1.0)	8.5 (5–15.5)	"
6–12 yr	13.5 (11.5)	40 (35)	86 (77)	34.0 (31.0)	(0.5–1.0)	8.1 (4.5–13.5)	"
12–18 yr Male	14.5 (13)	43 (36)	88 (78)	34.0 (31.0)	(0.5–1.0)	7.8 (4.5–13.5)	"
Female	14.0 (12)	41 (37)	90 (78)	34.0 (31.0)	(0.5–1.0)	7.8 (4.5–13.5)	"
Adult Male	15.5 (13.5)	47 (41)	90 (80)	34.0 (31.0)	(0.8–2.5)	7.4 (4.5–11)	"
Female	14.0 (12)	41 (36)	90 (80)	34.0 (31.0)	(0.8–4.1)	7.4 (4.5–11)	"

*Values are from fetal samplings.
†Under 1 m/o, capillary Hgb exceeds venous: 1 hr–3.6 g difference; 5 days–2.2 g difference; 3 wks–1.1 g difference.
‡Mean (95% confidence limits.)

From Forestier F et al: *Pediatr Res* 20:342, 1986; Oski FA, Naiman JL: *Hematological problems in the newborn infant*, Philadelphia, 1982, WB Saunders; Nathan D, Oski FA: *Hematology of infancy and childhood*, Philadelphia, 1981, WB Saunders; Metoth Y et al: *Acta Paed Scand* 60:317, 1971; Wintrobe: *Clinical hematology*, Philadelphia, 1981, Lea & Febiger.

TABLE 15.11.

Age Specific WBC Differential: Number of leukocytes are in thousands per mm³; ranges are estimates of 95% confidence limits; and percentages refer to differential counts.

Age	Total Leukocytes		Neutrophils*			Lymphocytes			Monocytes		Eosinophils	
	Mean	Range	Mean	Range	%	Mean	Range	%	Mean	%	Mean	%
Birth	—†	—	4.0	2.0–6.0	—	4.2	2.0–7.3	—	0.6	—	0.1	—
12 hr	—	—	11.0	7.8–14.5	—	4.2	2.0–7.3	—	0.6	—	0.1	—
24 hr	—	—	9.0	7.0–12.0	—	4.2	2.0–7.3	—	0.6	—	0.1	—
1–4 wk	—	—	3.6	1.8–5.4	—	5.6	2.9–9.1	—	0.7	—	0.2	—
6 mo	11.9	6.0–17.5	3.8	1.0–8.5	32	7.3	4.0–13.5	61	0.6	5	0.3	3
1 yr	11.4	6.0–17.5	3.5	1.5–8.5	31	7.0	4.0–10.5	61	0.6	5	0.3	3
2 yr	10.6	6.0–17.0	3.5	1.5–8.5	33	6.3	3.0–9.5	59	0.5	5	0.3	3
4 yr	9.1	5.5–15.5	3.8	1.5–8.5	42	4.5	2.0–8.0	50	0.5	5	0.3	3
6 yr	8.5	5.0–14.5	4.3	1.5–8.0	51	3.5	1.5–7.0	42	0.4	5	0.2	3
8 yr	8.3	4.5–13.5	4.4	1.5–8.0	53	3.3	1.5–6.8	39	0.4	4	0.2	2
10 yr	8.1	4.5–13.5	4.4	1.8–8.0	54	3.1	1.5–6.5	38	0.4	4	0.2	2
16 yr	7.8	4.5–13.0	4.4	1.8–8.0	57	2.8	1.2–5.2	35	0.4	5	0.2	3
21 yr	7.4	4.5–11.0	4.4	1.8–7.7	59	2.5	1.0–4.8	34	0.3	4	0.2	3

*Neutrophils include band cells at all ages and a small number of metamyelocytes and myelocytes in the first few days of life.
†Insufficient data for a reliable estimate.

From Dallmann PR: Developmental changes in number. In Rudolph AM, *Pediatrics*, ed 18, Norwalk, 1987, Appleton and Lange. (Data on infants under the age of 1 month are derived from Monroe et al: *J Pediatr* 95:89, 1979; Ewinberg et al: *J Pediatr* 106:462, 1985. Other values are from Albritton EC, editor: *Standard value in blood*, Philadelphia, 1952, WB Saunders.)

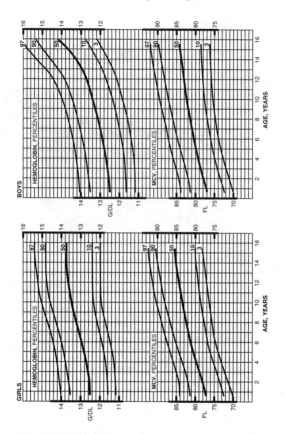

FIG. 15.2. Hemoglobin and mean corpuscular volume by age. *(Dallman PR, Siimes MA: J Pediatr 94:26, 1979.*

X. **BLOOD SMEAR FINDINGS**
   Color Plate 1. Normal smear   Round RBCs with central pallor about 1/3 of the cell's diameter, scattered platelets, occasional WBCs
   Color Plate 2. Iron deficiency   Hypochromic, microcytic RBCs, poikilocytosis, plentiful platelets, occasional ovalocytes and target cells
   Color Plate 3. Spherocytosis   Microspherocytes a hallmark (densely stained RBCs with no central pallor)
   Color Plate 4. Basophilic Stippling   Due to staining of ribosomal complexes containing RNA throughout the cell; seen with heavy metal intoxication, thalassemia, pyrimidine 5' nucleotidase deficiency, iron deficiency, and other states associated with ineffective erythropoiesis
   Color Plate 5. Hgb SS Disease   Sickled cells, target cells, hypochromic, poikilocytosis, Howell-Jolly bodies, nucleated RBCs common (not shown)
   Color Plate 6. Hgb SC Disease   Target cells, "oat cells," poikilocytosis; sickle forms rarely seen
   Color Plate 7. Microangiopathic Hemolytic Anemia   RBC fragments, anisocytosis, polychromasia, decreased platelets
   Color Plate 8. Toxic Granulations   Prominent dark blue primary granules; commonly seen with infection and other toxic states
   Color Plate 9. Howell-Jolly Body   Small, dense nuclear remnant in an RBC; suggests splenic dysfunction or asplenia
   Color Plate 10. Leukemia   Blasts showing large nucleus: cytoplasm ratio, may be little differentiation between blasts
   Color Plate 11. Polychromatophilia   Diffusely basophilic because of RNA staining; seen with early release of reticulocytes from the marrow
   Color Plate 12. Intraerythrocytic parasites   Malaria

IMMUNOLOGY 16

I. LABORATORY EVALUATION OF A SUSPECTED IMMUNODEFICIENCY (Table 16.1)

II. IMMUNE GLOBULIN (IVIG and IMIG)
A. General Information
1. Separated from pooled human plasma by alcohol fractionation and modified for IV administration
2. Protein content is $\geq$ 95% IgG but contains trace amounts of IgA and IgM.
3. Standard dosing provides immediate antibody levels with a half-life of 3–4 weeks.
4. Recommended only for those indications for which clinical efficacy has been established (see below)
5. Adverse reactions to both IVIG and IMIG
   a. Systemic symptoms include the following:
      1) High fever
      2) Hemodynamic changes (hypertension, hypotension, tachycardia)
      3) Hypersensitivity reactions (urticaria, anaphylaxis)
      4) See following information specific to IVIG or IMIG.
   b. Immune globulin and all other blood products containing IgA are relatively contraindicated in patients with complete IgA deficiency since they may rarely develop anti-IgA antibodies. But because systemic reactions are very rare, routine screening for IgA deficiency is not recommended. Products depleted in IgA are available.
   c. Serious systemic reactions are rare; however, trained personnel, equipment, epinephrine, and other necessary drugs for treating an acute reaction should be immediately available.

TABLE 16.1.

Laboratory Evaluation of a Suspected Immunodeficiency

Suspected abnormality	Clinical findings	Initial tests	More advanced tests
Antibody	Sinopulmonary infection (pyogenic bacteria) Gastroenteritis (enterovirus, other viruses, Giardia) Autoimmune disease (ITP, hemolytic anemia, inflammatory bowel disease)	Immunoglobulin levels (IgG, IgM, IgA) Antibody levels to protein vaccines (diphtheria, tetanus) Antibody titers to polysaccharide vaccines (pneumococcus)	B cell enumeration Immunofixation electrophoresis IgG antibody subclass levels
Cell-mediated immunity	Pneumonia (pyogenic bacteria, P. carinii, viruses) Gastroenteritis (viruses) Dermatitis/mucositis (fungi)	Total lymphocyte counts HIV ELISA / Western blot Delayed-type hypersensitivity skin test (Candida, tetanus toxoid, mumps, trichophyton)	T lymphocyte enumeration (CD2 or CD3) T lymphocyte subset enumeration (CD4, CD8) In vitro T lymphocyte proliferation to mitogens antigens or allogeneic cells
Phagocytosis	Cutaneous infections, abscesses, lymphadenitis (staphylococcus, enteric bacteria, fungi, mycobacteria)	WBC/neutrophil count and morphology	Nitroblue tetrazolium (NBT) test Chemotactic assay Phagocytic and bactericidal assay
Spleen	Bacteremia/hematogenous infection (pneumococcus, other streptococci, Neisseria)	Peripheral blood smear for Howell-Jolly bodies Hemoglobin electrophoresis (HgbSS)	Technetium-99 spleen scan
Complement	Bacterial sepsis Autoimmune disease (Lupus, glomerulonephritis)	CH_{50} (total hemolytic complement)	Classic and alternative pathway assays Individual component assays

ELISA, Enzyme-linked immunosorbent assay; *ITP,* idiopathic thrombocytopenic purpura.

B. Intravenous Immune Globulin (IVIG)
1. Available as 5%–12% solutions (50–120 mg/ml)
2. Indications for IVIG
   a. Antibody deficiency disorders (replacement therapy):
      Dosage: 300–400/mg/kg IV per month. Determine
      optimal frequency and dose of IVIG by monitoring
      clinical response.
   b. Idiopathic thrombocytopenic purpura (ITP)
      1) Initial therapy for acute ITP: 0.8–1.0 g/kg IV in
         1–2 doses
      2) Alternatively for acute ITP, prednisone may be
         added or substituted, 2mg/kg/day
      3) Maintenance therapy for chronic ITP is individual-
         ized to patient
   c. Kawasaki disease
      1) Recommended dosage: 2 g/kg IV as a single dose
         over 10–12 hours
      2) See Chapter 18 for further information.
3. Possible indications for IVIG: (Data is limited or shows
   only marginal benefit from therapy)
   a. Bone marrow transplantation
   b. Pediatric HIV infection
   c. Low birthweight infants

Adapted from 1994 Report of the Committee of Infectious Disease (Red Book).

   d. Autoimmune diseases: Polymyositis, dermatomyosi-
      tis, other auto-immune diseases
4. Adverse reactions to IVIG
   a. Minor systemic reactions may include the following:
      headache, myalgia, fever, chills, nausea, and vomiting.
      These can usually be alleviated by reducing the rate of
      infusion. Prophylaxis with antihistamines or IV hy-
      drocortisone may be of benefit if ongoing therapy is
      required.
   b. Aseptic meningitis
   c. Transmission of viral illness (e.g., hepatitis C)

C. Intramuscular Immune Globulin (IMIG)
1. Available as 16.5% solution (165 mg/ml)
2. Indications for IMIG
   a. IMIG is not the drug of choice for antibody deficiency,
      ITP, or Kawasaki disease. Recommended doses for

IVIG cannot be applied to IMIG because insufficient amounts of IgG can be delivered by this route.

b. Hepatitis A prophylaxis

1) Give to susceptible individuals 0.02 ml/kg up to 2 ml immediately if possible and within 14 days of exposure.

2) See Red Book* for details of dosing for preexposure prophylaxis

c. Measles prophylaxis

1) Nonvaccinated normal individuals (especially < 6 m/o): Dose of 0.25 ml/kg up to 15 ml IM given immediately if possible and within 6 days of exposure

2) Immunocompromised individuals or risk of severe morbidity: Dose of 0.5 ml/kg up to 15 ml IM

3) See Red Book for recommendations for subsequent immunization.

3. Adverse reactions to IMIG

a. Local pain, discomfort, or bleeding

b. Acrodynia with repeated use

c. Anaphylactoid reaction from IgG aggregates if injected into bloodstream

4. Precautions with IMIG

a. IMIG preparations should *never* be given intravenously since they contain IgG aggregates.

b. Only inject into a large muscle mass.

c. No more than 5 ml should be injected into one site.

D. Specific Immune Globulins

1. Hyperimmune globulins are prepared from donors known to have high antibody titers to antigens from specific sources.

2. Examples used in infectious diseases include the following: hepatitis B (HBIG), rabies (RIG), tetanus (TIG), varicella-zoster (VZIG), and cytomegalovirus (CMV IVIG).

---

*Peter G, editor: *1994 Red Book: report of the committee on infectious diseases,* ed 23, Elk Grove, Il, 1994, American Academy of Pediatrics.

III. IMMUNOLOGIC REFERENCE VALUES
A. Serum IgG, IgM, IgA Levels: Mean (95th % confidence interval) (Table 16.2)

TABLE 16.2.

Age	IgG (mg/dl)	IgM (mg/dl)	IgA (mg/dl)
Cord blood	1121 (636–1606)	13 (6.3–25)	2.3 (1.4–3.6)
1 mo	503 (251–906)	45 (20–87)	13 (1.3–53)
2 mo	365 (206–601)	46 (17–105)	15 (2.8–47)
3 mo	334 (176–581)	49 (24–89)	17 (4.6–46)
4 mo	343 (196–558)	55 (27–101)	23 (4.4–73)
5 mo	403 (172–814)	62 (33–108)	31 (8.1–84)
6 mo	407 (215–704)	62 (35–102)	25 (8.1–68)
7–9 mo	475 (217–904)	80 (34–126)	36 (11–90)
10–12 mo	594 (294–1069)	82 (41–149)	40 (16–84)
1 yr	679 (345–1213)	93 (43–173)	44 (14–106)
2 yr	685 (424–1051)	95 (48–168)	47 (14–123)
3 yr	728 (441–1135)	104 (47–200)	66 (22–159)
4–5 yr	780 (463–1236)	99 (43–196)	68 (25–154)
6–8 yr	915 (633–1280)	107 (48–207)	90 (33–202)
9–10 yr	1007 (608–1572)	121 (52–242)	113 (45–236)
Adult	994 (639–1349)	156 (56–352)	171 (70–312)

From Joliff CR et al: *Clin Chem* 28:126, 1982.

B. Serum IgG Subclass Levels: Mean (95th % confidence interval) (Table 16.3)

TABLE 16.3.

Age (yr)	IgG1 (mg/dl)	IgG2 (mg/dl)	IgG3 (mg/dl)	IgG4 (mg/dl)*
0–1	340 (190–620)	59 (30–140)	39 (9–62)	19 (6–63)
1–2	410 (230–710)	68 (30–170)	34 (11–98)	13 (4–43)
2–3	480 (280–830)	98 (40–240)	28 (6–130)	18 (3–120)
3–4	530 (350–790)	120 (50–260)	30 (9–98)	32 (5–180)
4–6	540 (360–810)	140 (60–310)	39 (9–160)	39 (9–160)
6–8	560 (280–1120)	150 (30–630)	48 (40–250)	81 (11–620)
8–10	690 (280–1740)	210 (80–550)	85 (22–320)	42 (10–170)
10–13	590 (270–1290)	240 (110–550)	58 (13–250)	60 (7–530)
13–Adult	540 (280–1020)	210 (60–790)	58 (14–240)	60 (11–330)

*10% of individuals appear to have absent IgG4 levels.
From Schur PH: *Ann Allergy* 58:89, 1987.

C. **Serum IgE Levels:** Geometric mean (95th % confidence interval)* (Table 16.4)

TABLE 16.4.

Age	IgE (IU/ml)
0 days	0.22 (0.04–1.28)
6 wk	0.69 (0.08–6.12)
3 mo	0.82 (0.18–3.76)
6 mo	2.68 (0.44–16.3)
9 mo	2.36 (0.76–7.31)
1 yr	3.49 (0.80–15.2)
2 yr	3.03 (0.31–29.5)
3 yr	1.80 (0.19–16.9)
4 yr	8.58 (1.07–68.9)
7 yr	12.89 (1.03–161.3)
10 yr	23.66 (0.98–570.6)
14 yr	20.07 (2.06–195.2)
17–85 yr†	13.20 (1.53–114.0)

*From Kjellman N-IM: *Clinical Allergy* 6: 51, 1976; †Zetterstrom O: *Allergy* 36(8):537, 1981.

D. **Lymphocyte Enumeration**
1. T cells: Normal values (5th–95th percentile) for T lymphocytes in peripheral blood (Table 16.5)

TABLE 16.5.

Age	CD3 (Total T-cells)	CD4 (T-helper/ inducer)	CD8 (T-suppressor/ cytotoxic)	CD4/CD8 ratio
2–3 mo	60%–87% (2070–6540)	41%–64% (1460–5110)	16%–35% (650–2450)	1.32–3.47
4–8 mo	57%–84% (2280–6450)	36%–61% (1690–4600)	16%–34% (720–2490)	1.20–3.48
12–23 mo	53%–81% (1460–5440)	31%–54% (1020–3600)	16%–38% (570–2230)	0.95–2.95
2–6 yr	62%–80% (1610–4230)	35%–51% (900–2860)	22%–38% (630–1910)	1.05–2.07
Adult	59%–81% (558–1948)	31%–55% (350–1334)	17%–38% (147–812)	0.84–3.05

Numbers in parentheses are absolute number of T cells/mm³
From Denny T et al: *JAMA* 267:1484, 1992.

2. B cells: Normal values (25th–75th percentile)* for B lymphocytes in peripheral blood (Table 16.6)

TABLE 16.6.

Age	CD19 (B cells)	Age	CD19 (B cells)
2–6 mo	21%–35%† (1300–2500)	37–48 mo	15%–23% (400–600)
7–18 mo	21%–32% (800–1600)	49–60 mo	14%–23% (300–900)
19–36 mo	21%–26% (600–900)	Adult	7%–23%‡ (n/a)

Numbers in parentheses are absolute number of B cells/mm³
*Please note values are 5th–95th percentile for the adult data.
†Ref. Becton-Dickinson Medical Dept, San Jose, CA, unpublished data.
‡Ref. Richert T et al: *Clin Immunol Immunopathol* 60:190, 1991.

E. Serum Complement Levels: Geometric mean (95th % confidence interval) (Table 16.7)

TABLE 16.7.

Age	C3 (mg/dl)	C4 (mg/dl)
Cord blood	83 (57–116)	13 (6.6–23)
1 mo	83 (53–124)	14 (7.0–25)
2 mo	96 (59–149)	15 (7.4–28)
3 mo	94 (64–131)	16 (8.7–27)
4 mo	107 (62–175)	19 (8.3–38)
5 mo	107 (64–167)	18 (7.1–36)
6 mo	115 (74–171)	21 (8.6–42)
7–9 mo	113 (75–166)	20 (9.5–37)
10–12 mo	126 (73–180)	22 (12–39)
1 yr	129 (84–174)	23 (12–40)
2 yr	120 (81–170)	19 (9.2–34)
3 yr	117 (77–171)	20 (9.7–36)
4–5 yr	121 (86–166)	21 (13–32)
6–8 yr	118 (88–155)	20 (12–32)
9–10 yr	134 (89–195)	22 (10–40)
Adult	125 (83–177)	28 (15–45)

From Joliff CR et al: *Clin Chem* 28:126, 1982.

IV. COMPLEMENT CASCADE (Fig. 16.1)

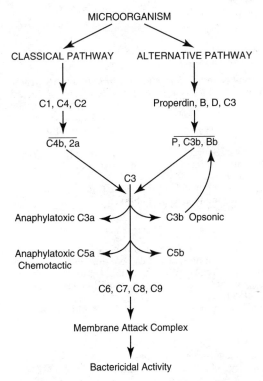

FIG. 16.1. Complement cascade *(From Oski FA et al:* Principles and practice of pediatrics, *ed 2, Philadelphia, 1994, JB Lippincott.)*

IMMUNOPROPHYLAXIS *17*

Note: For more detailed and updated information on immunizations, please refer to the following:

1. Current issues of *Morbidity and Mortality Weekly Report,* the package inserts of individual vaccines, or the current edition of the *Report of the Committee on Infectious Diseases of the American Academy of Pediatrics* (the *"Red Book**"*). Except where noted, the source for information in this chapter is the 1994 edition of the Red Book.
2. The list of Sources of Vaccine Information (pp. 7–9) and Directory of Telephone Numbers (p. 601) in the 1994 *Red Book*
3. An updated schedule of Red Book Committee immunization recommendations published in each January edition of *Pediatrics*

Note: Resources of Centers for Disease Control (CDC)

1. Voice Information System (VIS) of the National Immunization System of the CDC can provide consultation and printed material on immunizations. Up-to-date information can be provided by voice, mail, or fax. Ph. (404) 332-4553.
2. CDC home page address on the World Wide Web: http://www.cdc.gov/cdc.html.

I. IMMUNIZATION SCHEDULES
A. Routine Immunization Schedules
1. Standard childhood immunization schedule (Table 17.1)
2. *Haemophilus influenzae* type b: Primary series and booster schedule for multiple vaccine preparations in detail (Table 17.2)

---

*Peter G, editor: *1994 Red Book: report of the committee on infectious diseases,* ed 23, Elk Grove, Il, 1994, American Academy of Pediatrics.

TABLE 17.1.

Standard Childhood Immunization Schedule

	Birth	2 mo	4 mo	6 mo	12 mo	15 mo	18 mo	4–6 yr	11–12 yr	14–16 yr
Hepatitis B	HBV-1[1]	HBV-2[1]		HBV-3					(HBV)	
DTP		DTP[2,3]	DTP[3]	DTP[3]	DTP or DTaP at ≥ 15 mos			DT(a)P	Td[4]	
Hib		Hib[5]	Hib	HbOC[6]	Hib[5]					
Polio		OPV[2,7] IPV[7]	OPV IPV	OPV	IPV			OPV IPV		
MMR					MMR			MMR	MMR or (Var)	
Varicella					Var				(Var)	

[1] Give the 1st and 2nd hepatitis B vaccines at a 1–2 month interval.
[2] The first DTP and OPV vaccines may be given as early as 4 weeks.
[3] Acellular vaccines are likely to be licensed in 1996 for the primary series.
[4] Td boosters are routinely indicated 5 years after 5th DT(a)P dose and thereafter every 10 years.
[5] See sections I.A.2. and I.B.2.c for HIB vaccine available brands and detailed standard and alternative schedules; attempt to use same preparation for primary series; any may be used for booster.
[6] If HbOC is used for primary series.
[7] Expect OPV/IPV revised schedule in 1997; minimum intervals sequentially are 4 weeks and 6 months.
For catch-up immunization, see Section III.
Adapted From: *Pediatrics* 97:143, 1996.

TABLE 17.2.

Haemophilus Influenzae Type B: Primary Series and Booster Schedule for Multiple Vaccine Preparations in Detail

Vaccine type	Brands*	2 mo	4 mo	6 mo	12 mo†	15 mo
PRP-OMP	PedvaxHIB	PRP-OMP	PRP-OMP	—	PRP-OMP········	
HbOC	HIBTITER	HbOC	HbOC	HbOC	HbOC········	
PRP-T	ActHIB‡ OmniHIB	PRP-T	PRP-T	PRP-T	PRP-T········	
HbOC-DTP	Tetramune	HbOC-DTP	HbOC-DTP	HbOC-DTP	HbOC-DTP········	

*Please note that current brand names are included for ease of reference and no particular brand is recommended.
†PRP-D (ProHIBit) is only recommended in children ≥ 12 months old.
‡PRP-T (ActHIB) may be reconstituted in office with DTP (Connaught).
Adapted From: 1994 Red Book.

B. Alternative Immunization Schedules

1. Immunization schedule for children with lapsed immunizations
   a. Children should resume immunization schedule as if the expected interval had occurred
   b. Repeating doses is not indicated
2. Immunization schedules for children unimmunized in the first year of life (see schedule C below for Hib alternative schedule)
   a. Children 1–7 years old (Table 17.3)
   b. Children Over 7 years old (Table 17.3)
   c. *Haemophilus influenzae* type b (Hib): Alternative immunization schedule (for unimmunized children and children whose immunizations have lapsed) (Table 17.4)

TABLE 17.3.

		Months after first visit			Chronological age		
	1st visit	1 mo	2 mo	≥8 mo	4–6 yr	11–12 yr	10 yr later
Children 1–7							
Hepatitis B	HBV	HBV		HBV			
DTP	DTP[1]	DTP[1]	DTP[1]	DT(a)P	DT(a)P[2]		Td
Hib	Hib[3]		Hib[4]				
Polio	OPV	(OPV)[5]	OPV	OPV	OPV[6]		
MMR	MMR				MMR[7]	MMR[7]	
Varicella	Var · · · · · · · · · · · · ·|		or			Var	
Children >7							
Hepatitis B	HBV		HBV	HBV			
Td	Td	(Td)[5]	Td	Td			Td
Polio	OPV	(OPV)[5]	OPV	OPV			
MMR	MMR					MMR[7]	
Varicella	Var		Var[8]			or Var[8]	

[1]Acellular pertussis vaccines are likely to be licensed soon for the primary series.
[2]Dose not necessary if 4th dose given after 4 years old; if total doses D/T would exceed 6, give monovalent pertussis.
[3]Give 1st HIB if child is <5 years old.
[4]Give 2nd HIB if 1st HIB given at <15 months old.
[5]Second OPV and Td may be given at a 1 month interval.
[6]Give 4th dose OPV when the child enters school at 4–6 years old unless 3rd dose is given after 4 years old.
[7]Give 2nd dose MMR at 4–6 yrs or 11–12 yrs or at ≥1 mo interval.
[8]Give 2nd Varicella if ≥13 years old.
Adapted From: 1994 Red Book.

TABLE 17.4.

Haemophilus Influenzae Type B Alternative Immunization Schedule

Age	Immunization status	Conjugate vaccine[1]	Total doses yet to be given[2]	Age at booster[2]
2–6 mo	Unimmunized	PRP-OMP	3	12–15 mo
		PRP-T or HbOC	4	12–15 mo
7–11 mo	Unimmunized	Any[3]	3	12–18 mo
	Lapsed	Any[3]	2	12–15 mo
12–14 mo	Unimmunized	Any	2	—
	Lapsed	Any	1 or 2[4,5]	—
15–59 mo	Not UTD	Any	1	—
>60 mo	Unimmunized	Any	1 or 2[5,6]	—

[1]Attempt to use same type of vaccine in primary series before booster. The booster dose may be any conjugate vaccine; currently licensed vaccines are in Table 17.2.
[2]Includes both primary series and booster doses. All doses should be given at 2-month intervals except where a longer interval is indicated by the age at booster dose; however, in the primary series, a minimum of 1-month intervals may be allowed for "catch-up" immunization.
[3]Except PRP-D.
[4]The complete series is 3 doses.
[5]Both doses may be any conjugate vaccine.
[6]Give 1 dose if chronic illness at high risk for *H. influenzae* type b disease; 2 doses if illness also associated with impaired antibody response.
Adapted From: 1994 Red Book.

II. GENERAL INFORMATION: IMMUNIZATION GUIDELINES

A. Vaccine Administration

1. Volume/Dose: Unless otherwise specified all pediatric immunization doses are 0.5 ml, including for preterm infants.
2. Site: Administration of intramuscular (IM) and subcutaneous (SC) vaccines:
   a. Children ≤ 18 months old: Anterolateral thigh
   b. Toddlers: Anterolateral thigh or deltoid (deltoid preferred if large enough)
   c. Older children: Deltoid preferred
3. Route
   a. IM: Deep into muscle to avoid tissue damage from adjuvants, usually with a 22–23-gauge needle, which must be 7/8 inch (>2 cm).
   b. SC: Into pinched skin fold with a 25-gauge and 5/8-3/4 in (<2 cm) needle.

4. Multiple simultaneous administration: All routinely recommended vaccines for infants and children may be given simultaneously at different sites.
B. **General Contraindications and Precautions for All Vaccines**
 1. True contraindications
  a. Anaphylactic reaction to vaccine or vaccine constituent (see MMR and influenza sections for specific guidelines)
  b. Moderate or severe illness *regardless of fever*
  c. For atypical hosts see Section II.C.
 2. Not true contraindications or precautions (vaccine may be given)
  a. Mild acute illness *regardless of fever*
  b. Mild to moderate local reaction to previous dose of vaccine (soreness, redness, swelling)
  c. Current antimicrobial therapy
  d. Convalescent phase of illness
  e. Recent exposure to infectious disease
  f. Prematurity (same dosage and indications) (See specific guidelines for immunizations given before 2 months age.)
  g. Malnutrition
  h. Personal or family history of penicillin or allergies other than those in Section II.B.1.a.
Adapted From: 1994 Red Book.
C. **Special Hosts**
 1. Immunocompromised hosts and their contacts
  a. Contraindications for live virus vaccines
   1) Children with congenital disorders of immune function; live-virus and live-bacteria vaccines are contraindicated.
   2) Immunosuppressive therapy
    a) Live-virus vaccines are generally contraindicated, especially high-dose (≥ 2 mg/kg/24 hr) corticosteroids or chemotherapy
    b) Give live viral vaccines 3 or more months after immunosuppressive treatment has been discontinued.
   3) Patients treated with immune globulin and other blood products
    a) Immune globulin: Delay of immunizations varies with dose and indication from 3–11 months

(see Peter G, editor: *1994 Red Book: report of the committee on infectious diseases,* ed 23, Elk Grove, IL, 1994, American Academy of Pediatrics for details)

    b) Packed RBCs: Delay immunizations 3 months.

    c) Plasma/platelet products: Delay immunizations 7 months.

  4) Vaccinees who are household **contacts** of persons with an immunologic deficiency

    a) Do not give OPV.

    b) Give IPV, MMR, varicella vaccines routinely.

b. Immunization of children with known or suspected HIV disease

  1) Pneumococcal vaccine at 2 years of age

  2) Meningococcal vaccine may be given

  3) Influenza vaccine should be given to HIV-infected children who are symptomatic and considered in those who are asymptomatic beginning at 6 months of age.

  4) Give MMR regardless of clinical status.

  5) Do not give other live viral vaccines (OPV, VZV) or BCG; the only reported complications novel to HIV-infected vaccinees are with BCG.

  6) Regardless of immunization status, give passive immunization with specific immune globulin when exposed to measles, varicella, or tetanus (see specific disease guidelines in this chapter).

c. Immunization of children with Hodgkin's disease: Give pneumococcal and *H. influenzae* type b (Hib) vaccines appropriately.

d. Immunization of children with transplanted organs (Please see the Red Book for details.)

2. Asplenic children

a. Give pneumococcal and meningococcal vaccines appropriately.

b. Chemoprophylax for pneumococcus in selected groups (see Section III.H.5.b for details)

3. Preterm infants

a. Immunize based on chronologic age with standard dose.

b. Polio vaccine at appropriate ages: give IPV if patient remains hospitalized, or give OPV upon discharge.

    c. Influenza vaccine to infants with chronic respiratory disease (at age ≥6 months) and to their caretakers

  4. Pregnant women: All live-virus vaccines are relatively contraindicated in pregnancy; consider the risk of vaccine-associated infection and the threat of natural infection of the mother and fetus if unvaccinated.

D. Active Immunization in Postexposure Prophylaxis: Indicated in susceptible hosts for significant exposure to hepatitis B, measles, DTP, mumps, rabies, rubella and tetanus; may be used in meningococcus.

III. IMMUNOPROPHYLAXIS GUIDELINES FOR SPECIFIC DISEASES

A. Diphtheria/Tetanus/Pertussis Vaccine and Tetanus Immunoprophylaxis

  1. Description

    a. DTP: Adsorbed triple vaccine containing whole cells; dose, 0.5 ml IM

    b. DTaP: Contains an acellular pertussis component; recommended only for the fourth and fifth doses of the series at the time of publication. Acellular vaccines are likely to be licensed in 1996 for the primary series.

Note: DTaP is not a substitute for DTP in children in whom there is a contraindication for the use of pertussis vaccine.

    c. DT: Adsorbed divalent vaccine without pertussis component

    d. Td: Adsorbed divalent vaccine with 1/3 to 1/6 the dose of diphtheria toxoid of the other preparations such as DTP, DT

  2. Vaccine indications

    a. DTP: Routine immunization for children under 7 years old

    b. Td: Booster every 10 years for all persons; every 5 years if person frequents places where Td may not be available

    c. See wound management Section III.A.5.e.

  3. Vaccine contraindications

    a. For general contraindications and precautions see Section II.B.

    b. Contraindications to pertussis immunization (use DT vaccine)

1) Encephalopathy within 7 days of previous DTP vaccine
2) An immediate anaphylactic reaction.
   c. Precautions: The following are now considered precautions and **not contraindications.** The patient should be reevaluated for possible immunization with DTP at each visit.
   1) Progressive neurologic disorders characterized by developmental delay or neurologic findings
   2) Neurologic conditions that predispose to seizures or to neurologic deterioration unless condition is resolved, corrected, or controlled
   3) History of recent seizures without specific diagnosis
   4) A history of severe reactions to DTP
      a) Unexplained fever > 40.5° C within 48 hours, unexplained by another cause
      b) Inconsolable screaming for ≥3 hours within 48 hours
      c) Collapse or shock within 48 hours
      d) Convulsions within 72 hours (with or without fever)

Adapted From: 1994 Red Book.

   d. Not contraindications or precautions (to DTP vaccinations)
   1) Family history of sudden infant death syndrome (SIDS), convulsions, or nonsevere adverse reactions to DTP vaccination
   2) High-pitched or unusual cry after immunization
   3) Pregnancy is not a contraindication to Td booster.
4. Vaccine side effects
   a. Common side effects of DTP vaccine occurring within 48 hours of vaccination (all ages) include the following: pain at site (51%), fever (47%), swelling at the injection site (40%), redness (37%), drowsiness (32%), anorexia (21%); convulsions and collapse with shock-like state are relatively uncommon (0.06%). Most common side effects occur significantly less frequently with DTaP vaccine including fever.
   b. Fever is common: Fever ≥38° C occurs in 44% of children with DTP and 20% of children with DTaP (all children 15–20 months old).

c. High fever is uncommon; 0.3% of children with DTP (all ages) had fevers ≥ 40.5° C and 0.3% of children with DTaP (15–20 months old) had fevers ≥39° C.

Adapted From: *MMWR* 41(RR–15):4, 1992; *Pediatrics* 68:650, 1981.

5. Special considerations
   a. Pertussis exposure
      1) Immunization for partially immunized children <7 years old who are close contacts
         a) Give 4th dose of DTP or DTaP if child received 3rd dose ≥6 months ago.
         b) Give booster dose of DTaP or DTP if last dose was >3 years ago.
         c) Continue schedule for all other children.
      2) Chemoprophylaxis for all household and other close contacts: Treatment to limit secondary transmission is with erythromycin regardless of vaccination status. Estolate preparation is recommended by some sources (see Formulary, Chapter 26, for dosing).
   b. Pertussis outbreak (See Red Book for information.)
   c. Tetanus immunoprophylaxis (Table 17.5)
      1) Passive immunization
         a) Give tetanus immunoglobulin (TIG) 250 U IM.
         b) Tetanus antitoxin (TAT) 3000–5000 U IM may be substituted if TIG is unavailable.
         c) Any child with AIDS should receive TIG for tetanus-prone wounds, regardless of vaccination status.
      2) Active immunization: Use vaccine preparations that include diptheria toxoid, as well as tetanus toxoid.
         a) DTP if <3 doses DTP given
         b) DTaP if ≥3 doses DTP given, and patient ≥ 15 months old
         c) DT if pertussis is contraindicated
         d) Td if ≥7 years old
   d. Treatment of clinical tetanus (see Red Book for information)
6. Vaccine administration (immunization with Td): Unimmunized pregnant women: Give 2 doses at ≥4-week interval so that second dose ≥2 weeks before delivery.

TABLE 17.5.

Prophylaxis of Tetanus in Wound Management

History of tetanus toxoid doses	Clean, minor wounds		All other wounds	
	Td*	TIG	Td*	TIG
Unknown or <3	Yes	No	Yes	Yes
≥3	Not†	No	Not‡	No

*See recommendations for form of tetanus vaccine. See III.A.5.c.2.
†Immunize if > 10 years since last dose.
‡Immunize if > 5 years since last dose.
From: 1994 Red Book.
TD, Tetanus and diphtheria; *TIG*, tetanus immunoglobulin.

B. *Haemophilus influenzae* Type B Vaccine
   1. Description: Currently four vaccines are licensed of PRP capsular polysaccharide antigen conjugated to a carrier. Use the same type of vaccine (PRP-OMP, HbOC, or PRP-T) throughout the primary series. HbOC-DTP may be interchanged with HbOC.
   2. Indications
      a. Routine
      b. Any child who has had invasive *H. influenzae* type b disease at age <24 months should begin Hib immunization one month after the acute illness and continue immunization as if previously unimmunized.
   3. Contraindications
      a. General contraindications apply (see Section II.B).
      b. Children older than 24 months who have had invasive *H. influenzae* type b disease at age ≥24 months require no further Hib immunization.
   4. Side Effects: Few vaccine-related side effects except for local reactions such as pain, redness, and swelling in ≤ 25% recipients. Frequency of fever and irritability when given with DTP are same as DTP alone.
   5. Special Considerations (*H. influenzae* type b chemoprophylaxis): Prophylax household and child care contacts with rifampin; see Formulary, Chapter 26, for dosing, and see Red Book for details.
C. Hepatitis A Vaccine
   Primary methods of prevention of disease include adequate sanitation, hand washing, and avoidance of potentially contaminated foods.

1. Description
   a. Inactivated adsorbed vaccine
   b. Efficacy 94% after 2 doses and 100% after 3 doses, though long-term efficacy is unknown.
2. Indications
   a. Travelers to or residents of areas of intermediate or high endemicity (note that IMIG may be substituted for vaccine if short-term exposure is anticipated)
   b. Ethnic and geographic populations that experience cyclic epidemics
   c. Postexposure to Hepatitis A
   d. Military personnel
   e. Other individuals deemed to be at high risk of infection (homosexual or bisexual males, users of illicit IV drugs) or severe disease (including those with chronic liver disease)
   f. Healthy individuals ≥ 2 years old, at the discretion of the physician
   g. Immunocompromised individuals may be immunized, though efficacy is not established in children.
   h. In addition, the vaccine may be considered in the staff of child care centers with ongoing or recurrent outbreaks.
   i. The presence of Hepatitis A antibody indicates adequate immunity, but its absence may not correlate with lack of immunity; routine serology is not recommended in children.
3. Contraindications: Only general contraindications apply (see Section II.B).
4. Side effects: The following have been reported: local reactions including induration, redness, swelling (18%); headache (12%), fever (6%), fatigue, malaise, anorexia, nausea (1–10%). No serious adverse effects have been reported.
5. Special considerations for postexposure prophylaxis
   a. Significant exposure includes household and sexual contact, newborns of infected mothers, and some cases of child care center exposure (see Red Book for details).
   b. Give 0.02 ml/kg of immune globulin (Ig), IM min 0.25 ml to max 2 ml if within 2 weeks of exposure.

    c. May begin concomitant immunization schedule (esp. if future exposure is likely), but immunization alone is not adequate.

    d. For continuous exposure, see Red Book for detailed dosing information.

  6. Vaccine administration

    a. Primary series in children 2–18 years old: Two 360 U/0.5 ml doses of 0.5 ml IM given at least 1 month apart.

    b. Primary series in adults: One 1440 U/ml dose of 1 ml IM.

    c. A single equivalent booster dose may be given in children or adults 6 to 12 months after primary series.

    d. A single dose usually provides adequate immunity if time does not permit subsequent dosing before travel exposure.

    e. Hepatitis A vaccines may be administered with other vaccines.

D. Hepatitis B Immunoprophylaxis

  1. Description

    a. Hepatitis B immune globulin: Prepared from plasma known to contain a high titer of anti-Hepatitis B antibodies and to be negative for antibody to HIV

    b. Hepatitis B vaccines

      1) Adsorbed Hepatitis B surface antigen (HBsAg) (produced by recombinant methods)

      2) Recombinant vaccines are similar and may be used interchangeably.

  2. Vaccine indications

    a. Recommended as routine immunization for the following:

      1) All infants (see following text for infants of mothers who are HBsAg-positive)

      2) Infants in high-risk populations should be immunized by 6–9 months of age if possible.

      3) All adolescents and preadolescents not previously immunized, especially those in out-of-home child care

      4) Children and staff of institutions for the developmentally disabled or of nonresidential programs where individuals attend who are known HBV carriers

5) Health professionals or others with occupational exposure to human blood
6) Hemodialysis patients
7) Users of IV drugs
8) Sexually active homosexual or bisexual males
9) Sexually active heterosexual individuals with greater than one partner in the previous 6 months or with a sexually transmitted disease
10) Individuals with bleeding disorders and others who receive certain blood products
11) Household contacts and sexual partners of HBV carriers
12) Member of households with adopted individuals from countries where HBV infection is endemic if adopted individual is HBsAg-positive on screening

From: 1994 Red Book.

13) Travelers expecting to live >6 months in or likely to have blood or sexual contact in areas of high HBV endemicity
14) Inmates of long-term correctional facilities

   b. Booster doses are not recommended routinely
   c. Routine serologic evaluation is not indicated.
3. Vaccine contraindications: Only general contraindications apply (see Section II.B).
4. Vaccine side effects: Between 1% and 6% of recipients may experience pain at the injection site or a low-grade fever.
5. Special considerations
   a. Dosing of HBIG: Give IM: 0.5 ml in infants or 0.06 ml/kg in older children for any significant exposure
   b. Management of neonates
      1) Preterm infants weighing <2 kg born to HBsAg-negative mothers
         a) Immunize at discharge if age is <2 months and weight is >2 kg *or*
         b) Immunize at 2 months of age.
      2) Infants whose mothers serologic status is unknown at birth
         a) Begin routine vaccine schedule within 12 hours of birth.

      b) Only if mother found to be HBsAg-positive: HBIG as soon as possible, within 7 days of life, and continue subsequent immunization at 1 and 6 months.

   3) Infants born to mother known to be HBsAg-positive

      a) Vaccine and HBIG within 12 hours of birth

      b) Subsequent vaccination at 1 and 6 months

  c. Postexposure prophylaxis

   1) HBIG + immunization

      a) Perinatal

      b) Sexual: Acute infection

      c) Household contact: Acute case with identifiable blood exposure

      d) Infant (<12 mo): Acute case in primary caregiver

   2) HBIG ± immunization (depending on vaccination status of host; see Red Book, p. 237–8): Accidental—percutaneous/permucosal

   3) Immunization only (no HBIG)

      a) Sexual: Chronic carrier

      b) Household contact: Chronic carrier

6. Vaccine administration (Table 17.6)

TABLE 17.6.

Recommended Dosages of Hepatitis B Vaccines (all doses IM)

	Recombivax HB Dose		Engerix-B Dose	
	mcg	(ml)	mcg	(ml)
Infants and <11 y/o	2.5	(0.5)*	10	(0.5)
Infants of HBsAg(+) mothers	5	(0.5)† or (1.0)*	10	(0.5)
Children 11–19 y/o	5	(0.5)†	10	(0.5)
Adults ≥20 y/o	10	(1.0)†	20	(1.0)
Dialysis patients Immunosuppressed adults	40	(1.0)‡	40	(2.0)

*Pediatric formulation (5 mcg/ml).
†Adult formulation (10 mcg/ml).
‡Special formulation for dialysis patients (40 mcg/ml).
Adapted from Table 3.12 "Recommended Doses of Hepatitis B Vaccines" Red Book. 1994:229.

E. Influenza Vaccine and Chemoprophylaxis
1. Description
    a. Preparations
        1) Whole inactivated virus vaccine grown in eggs
            a) Prepared from intact purified virus particles
            b) Not used in children <13 years old
        2) "Split" vaccines
            a) Subvirion: Additional step of denaturing lipid membrane of virus
            b) Purified surface antigen vaccine
    b. Protective response in 70%–80% hosts
2. Indications
    a. Recommended immunization for targeted high-risk children
        1) Chronic pulmonary disease including asthma
        2) Hemodynamically significant cardiac disease
        3) Hemoglobinopathies including sickle cell anemia
        4) Immunosuppressive therapy
    b. Consider immunization for other high-risk children
        1) HIV infection
        2) Chronic renal diseases
        3) Chronic metabolic diseases
        4) Diabetes
        5) Children on long-term aspirin therapy (Reye's syndrome)
    c. Recommended immunization for close contacts of high-risk patients
        1) Hospital personnel in contact with pediatric patients
        2) Child and adult household contacts of high risk children
        3) Child household contacts of high risk adults
    d. May consider immunization of the following:
        1) Members of residential or academic institutions where close contact facilitates rapid transmission
        2) Children of parents requesting immunization
        3) International travel
Adapted From: 1994 Red Book.
3. Contraindications
    a. For general contraindications and precautions, see Section II.B.

   b. Anaphylactic reaction to chicken or eggs
   c. Not routinely recommended for children <6 months old
   d. Precautions
      1) Immunosupressed children receiving chemotherapy do not have high seroconversion rates until chemotherapy is discontinued for 3–4 weeks and peripheral absolute neutrophil and lymphocyte counts are >1000/mm^3.
      2) Immunization may be deferred in patients receiving high-dose steroids (equivalent of 2 mg/kg/day or 20 mg/day prednisone) only if time allows before influenza season.
4. Side effects
   a. Fever 6–24 hours after immunization in children <2 years old
   b. Local reactions rare in children <13 years old; ~ 10% vaccinees ≥ 13 years old
   c. Side effects and immunogenicity are similar for whole and split vaccine in individuals >12 years old.
   d. Guillain-Barré syndrome (GBS) has not been clearly associated with influenza vaccine preparations since 1977 ("swine flu") and has not been reported in children.
5. Special considerations
   a. Chemoprophylaxis for Influenza A
      1) Amantidine and rimantidine can effectively reduce symptoms and transmission of influenza.
      2) See Formulary, Chapter 26, for dosing.
      3) Indications for amantidine or rimantidine chemoprophylaxis
         a) Children and adults immunized after influenza is present in community: Give for 2 weeks after completion of immunization to reduce risk of infection before vaccine response.
         b) Unimmunized persons providing care to high-risk individuals
         c) Immunodeficient individuals unlikely to have adequate protection after immunization
         d) Individuals at high risk for influenza infection with contraindication to vaccine (e.g., allergy)
      4) Precaution: Neither drug has been evaluated in children <12 months old.

6. Vaccine administration
   a. Antigenic makeup varies from year to year; administer during autumn in preparation for winter influenza season beginning in December.
   b. Schedule including dosage (Table 17.7)

TABLE 17.7.

Influenza Immunization Schedule (IM)

Age	Vaccine type	Volume/route	Number of doses
6–35 months	Split virus only	0.25ml IM	1 or 2*
3–8 years	Split virus only	0.5 ml IM	1 or 2*
9–12 years	Split virus only	0.5 ml IM	1
> 12 years	Whole or split virus	0.5 ml IM	1

*2 doses at 1-month interval indicated for first-time immunization.
Adapted From: 1994 Red Book.

F. Measles/Mumps/Rubella Immunoprophylaxis
   1. Description
      a. Measles/mumps/rubella (MMR) Vaccine: A combined vaccine composed of live, attenuated viruses. Measles and mumps vaccines prepared in chicken embryo cell culture; rubella vaccine prepared in human diploid cell culture. Dose, 0.5 ml SC. Each is available in monovalent form.
      b. Measles (monovalent) and MR combination is also available.
      c. Immune globulin (IG, also known as IMIG): Similar concentration of measles antibody to IVIG
   2. Vaccine indications
      a. All persons susceptible to measles, > 12 months old
         1) A person is considered *susceptible* to measles unless they have had physician-documented measles episode, have laboratory evidence of immunity, were born before 1957, or are documented to have completed appropriate live-virus immunization without concomitant IG.
         2) May include persons who have previously received some form of measles vaccination.
         3) Reimmunization with 2 doses MMR at ≥ 1 month interval indicated for susceptible students at educational institutions beyond high school (typically identified by low antibody titers on screening)

      b. Postexposure prophylaxis within 72 hours for susceptible persons (if household contact consider IG instead)

      c. Control of school-based measles outbreaks (see Section III.F.5.a.1. and Red Book for details)

      d. Susceptible contacts of persons with altered immunity (other than HIV infection)

      e. The combined MMR vaccine should be used in all situations where the host is likely to be susceptible to mumps or rubella.

3. Vaccine contraindications: General contraindications and special host considerations for live-virus vaccines apply (see Section II).

      a. Contraindications

         1) Altered immunity (except HIV infection)

         2) Egg or neomycin *anaphylactic* allergy: Although of uncertain predictive value, skin testing with the vaccine is recommended for patients with history of anaphylaxis after egg ingestion before immunization.

      b. Precautions: Immunization after transfusion of blood products or IG (see Section II.C.1.a.3 and Red Book for details)

      c. Not contraindications:

         1) Nonanaphylactic allergic reaction after egg ingestion

         2) Allergy to penicillin (vaccines do not contain penicillin)

         3) Exposure to measles

         4) Tuberculosis

         5) HIV infection

4. Vaccine side effects

      a. Fever $\geq 39.4°$ C or $103°$ F, usually beginning 7–12 days after immunization, lasting 1–5 days (~5%–15%)

      b. Transient rashes (5%)

      c. Transient thrombocytopenia (reported)

      d. Subacute sclerosing pancephalitis (SSPE) (rarely reported; unclear association)

      f. Seizure: Increase in frequency in children already at increased risk to have seizure and likely related to fever; no permanent neurologic damage associated

5. Special considerations
   a. Measles postexposure immunoprophylaxis
      1) Vaccine
         a) Live measles vaccine given within 72 hours of exposure can effectively prevent disease.
         b) Monovalent vaccine may be given to infants 6–12 months old especially in an outbreak setting and is preferred to IG.
         c) MMR may be given to infants age 6–12 months old if monovalent vaccine is unavailable.
         d) Immunize susceptible (see Section F.2.a.1) siblings of patient exposed during outbreak at nonmedical institutions; dose at ≥ 1-month interval
      2) Immune globulin (IG)
         a) For susceptible (see Section F.2.a.1) household contacts or any HIV-infected contacts
         b) May consider deferring in infants less than 5 months old unless mother is infected
         c) Standard dose IG

            • Indicated for children or pregnant women
            • 0.25 ml/kg (max 15 ml) IM within 6 days of exposure.
            • Immunization should be given no sooner than 5 months after standard-dose IG administration.

         d) High dose IG

            • Indicated for immunocompromised children
            • Give 0.5 ml/kg (max 15 ml) IM
            • Not required if IVIG received within 3 weeks of exposure in patient who regularly receives IVIG.
            • Immunization should be given no sooner than 5 months after high-dose IG administration.

   b. Rubella postexposure immunoprophylaxis: IG may modify rubella disease. Not generally recommended for children or in women <13 weeks pregnant. Dose is 0.55 ml/kg IM of immune globulin.

6. Vaccine administration: Immunize ≥ 2 weeks before any necessary administration of IG, such as for international travel.

G. Meningococcus Prophylaxis

1. Description: Quadrivalent serogroup-specific vaccine made from purified capsular polysaccharide antigen from groups A, C, Y, and W-135

2. Vaccine indications
   a. Children ≥ 2 years at high risk
      1) Functional or anatomic asplenia
      2) Terminal complement deficiencies
      3) Revaccination may be indicated in children at high risk especially if immunized before 4 years old; need for revaccination in older children and adults is uncertain.
   b. As an adjunct to postexposure chemoprophylaxis (see Section G.5.a.)
   c. Travelers to areas with endemic or hyperendemic disease
   d. Outbreaks of a serogroup contained in vaccine
   e. Immunogenicity of serogroup antigens varies in children <4 year old (especially <2y/o) (see Red Book for details).

3. Vaccine contraindications: Only general contraindications apply (see Section II.B).

4. Vaccine side effects Localized erythema for 1–2 days occurs infrequently.

5. Special considerations
   a. Postexposure chemoprophylaxis
      1) Antibiotic chemoprophylaxis should be given to exposed individuals within 24 hours of diagnosis of primary case.
      2) Persons considered exposed include the following:
         a) Household child care and nursery school contacts
         b) Anyone with potential contact with oral secretions of infected patient
         c) **Do not consider medical staff exposed unless there is contact with oral secretions.**
      3) Drug of choice is rifampin (see Chapter 26 for dosing).

4) In persons over 18, ciprofloxacin (500 mg PO as a single dose) is effective.
5) For Group A meningococcus exposure, single dose ceftriaxone (125 mg IM/IV<12 y/o, 250 mg IM/IV ≥ 12 y/o) may be substituted for rifampin; this may be more efficacious in reducing nasal carriage.
6) For isolates known to be sensitive, sulfisoxazole is recommended (500 mg/24 hr ÷ QD PO for <1 y/o, 1000 mg/24 hr ÷ Q12 hr PO for 1–12 y/o, and 2000 mg/24 hr ÷ Q12 hr PO for >12 y/o). All regimens consist of a 2-day course.

Adapted From: 1994 Red Book.

b. Treatment: Exposed individuals should be observed for the first signs of febrile illness, in which case prompt medical evaluation for treatment of invasive disease should follow.
6. Vaccine administration: Give 0.5 ml SC; if second dose is indicated (see Section G.2.a.3), give 2–3 years after first immunization.

H. Pneumococcal Vaccine
1. Description
   a. Purified capsular polysaccharide antigen from 23 serotypes of *Streptococcus pneumoniae*
   b. Effective against serotypes causing bacteremia and meningitis; however, protection is not 100%, and fatal infection may still occur.
2. Indications
   a. Children >2 years of age with increased risk of acquiring infection or developing severe infection with pneumococcus.
      1) Sickle cell disease
      2) Functional or anatomic asplenia
      3) Chronic renal failure
      4) Nephrotic syndrome
      5) Immunosuppression including organ transplantation or cytoreduction therapy
      6) CSF leaks
      7) HIV infection
   b. Consider revaccination for certain patients (see Red Book for details).
3. Contraindications Only general contraindications apply (see Section II.B).

4. Side effects: Mild local reactions including local pain and erythema at injection site are common; fever is uncommon.
5. Special considerations
   a. Passive immunoprophylaxis: IVIG or IMIG for children with congenital or acquired immunodeficiency states and recurrent pneumococcal infections
   b. Chemoprophylaxis: Oral penicillin
      1) Indicated in patients with functional or anatomic asplenia
      2) Consider especially in patients not likely to respond to immunization: ≤ 2 years old or receiving intensive chemotherapy or cytoreduction therapy.
      3) See Formulary, Chapter 26: dosing for sickle cell patients should be used.
      4) Begin before 4 months old for patients with sickle cell disease.
6. Vaccine administration
   a. Dose is 0.5 ml SC or IM.
   b. May be given concurrently with other vaccines.
   c. Give vaccine 2 weeks or more before elective splenectomy, chemotherapy, radiation therapy, or immunosuppressive therapy; or give 3 months after chemotherapy or radiation therapy.

I. Poliomyelitis Vaccine

1. Description
   a. Oral polio virus vaccine (OPV): Trivalent vaccine of live poliovirus types 1, 2, and 3 grown in monkey kidney cells
   b. Inactivated polio virus vaccine (IPV)
      1) Trivalent enhanced vaccine of live poliovirus types 1, 2, and 3 grown in human diploid or Vero cells and inactivated with formalin
      2) Seroconversion equal to or greater than OPV
   c. In the case of lapsed immunizations or change in the indication status of the host, IPV or OPV may be used to complete immunization series.
2. Indications
   a. IPV is currently advocated by some as preferable to OPV in all hosts. Check with latest Committee on Infectious Diseases (Red Book Committee) recommendations before administering OPV or IPV.

  b. Indications for OPV
    1) Healthy infants and children receiving routine immunization
    2) Unimmunized or partially immunized individuals who are at imminent risk of exposure to poliovirus (dose interval may be 4 weeks)
    3) Adults at future risk of exposure to poliomyelitis who previously received one or more doses of OPV or IPV (IPV is also acceptable)
    4) Adults at imminent (within 4 weeks) risk of exposure to poliomyelitis who are unimmunized
  c. Indications for IPV
    1) Persons with compromised immunity or partial immunity who are unimmunized or partially immunized
    2) Symptomatic and asymptomatic persons known to be infected with HIV
    3) Household contacts of an immunocompromised individual, including those known to be HIV infected
    4) Partially immunized or unimmunized adults or other close contacts in household of children to be given OPV
    5) Unimmunized adults at future risk of exposure to poliomyelitis
    6) Adults at future risk of exposure to poliomyelitis who have been partially immunized with IPV or OPV (OPV is also acceptable)
    7) Adults at future risk of exposure to poliomyelitis who have had a primary series of IPV
    8) Individuals refusing OPV immunization

Adapted From: 1994 Red Book.

  3. Contraindications: General contraindications and special host considerations apply (see Section II.B.).
    a. Contraindications for OPV
      1) Immunodeficiency disorders
      2) Household contacts of persons with immunodeficiency disease, altered immune states, immunosuppression due to therapy for another disease, or known HIV infection

3) If vaccinee is child of parent with one or more immunodeficient children, use IPV until immune status of vaccinee is known.
   b. Contraindication for IPV: Anaphylactic reaction to streptomycin or neomycin
   c. Not contraindications for OPV or IPV: Diarrhea, current antimicrobial therapy or breastfeeding.
4. Side effects
   a. Risk of paralytic disease from OPV in vaccinees is 1 per 6.8 million doses distributed and in contacts is 1 per 6.4 million doses distributed
   b. Possible local irritation with IPV
5. Special considerations
   a. If protection against poliomyelitis is needed urgently and
      1) >2 months available: Give 3 doses IPV at least 1-month intervals.
      2) 1–2 months available: Give 2 doses IPV at 1 month apart.
      3) <1 month available: Give 1 dose of IPV or OPV (preferable).
      4) The primary series should be completed if the person remains at risk.
6. Vaccine administration: IPV: Route is SC or IM; see package insert.

J. Rabies Immunoprophylaxis
   1. Description
      a. Human diploid cell vaccine (HDCV)
      b. Rabies vaccine adsorbed (RVA) (rhesus diploid cell vaccine)
   2. Indications
      a. Preexposure prophylaxis: Indicated for high-risk groups including veterinarians, animal handlers, laboratory workers, children living in high-risk environment, persons traveling to live in high-risk areas.
      b. Postexposure prophylaxis (see Section J.5.)
   3. Contraindications: Only general contraindications apply (see Section II.B).

4. Side Effects (to HDCV)
    a. Local reactions in 25% vaccinees
    b. Mild systemic reactions in 20% vaccinees: headache, nausea, abdominal pain, myalgias, and dizziness
    c. Neurologic illness 1 in 150,000: Illness resembling Guillain-Barré or a focal, subacute CNS disorder; no neurologic sequelae reported
    d. Immune complexlike reaction in up to 6% of vaccinees receiving booster dose; symptoms begin 2–21 days after immunization.
5. Special considerations
    a. Postexposure prophylaxis
        1) General wound management
            a) All wound care should begin with an immediate and thorough cleansing with soap and water.
            b) Avoid suturing wound.
            c) Consider tetanus prophylaxis and antibacterial management if indicated.
        2) Consideration of prophylaxis: Risk of exposure
            a) More likely infected animals: Skunks, raccoons, and bats
            b) Occasionally infected animals: Foxes, coyotes, cattle, dogs, and cats
            c) Rarely infected: Rodents (squirrels, rats or mice), lagomorphs (rabbits and hares)
            d) Exposures other than bites or scratches almost never infect, but consider contamination of open wound or mucous membrane with body fluid or brain tissue of animal.
            e) Also consider vaccination status of animal, prevalence of rabies in locale, and nature of the attack.
            f) Decision to immunize should be made in conjunction with local health officials.
        3) Prophylaxis is recommended for the following:
            a) Bite or scratch by animal (wild or domestic) that may be infected
            b) Potentially infectious exposure to human with rabies
    b. Rabies postexposure prophylaxis recommendations (Table 17.8)

6. Vaccine (and rabies immune globulins [RIG]) administration
   a. Vaccine for postexposure prophylaxis
      1) HDCV or RVA may be used interchangeably, especially if severe allergic reaction develops to one type.
      2) Deltoid muscle except in infants
      3) Routine serologic testing is not indicated.
      4) Unimmunized: Vaccine dose is 1 ml IM given on days 0, 3, 7, 14, and 28: consider RIG.
      5) Previously immunized: Give 1 ml IM on days 0 and 3: *do not give RIG.*
   b. Vaccine for preexposure prophylaxis: 3 doses of RVA (1 ml IM) or HDCV (1 ml IM or 0.1 ml intradermal) on days 0, 7, and 28.

TABLE 17.9.

Rabies Postexposure Prophylaxis

Animal type	Evaluation and disposition of animal	Postexposure prophylaxis recommendations
Dogs and cats	Healthy and available for 10 days observation	Do not begin prophylaxis unless animal develops symptoms of rabies
	Rabid or suspected rabid	Immediate immunization and RIG*
	Unknown (escaped)	Consult public health officials
Wild animal	Available for examination	Immediate immunization and RIG*
Skunk, raccoon, bat, fox, most other carnivores; woodchucks	Regard as rabid unless local area known to be free of rabies or until animal has negative fluorescent Ab	Immediate immunization and RIG* (Animal should be killed and brain tissue tested as soon as possible)
Livestock, ferrets, rodents, and lagomorphs	Consider individually	Consult public health officials; these bites rarely require treatment

*Treatment may be discontinued if animal fluorescent antibody is negative; do *not* give RIG if patient previously immunized
Adapted From: 1994 Red Book.

    c. Human rabies immune globulin (HRIG)
       1) HRIG is given in postexposure prophylaxis with the vaccine to unimmunized hosts as soon as possible after exposure, but no later than the seventh day of vaccine schedule (if possible).
       2) For persons not previously immunized, give HRIG 20 IU/kg, infiltrate one-half dose at site of bite/wound, if possible. Give remainder IM. Never give vaccine in same body part as HRIG.
       3) RIG is not recommended for the following:
          a) Individuals with adequate rabies vaccination before exposure (see Red Book for details)
          b) Individuals with documented protective rabies titer

K. Varicella Immunoprophylaxis
  1. Vaccine description
    a. Vaccine: Cell-free live attenuated varicella virus vaccine
    b. Measles-mumps-rubella-varicella (MMRV) is expected in the future, but in their present forms the vaccines may not be mixed.
    c. Efficacy: 70% after 1 year, 95% against severe disease; annual prevalence in vaccinees over 8 years was 1%–4% vs. 7%–8% for unvaccinated children.
  2. Vaccine indications
    a. All children, adolescents, and **young** adults not previously infected with chickenpox
    b. No data support the use of postexposure immunization to prevent disease occurrence.
    c. Serologic evaluation may be used to determine if vaccine is indicated in immune competent hosts or to guide postexposure management.
  3. Vaccine contraindications
    a. General contraindications and special host considerations apply (see Section II).
    b. Patients with altered immunity, children on steroid or salicylate therapy, and pregnant women
    c. Asymptomatic HIV-infected children should not be immunized (see Red Book for details).
    d. Certain children with acute lymphoblastic leukemia (ALL), usually in remission > 1 year, may be immunized.

e. Not contraindicated: Immunization is not contraindicated in vaccinees with immunocompromised household contacts; precautions are only necessary if a rash develops.

4. Vaccine side effects
   a. Most frequently reported side effects included: local reaction (erythema, swelling, soreness) (20%–35%), fever 1 to 42 days postvaccination (15%, comparable with placebo), varicellalike rash (local and systemic) (7%–8%), and zosterlike illness (<0.1%).
   b. Vaccine varicella rash may be so mild as to be mistaken for insect bites clinically, but patient is still infectious.

5. Vaccine administration
   a. Dose 0.5 ml given SC; may be given simultaneously with MMR.
   b. Avoid giving for 5 months after VZIG administration, and do not give concurrently.
   c. Avoid use of salicylates for 6 weeks after vaccine administration (theoretical risk of Reye's syndrome).

Adapted From: 1994 Red Book.

6. Special considerations
   a. Passive immunization with varicella zoster immunoglobulin (VZIG)
      1) Indications for VZIG
         a) Candidates for VZIG provided significant exposure
            - Immunocompromised children without history of chickenpox
            - Susceptible, pregnant women
            - Newborn infant; Onset of varicella (other than zoster) in mother of newborn infant ≤5 days before delivery or ≤48 hours after delivery (even if mother received VZIG during pregnancy)
            - Hospitalized premature infant (≥28 weeks gestation); no maternal history of chickenpox at any time
            - Hospitalized premature infant (<28 weeks gestation); regardless of maternal history

b) Significant exposures
- Household (residing in the same household)
- Playmate (face to face indoor play)
- Onset of varicella (other than zoster) in mother of newborn infant ≤5 days before delivery or ≤48 hours after delivery (even if mother received VZIG during pregnancy)
- Hospital:
   Varicella
   Rooming with infected patient
   Nontransient face to face contact with infectious individual
   Visit by contagious individual
   Zoster
   Intimate contact (touching or hugging) with contagious individual

2) Contraindications of VZIG: VZIG is not recommended in normal nonpregnant adults (use acyclovir, see Section K.5.b).
3) Dosing of VZIG
   a) Give 1 vial (125 units, IM) for each 10 kg body weight (min 125 units, max 625 units).
   b) Optimal if given within 48 hours, effective if given within 96 hours
   c) Efficacy felt to last up to 3 weeks

b. Chemoprophylaxis: Oral acyclovir
1) Adults over 12 years old and not pregnant may be treated with oral acyclovir once infection is manifest.
2) Oral acyclovir is not usually recommended in healthy children (see Red Book for exceptions and details).

Adapted From: 1994 Red Book.

INFECTIOUS DISEASES   *18*

I. **HUMAN IMMUNODEFICIENCY VIRUS (HIV) AND THE ACQUIRED IMMUNODEFICIENCY SYNDROME (AIDS):** For the most recent information in the diagnosis and management of children with HIV infection, check the most recent recommendations in *Morbidity and Mortality Weekly Report.* [http://www.cdc.gov/]

A. **Counseling and Testing:** Legal requirements vary by state. Counseling should include informed consent for testing, implications of positive test results, and prevention of transmission. All pregnant women should be offered counseling and testing in order to make an informed decision regarding therapy aimed at reducing transmission to the infant.

B. **Diagnosis of HIV Infection in Children**
   1. Diagnosis: HIV Infected
      a. A child <18 months old who is known to be HIV seropositive or born to an HIV-infected mother **and**
         1) Has positive results on two separate determinations (excluding cord blood) from one or more of the following HIV detection tests:
            a) HIV culture
            b) HIV polymerase chain reaction (PCR)
            c) HIV antigen (p24)
            or
         2) Meets criteria for AIDS diagnosis based on 1987 AIDS surveillance case definition; (from revision of the Centers for Disease Control (CDC) surveillance case definition for AIDS, *MMWR* 36(suppl), 1–15s 1987)
      b. A child ≥ 18 months old born to an HIV-infected mother or any child infected by blood, blood products, or other known modes of transmission who

1) Is HIV-antibody positive by repeatedly reactive enzyme immunoassay (EIA) and confirmatory test (e.g., Western blot or immunofluorescence assay [IFA]);
   or

2) Meets any of the criteria in a. on previous page

2. Diagnosis: Perinatally exposed: A child who does not meet the aforementioned criteria who:
   a. Is HIV seropositive by EIA and confirmatory test (e.g., Western blot or IFA) and who is <18 months old at the time of test;
      or
   b. Has unknown antibody status but was born to a mother known to be infected with HIV.

3. Diagnosis: Seroreverter (SR): A child who is born to an HIV-infected mother and who:
   a. Has been documented as HIV-antibody negative (i.e., two or more negative EIA tests performed at 6–18 months of age or one negative EIA test after 18 months of age);
      and
   b. Has no other laboratory evidence of infection (has not had two positive viral detection tests, if performed—see B.1.a.[1]);
      and
   c. Has not had an AIDS-defining condition.

C. **Classification of Diagnosed Pediatric HIV** (Table 18.1)
D. **Immunologic Categories Based on Age-specific CD4 Count (#/mcL) and Percent of Total Lymphocytes (%)** (Table 18.2)
E. **Clinical Categories for Children with HIV**
   1. **Category N:** Not symptomatic; children who have no signs or symptoms considered to be the result of HIV infection or who have only one of the conditions listed in category A
   2. **Category A:** Mildly symptomatic; children with two or more of the conditions listed below but none of the conditions listed in categories B and C
      a. Generalized lymphadenopathy
      b. Hepatomegaly
      c. Splenomegaly

TABLE 18.1.

Immunologic categories	Clinical categories*			
	N: No signs/ symptoms	A: Mild signs/ symptoms	B: Moderate signs/ symptoms	C: Severe signs/ symptoms
1) No evidence of suppression	N1	A1	B1	C1
2) Evidence of moderate suppression	N2	A2	B2	C2
3) Severe suppression	N3	A3	B3	C3

*See I.E. clinical categories.
Both category C and lymphoid interstitial pneumonitis in category B are reportable to state and local health departments as AIDS.
Children whose HIV-infection status is not confirmed are classified by using the above grid with a letter E (for perinatally exposed) placed before the appropriate classification code (e.g., EN2)

TABLE 18.2.

Immunologic category	Age of child					
	<12 mo		1–5 yr		6–12 yr	
	#/mcL	%	#/mcL	%	#/mcL	%
1) No evidence of suppression	≥ 1500	(≥25)	≥1,000	(≥25)	≥500	(≥25)
2) Evidence of moderate suppression	750–1499	(15–24)	500–999	(15–24)	200–499	(15–24)
3) Severe suppression	<750	(<15)	<500	(<15)	<200	(<15)

     d. Dermatitis

     e. Parotitis

     f. Recurrent or persistent upper respiratory infection, sinusitis, or otitis media

  3. **Category B:** Moderately symptomatic; children who have symptomatic conditions other than those listed for category A or C that are attributed to HIV infection, including, but not limited to, the following:

     a. Anemia, neutropenia, or thrombocytopenia for ≥ 30 days

     b. Bacterial meningitis, pneumonia, or sepsis (single episode)

    c. Candidiasis, oropharyngeal, persisting >2 months in children >6 months old

    d. Cardiomyopathy

    e. Cytomegalovirus (CMV) infection with onset <1 month old

    f. Diarrhea, recurrent or chronic

    g. Hepatitis

    h. Herpes simplex virus (HSV) stomatitis, recurrent (>2 episodes in 1 year)

    i. HSV bronchitis, pneumonitis, or esophagitis with onset <1 month old

    j. Herpes zoster involving at least 2 distinct episodes or >1 dermatome

    k. Leiomyosarcoma

    l. Lymphoid interstitial pneumonia or pulmonary lymphoid hyperplasia complex

    m. Nephropathy

    n. Nocardiosis

    o. Persistent fever (>1 month)

    p. Toxoplasmosis, onset <1 month old

    q. Varicella, disseminated

4. **Category C:** Severely symptomatic

    a. Serious bacterial infections, multiple or recurrent

    b. Candidiasis, esophageal or pulmonary (bronchi, trachea, lungs)

    c. Coccidioidomycosis, disseminated

    d. Cryptococcus, extrapulmonary

    e. Cryptosporidiosis or isosporiasis with diarrhea >1-month duration

    f. CMV disease (other than liver, spleen, nodes) onset at >1 month old

    g. Encephalopathy (including progressive developmental or cognitive deficits, impaired brain growth, and motor deficits)

    h. HSV ulcer, chronic (>1 month duration) or pneumonitis or esophagitis onset at >1 month of age

    i. Histoplasmosis, disseminated or extrapulmonary

    j. Kaposi's sarcoma

    k. Lymphoma, primary, in brain

    l. Lymphoma (Burkitt's, large cell, or immunoblastic sarcoma)

    m. *Mycobacterium tuberculosis,* disseminated or extrapulmonary

n. Mycobacterium, other species or unidentified species, disseminated or extrapulmonary

o. *Mycobacterium avium* complex or *M. kansasii,* disseminated or extrapulmonary

p. *Pneumocystis carinii* pneumonia (PCP)

q. Progressive multifocal leukoencephalopathy

r. Salmonella (nontyphoid) septicemia, recurrent

s. Toxoplasmosis of brain, onset after 1 month of age

t. Wasting syndrome due to HIV

F. **Guidelines for Prophylaxis Against First Episode of Opportunistic Infections**

1. *Pneumocystis carinii* pneumonia

a. Indications for prophylaxis (Table 18.3)

b. For recommended chemoprophylaxis regimens for first episode of opportunistic disease in HIV-infected infants and children. See references at the end of this section on p. 355.

G. **Antiretroviral Therapy:** Recommendations provided are current at time of publication; please check most recent recommendations for most current therapy. [http//www.hivatis.org]

1. Treatment

a. Recommended for all children who are HIV infected or perinatally-exposed to HIV, except those categorized as N1 outside the neonatal period

b. Agents labeled for use in children: zidovudine (ZDV, AZT), didanosine (ddI), and lamivudine (3TC)

c. Agents approved for use in adolescents and adults: AZT, ddI, ddC, D4T, 3TC, niverapine, protease inhibitors (saquinavir, indinavir, ritonavir)

d. If patient intolerant of agent, consider supportive measures (e.g., granulocyte colony stimulating factor [GCSF] for bone marrow suppression); if agent fails to halt progression of the disease, consider changing or combining antiretroviral agents.

e. In general, research supports the increasing trend toward combination therapy.

TABLE 18.3.

Indications for PCP Prophylaxis

Age/HIV infection status	PCP prophylaxis	CD4 monitoring at age:
Birth to 4–6 wk, HIV exposed	No prophylaxis	1 mo
4–6 wk to 4 mo, HIV exposed	Prophylaxis	3 mo
4–12 mo		
HIV infected or indeterminate	Prophylaxis	6, 9, and 12 mo
HIV infection reasonably excluded	No prophylaxis	None
1–5 yr, HIV infected	Prophylaxis if CD4 count (#/mcL) <500 or CD4 percentage is <15%	Every 3–4 mo
6–12 yr, HIV infected	Prophylaxis if CD4 count (#/mcL) <200 or CD4 percentage is <15%	Every 3–4 mo

> **Recommended regimen:**
>
> Trimethoprim/sulfamethoxazole
>
> (TMP/SMX) 150 mg
>
> TMP/m^2/24 hr and 750 mg
>
> SMX/m^2/24 hr PO divided Q12 hr
>
> 3 days/wk on consecutive days
>
> **Alternative TMP-SMX regimens:**
>
> (1) Same 24-hr dose as above given Q24 hr rather than
>
>   Q12 hr
>
> (2) Same dose as above given Q12 hr 7 days/wk
>
> (3) Same dose as above given Q12 hr on alternate days 3
>
>   days/wk
>
> **Alternate regimens if TMP-SMX is not tolerated:**
>
> (1) Dapsone 2 mg/kg (max 100 mg) PO Q24 hr
>
> (2) Aerosolized pentamidine (children ≥ 5 y/o) 300 mg via
>
>   Respiragard II inhaler monthly

Children who have had *Pneumocystis carinii* pneumonia (PCP) should receive lifelong prophylaxis

2. Prophylaxis: Use of ZDV therapy during pregnancy and in infancy to reduce perinatal HIV transmission
   a. ZDV 100 mg PO 5x/24 hr initiated at 14–34 weeks gestation and continued throughout pregnancy
   b. During labor, intravenous (IV) ZDV in a loading dose of 2 mg/kg over 1 hour, followed by continuous infusion of 1 mg/kg/hr until delivery
   c. For the newborn, ZDV 2 mg/kg/dose PO Q6 hr for first 6 weeks of life beginning 8–12 hours post-partum

H. Routine Childhood Immunizations in HIV-exposed or Infected Infants and Children (Specific guidelines are discussed in Chapter 17.)

From CDC: USPHS/IDSA guidelines for the prevention of opportunistic infections in persons infected with human immunodeficiency virus: a summary, *MMWR* 44 [No. RR-8], 1995; CDC: 1994 revised classification system for human immunodeficiency virus infection in children less than 13 years of age, *MMWR* 43 [No. RR-12], 1994; CDC: 1995 revised guidelines for prophylaxis against *Pneumocystis carinii* pneumonia for children infected with or perinatally exposed to human immunodeficiency virus, *MMWR* 44 (No. RR-4), 1995; CDC: recommendations of the U.S. Public Health Service Task Force on the use of zidovudine to reduce perinatal transmission of human immunodeficiency virus, *MMWR* 43 [No. RR-11], 1994)

II. SEXUALLY TRANSMITTED DISEASES (STDs)
A. Pelvic Inflammatory Disease (PID)
1. Diagnostic criteria: Minimum criteria (must have all of the following):
   a. Lower abdominal tenderness
   b. Adnexal tenderness
   c. Cervical motion tenderness
   d. Absence of an established etiology other than PID
2. Additional criteria (presence of these criteria increases the specificity of the diagnosis)
   a. Routine criteria
      1) Oral temperature >38.3° C
      2) Abnormal cervical or vaginal discharge
      3) Elevated erythrocyte sedimentation rate (ESR)
      4) Elevated C-reactive protein
      5) Laboratory documentation of cervical infection with *N. gonorrhoeae* or *C. trachomatis*

b. Elaborate criteria
   1) Histopathologic evidence of endometritis on endometrial biopsy
   2) Tuboovarian abscess on sonography or other radiologic tests
   3) Laparoscopic abnormalities consistent with PID
2. Criteria for hospitalization
   a. The diagnosis is uncertain, and surgical emergencies such as appendicitis and ectopic pregnancy cannot be excluded.
   b. Pelvic abscess is suspected.
   c. The patient is pregnant.
   d. The patient is an adolescent.
   e. The patient has HIV infection.
   f. Severe illness or nausea and vomiting preclude outpatient management.
   g. The patient has failed to respond to outpatient therapy.
   h. Clinical follow-up within 72 hours of starting antibiotic treatment cannot be arranged.
3. Treatment
   a. Inpatient treatment
      1) Regimen A: Cefoxitin 2 g IV Q6 hr or cefotetan 2 g IV Q12 hr **plus** doxycycline 100 mg IV/PO Q12 hr
      2) Regimen B: Clindamycin 900 mg IV Q8 hr (15–40 mg/kg/24 hr ÷ Q8 hr) **plus** gentamicin 2 mg/kg IV/IM loading dose followed by 1.5 mg/kg/dose Q8 hr maintenance dose
      3) The above regimens should be continued for at least 48 hours after the patient demonstrates substantial clinical improvement, then followed with doxycycline 100 mg PO Q12 hr **or** clindamycin 450 mg PO Q6 hr to complete a total of 14 days of therapy.
   b. Outpatient treatment
      1) Regimen A
         a) Cefoxitin 2 g IM x 1 dose **plus** probenecid 1 g PO x 1 dose concurrently **or**
         b) Ceftriaxone 250 mg intramuscular (IM) or other parenteral 3rd generation cephalosporin **plus** doxycycline 100 mg PO BID x 14 days

2) Regimen B (>18 years of age): Ofloxacin 400 mg PO Q12 hr x 14 days **plus** clindamycin 450 mg PO Q6 hr **or** metronidazole 500 mg PO Q12 hr x 14 days

From Centers for Disease Control and Prevention: 1993 Sexually transmitted diseases treatment guidelines, *MMWR* 42:75, 1993.

B. **Therapy for Chlamydia, Gonorrhea, and Syphilis** (Table 18.4)

C. **Congenital Syphilis**

    1. Evaluation

        a. All pregnant women should be screened with a nontreponemal antibody test early in pregnancy and early in the third trimester. Treat if evidence of infection and follow serologies to assess the efficacy of therapy.

        b. Evaluate any infant with clinical evidence of syphilis who has a reactive cord blood test or who is born to a serologically positive mother. Determine adequacy of maternal treatment. Consider treatment inadequate if mother:

            1) Was not treated

            2) Had treatment but course was poorly documented

            3) Received inadequate doses or duration of treatment

            4) Was treated with nonpenicillin regimen (e.g., erythromycin)

            5) Was treated <1 month before delivery

            6) Had insufficient serologic follow-up to assure that she responded appropriately to treatment by demonstrating a four-fold or greater decrease in titer in 3 months with course of treatment

    2. Further evaluation

        a. Physical examination (e.g., rash [vesicobullous], hepatomegaly, generalized lymphadenopathy, persistent rhinitis)

        b. Serologic test on infant's venous blood (cord blood may give false positive results)

        c. Examine cerebrospinal fluid (CSF) for protein, cell count, and Venereal Disease Research Laboratory test (VDRL) (do not use rapid plasma reagin test (RPR) or fluorescent treponemal antibody absorption test (FTA-ABS) high false positive rate).

        d. Radiographic studies: Long bone films for diaphyseal periostitis, osteochondritis

        e. If available, antitreponemal IgM

Adapted from: 1994 Red Book.

TABLE 18.4.

Therapy for Chlamydia, Gonorrhea, and Syphilis

Type or stage	Firstline drug and dosage	Alternatives
Chlamydia trachomatis		
	Diagnostic techniques:	
	(1) Definitive diagnosis: Isolation of specimen in tissue culture; this is the only acceptable method when evaluating a child for sexual abuse. Specimen must include cells.	
	(2) Presumptive diagnosis: Specimen from site of suspected infection sent for rapid detection of antigen through direct fluorescent staining using monoclonal antibody (DFA), enzyme immunoassay (EIA), or DNA probe; these should not be used for testing rectal, vaginal, or urethral specimens from children because of fecal cross-contamination.	
	(3) Serologies are generally not available.	
Urethritis, cervicitis, or proctitis	Doxycycline 100 mg PO Q12 hr x 7 days (if >9 y/o) **or** Azithromycin 1 g PO x 1 dose	Erythromycin base 500 mg PO Q6 hr x 7 days **or** Erythromycin ethylsuccinate 800 mg PO Q6 hr x 7 days **or** Ofloxacin 300 mg PO Q12 hr x 7 days (if >18 y/o)
Infection in pregnancy	Erythromycin base 500 mg PO Q6 hr x 7 days **or** Erythromycin ethylsuccinate 800 mg PO Q6 hr x 7 days	Amoxicillin 500 mg PO Q8 hr x 10 days **or** Sulfisoxazole 500 mg PO Q6 hr x 10 days (contraindicated if near term)
Neonatal ophthalmia	Erythromycin 50 mg/kg/24 hr PO or IV ÷ Q6 hr x 14 days	Topical treatment is ineffective
Neonatal pneumonia	Erythromycin 50 mg/kg/24 hr PO or IV ÷ Q6 hr x 14 days	Sulfisoxazole 100 mg/kg/24 hr (max 2 g/24 hr) ÷ Q6 hr PO/IV x 14 days

(Continued.)

TABLE 18.4. (cont.)

Type or stage	Firstline drug and dosage	Alternatives
Gonorrhea		
	Diagnostic techniques:	
	(1) Definitive diagnosis: Direct culture is the only acceptable method in the context of a sexual abuse evaluation; specimens for *N. gonorrhoeae* culture inoculated immediately onto selective medium with CO_2 incubation before transport: chocolate agar for cultures from sterile sites (blood, CSF), and more selective agar (usually Thayer-Martin media).	
	(2) Presumptive diagnosis: Gram-negative intracellular diplococci on microscopic exam of smear, enzyme immunoassay (EIA), and DNA probe	
	(3) Therapy should include treatment for presumed concomitant chlamydial infection.	
NEWBORNS		
Sepsis, arthritis, meningitis, scalp abscess	Ceftriaxone 25–50 mg/kg/24 hr IV/IM ÷ Q24 hr x 7 days (10–14 days if meningitis) **or** Cefotaxime 50 mg/kg/24 hr IV/IM ÷ Q12 hr x 7 days (10–14 days if meningitis)	
Neonatal ophthalmia	Ceftriaxone 25–50 mg/kg (max 125 mg) IV/IM x 1 dose plus saline irrigation **or** Cefotaxime 50–100 mg/kg/24 hr IV/IM ÷ Q8–12 hr x 7 days plus saline irrigation	For known susceptible strains: Penicillin G 100,000 U/kg/24 hr IV in 4 doses x 7 days plus saline irrigation Note: For routine prophylaxis, silver nitrate, tetracycline, or erythromycin ointment is instilled into each eye within 1 hour of birth.

PREPUBERTAL CHILDREN WHO WEIGH <100 LB (45 KG)

Uncomplicated urethritis, vulvovaginitis, proctitis, or pharyngitis
Ceftriaxone 125 mg IM x 1 dose
Spectinomycin 40 mg/kg (max 2 g) IM x 1 dose

Bacteremia, peritonitis, or arthritis
Ceftriaxone 50 mg/kg/24 hr (max 1 g) IM/IV ÷ Q24 hr x 7–10 days

Meningitis
Ceftriaxone 50 mg/kg/24 hr (max 2 g/24 hr) IV/IM ÷ q12–24h x 10–14 days

CHILDREN WHO WEIGH ≥ 100 LB (45 KG) AND ARE ≥ 9 YEARS OLD

Uncomplicated endocervictis or urethritis
Ceftriaxone 125 mg IM x 1 dose
Cefixime 400 mg PO x 1 dose **or**
Ciprofloxacin 500 mg PO x 1 dose (if >18 y/o) **or**
Ofloxacin 400 mg PO x 1 dose (if >18 y/o) **or**
Spectinomycin 40 mg/kg (max 2 g) IM x 1 dose

Pharyngitis
Ceftriaxone 125 mg IM x 1 dose

Pelvic inflammatory disease
See p. 342

Disseminated gonococcal infections
Ceftriaxone 1 g/24 hr IV/IM ÷ Q24 hr x 7 days
Cefotaxime or Ceftizoxime 3 g/24 hr IV ÷ Q8 hr x 7 days **or** for persons allergic to betalactam drugs: Spectinomycin 4 g/24 hr IM ÷ Q12 hr x 7 days

Meningitis
Ceftriaxone 2–4 g/24 hr IV ÷ Q12 hr x 10–14 days

(Continued.)

TABLE 18.4. (cont.)

Type or stage	Firstline drug and dosage	Alternatives
SYPHILIS	Diagnostic tests:	
	(1) Definitive diagnosis: Microscopic darkfield exam or direct fluorescent antibody test of lesion exudate or tissue (not for oral or rectal sites)	
	(2) Nontreponemal antibody tests (VDRL, RPR, ART) are useful for screening and as indicators of disease activity; false positives with EBV, TB, connective tissue disease, endocarditis, and IV drug use.	
	(3) Serologic treponemal tests (FTA-ABS, MHA-TP) are useful in determining a provisional diagnosis; false positives in other spirochetal diseases. Reactive tests remain positive for life and are therefore not useful for identifying disease recurrence.	
Congenital syphilis (neonatal)	See text.	
Congenital syphilis (beyond neonatal period)	Aqueous crystalline PCN 200,000–300,000 U/kg/24 hr IV ÷ Q6 hr x 10–14 days	
Early acquired syphilis of <1 year	Benzathine PCN G 50,000 U/kg (max 2.4 million U) IM x 1 dose	Tetracycline 500 mg PO Q6 hr x 14 days or Doxycycline 4 mg/kg/24 hr (max 200 mg) PO ÷ Q12 hr x 14 days
Syphilis of >1 year (late syphilis)	Benzathine PCN G 50,000 U/kg/dose (max 2.4 million U) IM every week x 3 weeks Note: Must examine CSF.	Tetracycline 500 mg PO Q12 hr x 28 days or Doxycycline 4 mg/kg/24 hr (max 200 mg) PO ÷ Q12 hr x 28 days

Type or stage	Firstline drug and dosage	Alternatives
Neurosyphilis	Aqueous crystalline PCN G 50,000 U/kg IV Q4–6 hr (max 4 million U IV Q4 hr) x 10–14 days; May be followed by benzathine PCN 50,000 U/kg/dose (max 2.4 million U) IM every week x 3 weeks	Aqueous procaine PCN G 2.4 million U IM Q24 hr x 10–14 days **plus** Probenecid 500 mg PO Q6 hr x 10–14 days May be followed by benzathine PCN 50,000 U/kg/dose (max 2.4 million U) IM every week x 3 weeks

If PCN-allergic, especially if less than 9 years old, consider PCN desensitization and administration in an appropriate setting.
Adapted from 1994 Red Book.

f. HIV-antibody test: High incidence of coinfection with HIV and *T. pallidum*
g. Guide for interpretation of the syphilis serology of mothers and their infants (Table 18.5)

TABLE 18.5.

Guide for Interpretation of the Syphilis Serology of Mothers and Their Infants

Nontreponemal Test (VDRL, RPR, ART, RST, EIA)		Treponemal Test (MHA-TP, FTA-ABS)		Interpretation*
Mother	Infant	Mother	Infant	
−	−	−	−	No syphilis or incubating syphilis in the mother and infant
+	+	−	−	No syphilis in mother (false-positive nontreponemal test with passive transfer to infant)
+	+ or −	+	+	Maternal syphilis with possible infant infection; or mother treated for syphilis during pregnancy; or mother with latent syphilis and possible infection of infant†
+	+	+	+	Recent or previous syphilis in the mother; possible infection in infant
−	−	+	+	Mother successfully treated for syphilis before or early in pregnancy; or mother with Lyme disease, yaws, or pinta (i.e., false-positive serology)

*Table presents a guide and not the definitive interpretation of serologic tests for syphilis in mothers and their infants. Other factors that should be considered include the timing of maternal infection, the nature and timing of maternal treatment, quantitative maternal and infant titers, and serial determination of nontreponemal test titers in both mother and infant.
†Approximately 20% of mothers with latent syphilis have nonreactive nontreponemal tests.
Peter G, editor: *1994 Red Book: report of the committee on infectious diseases,* ed 23, Elk Grove, II, 1994, American Academy of Pediatrics.

3. Treatment
    a. Treat infants with clinical evidence suggestive of syphilis regardless of CSF results
        1) Aqueous crystalline penicillin G, 100,000–150,000 U/kg/24 hr administered as 50,000 U/kg IV Q12 hr during the first 7 days of life and every 8 hours thereafter for 10–14 days
            or
        2) Procaine penicillin G, 50,000 U/kg IM daily for 10–14 days.
            If more than 1 day of therapy is missed, the entire course should be restarted. Follow nontreponemal tests at 3, 6, and 12 months posttreatment until nonreactive.
    b. An infant whose complete evaluation was normal but whose mother received no treatment, had inadequate or undocumented treatment, or who was reinfected after treatment should receive aqueous crystalline penicillin G, 100,000–150,000 U/kg/24 hr administered as 50,000 U/kg IV Q12 hr during the first 7 days of life and Q8 hr thereafter for 10–14 days.
    c. An infant whose complete evaluation was normal but whose mother was treated for syphilis during pregnancy with erythromycin, treated for syphilis <1month before delivery, or treated with an appropriate regimen before or during pregnancy but did not yet have a fourfold decrease in titer of a nontreponemal serologic test should be treated with benzathine penicillin G 50,000 U/kg IM x 1 dose.

From CDC. 1993 sexually transmitted diseases, *MMWR* 42(RR-14), 1993; Committee on Infectious Diseases, 1994 Red Book (Elk Grove: American Academy of Pediatrics, 1994), pp. 445–55.

D. **Sexual Abuse:** Evaluate victims of sexual abuse for STDs and consider treatment. If abuse episode occurred within 72 hours of evaluation, the victim should have a complete forensic exam.
    1. Throat, rectal, urethral, vaginal, and/or endocervical cultures for *N. gonorrhoeae* and *C. trachomatis*
    2. Darkfield exam of any chancres for syphilis; serologic tests for syphilis

3. Consider evaluation for HIV, hepatitis B, HSV, trichomonas, bacterial vaginosis, and papillomavirus if suspected.

From Committee on Infectious Diseases, 1994 Red Book (Elk Grove: American Academy of Pediatrics, 1994) p. 109.

Note: For other STDs (herpes, trichomonas, chancroid, granuloma inguinale, and HPV) see Chapter 5.

IV.   **TUBERCULOSIS**
A.   **Recommended Tuberculosis Testing**
   1. Testing schedule
      a. Test in low-risk children at health visits. Recommended test at 12–15 months old, 4–6 years old, 14–16 years old. Previous bacille Calmette-Guérin (BCG) vaccine is never a contraindication to testing.
      b. Annual tuberculin testing in high-risk children
         1) Exposure-related risks
            a) Contacts of adults with infectious tuberculosis
            b) Those who are from, or whose parents are from, regions of the world with high prevalence of tuberculosis
            c) Incarcerated adolescents
            d) Children frequently exposed to adults who are HIV-infected, homeless, users of street drugs, medically indigent, residents of nursing homes, incarcerated, institutionalized, or migrant farm workers
         2) Evidence of tuberculosis infection
            a) Those with radiologic evidence of tuberculosis
            b) Those with clinical evidence of tuberculosis
         3) Medical risk factors
            a) Children with HIV or other immunosuppressive conditions
            b) Children with Hodgkin's disease, lymphoma, diabetes mellitus, chronic renal failure, malnutrition
      c. Test children exposed to someone with known active disease. If initial test is negative, repeat 8–10 weeks after separation from contact.

2. Standard tuberculin test: Mantoux test 5TU-PPD (0.1 ml). The tine test (MPT) is no longer recommended.
    a. Inject intradermally on volar aspect of forearm to form 6–10 mm wheal. All results (positive or negative) should be read at 48–72 hours by qualified medical personnel.
    b. Definition of positive Mantoux skin test (regardless of whether BCG has been previously administered)
        1) Reaction ≥ 5 mm
            a) Children in close contact with persons who have known or suspected infectious cases of tuberculosis
            b) Children suspected to have tuberculous disease based on chest films or other clinical evidence of tuberculosis
            c) Children with immunosuppressive conditions or HIV infection
        2) Reaction ≥ 10 mm
            a) Children at increased risk of dissemination based on young age (<4 yr) or on other medical risk factors, including Hodgkin's disease, lymphoma, diabetes melitis, chronic renal failure, and malnutrition
            b) Children with increased environmental exposure
                i. Born, or whose parents were born, in regions of the world where tuberculosis is highly prevalent
                ii. Frequently exposed to adults who are HIV infected, homeless, users of street drugs, medically indigent, residents of nursing homes, incarcerated, institutionalized, or migrant farm workers
        3) Reaction ≥ 15 mm: Children ≥ 4 years of age without any risk factors

B.   Drug Therapy
    1. Prophylaxis
        a. Indications
            1) Children with a positive tuberculin test but no evidence of clinical disease

       2) Recent contacts, especially HIV-positive contacts, of persons with infectious tuberculosis, even if tuberculin test and clinical evidence are not indicative of tuberculosis

  b. Recommendations (see Formulary for specific doses)

      1) Isoniazid 10 mg/kg (max 300 mg) PO Q24 hr x 9 months

      2) If patient is HIV-positive, give 12 months of isoniazid (INH).

      3) If patient is suspected to have been exposed to persons with isoniazid-resistant tuberculosis, treat with rifampin 10 mg/kg (max 600 mg) PO Q24 hr, in addition to isoniazid, until susceptibility test results are available on the isolate from the index case.

      4) If index case is known to be excreting INH-resistant tuberculosis, discontinue the INH and treat with rifampin for a total of 9 months.

      5) If adherence with daily preventive therapy cannot be assured, twice weekly directly observed therapy with INH can be considered, preferably after completion of 1–2 months of daily therapy. Directly observed therapy requires that a health care worker observe administration of INH to the patient. See Formulary for dosing.

  2. Treatment (For details, please see 1994 Red Book.) (Table 18.6)

C. **Management of Infants of Tuberculosis (TB)–infected Mother or Other Household Contact** (Table 18.7)

TABLE 18.6.

Infection/disease	Regimen	Comments
Asymptomatic infection (positive PPD, no disease)		
•INH-susceptible in HIV positive child	INH Q24 hr x 9 mo INH Q24 hr x 12 mo R Q24 hr x 9 mo	If daily, self-administered therapy is not reliable, twice-weekly, directly-observed therapy must be provided.
•INH-resistant in HIV positive child	R Q24 hr x 12 mo	
Pulmonary (including hilar adenopathy) **or** extrapulmonary other than meningitis, disseminated (miliary), or bone/joint	Standard 6 month regimen: INH, R, and Z Q24 hr x 2 mo followed by INH and R Q24 hr x 4 mo **or** INH, R, and Z Q24 hr x 2 mo followed by INH and R twice weekly x 4 mo Alternative 9 mo regimen: INH and R Q24 hr x 9 mo **or** INH and R Q24 hr x 1 mo followed by INH and R twice weekly x 8 mo	If possible drug resistance is a concern, another drug (ethambutol or S) should be added to the initial 3-drug therapy until drug susceptibility is known and the 2-drug 9-month regimen should not be used. Drugs can be given 2–3 times per week under direct observation in the initial phase if nonadherence is likely. For hilar adenopathy, regimens consisting of 6 months of daily INH and R or 1 month of daily INH and R followed by 5 months of INH and R twice weekly, have been successful in areas where drug resistance is rare.
Meningitis, disseminated (miliary), and bone/joint	INH, R, Z and S Q24 hr x 2 mo followed by INH and R Q24 hr x 10 mo **or** INH, R, Z and S Q24 hr x 2 mo followed by INH and R twice weekly x 10 mo	S is given in initial therapy until drug susceptibility is known. For patients who may have acquired TB in geographic areas where resistance to S is common, capreomycin, or kanamycin may be used instead of S.

Z, Pyrazinamide; *R*, rifampin, *S*, streptomycin.

TABLE 18.7.

Management of Infants of TB-infected Mother or Other Household Contact

Mother (contact)	Newborn	Comments
Positive PPD, no evidence of infection	No therapy if no evidence of contact or exposure; consider INH until all contacts cleared of active infection	Test infant with PPD at 3–4 months.
Newly diagnosed TB with minimal disease or disease that has been treated for at least 2 weeks and judged to be noncontagious at delivery	INH until negative PPD at 3–4 months and no active cases in household; if mother (contact) has positive sputum, is noncompliant, and supervision is impossible, separate infant from the contact and consider BCG vaccine	Examine infant monthly; check chest x-ray exam and PPD on infant at 3–4 months and at 6 months; mother may breastfeed if adherent with treatment.
Contagious TB	INH until negative PPD at 3–4 months and no active cases in household; if mother (contact) has positive sputum, is noncompliant, and supervision is impossible, consider BCG vaccine.	Separate mother and infant until the infant is receiving therapy or the mother is confirmed to be noncontagious. Examine infant monthly; check CXR and PPD on infant at 3–4 months and at 6 months, mother may breastfeed if adherent with treatment.
Hematogenously spread TB	1) INH if no evidence of congenital TB; repeat PPD at 3–4 months; if positive continue INH for total of 12 months. 2) If evidence of congenital TB, treat with INH, rifampin, pyrazinamide, and streptomycin; if positive diagnosis, treat using regimen for TB meningitis.	Infant at risk for congenital TB; do PPD and CXR at birth, at 3–4 months, and at 6 months. If no congenital TB, separate mother until no longer contagious. Examine infant monthly.

Adapted From: Committee on Infectious Diseases. 1994 Red Book (Elk Grove: American Academy of Pediatrics, 1994)

V.   KAWASAKI DISEASE

A.   Diagnosis: Should have fever for at least 5 days plus 4 of the following:
1. Discrete bulbar conjunctival injection without exudate
2. Erythematous mouth and pharynx, strawberry tongue, and red, cracked lips
3. A polymorphous generalized erythematous rash that can be morbilliform, maculopapular, or scarlatiniform, or may resemble erythema multiforme
4. Changes in the peripheral extremities consisting of induration or the hands and feet with erythematous palms and soles
5. A usually solitary, frequently unilateral cervical lymph node enlarged to more than 1.5 cm in diameter

B.   Associated features
1. Acute and subacute period (first 3 weeks): anterior uveitis (80%), sterile pyuria (70%), arthritis or arthralgias (35%), aseptic meningitis (5%), carditis (<5%), pericardial effusion or arrhythmias (20%), gallbladder hydrops (<10%)
2. Late (2–4 weeks): coronary aneurysms (20% if untreated); obtain echocardiogram early in the acute phase of the illness, 3 weeks after onset, and 8 weeks after onset.

C.   Treatment
1. Intravenous immunoglobin (IVIG) 2 g/kg over 10–12 hours x 1 dose
2. Aspirin
   a. Initial high-dose therapy: 80–100 mg/kg/24 hr divided Q6 hr until fever controlled
   b. Then, 3–5 mg/kg/24 hr (max 80 mg/24 hr) PO QD x 2 mo or until erythrocyte sedimentation rate (ESR) and platelet count are normal
   c. Follow serum salicylate level during high-dose therapy
   d. Consider immunization against influenza (seasonal) and varicella to minimize risk of Reye's syndrome while on aspirin.

D.   Follow-up recommendations (see Chapter 7)

From Committee on Infectious Diseases. 1994 Red Book (Elk Grove: American Academy of Pediatrics, 1994), pp. 284–287.

VI. **GROUP B STREPTOCOCCAL (GBS) INFECTIONS**
A. **Presentation**
  1. Early-onset disease (first 24 hr, up to 6th day of life): respiratory distress, apnea, shock, pneumonia, meningitis
  2. Late-onset disease (1 week to 3 months): bacteremia or meningitis; also osteomyelitis, septic arthritis, and cellulitis
B. **Maternal chemoprophylaxis**
  1. Recommendation: Maternal GBS carriers, identified either antepartum (at 26–28 weeks of gestation) or intrapartum, with one or more of the following risk factors:
    a. Preterm labor or premature rupture of membranes at less than 37 weeks gestation
    b. Fever during labor
    c. Multiple births (such as twins)
    d. Previous delivery of an infant with invasive GBS disease
    e. Prolonged rupture of membranes (>18 hr)
  2. Chemoprophylaxis regimens (maternal)
    a. Ampicillin 2 g IV, then 1–2 g IV Q4–6 hr
    b. Penicillin G 5 million U IV Q6 hr
    c. If penicillin-allergic: clindamycin or erythromycin IV
C. **Treatment of neonatal disease**
  1. Penicillin G or ampicillin, plus an aminoglycoside (See Formulary for dosing.)
  2. Duration
    a. Bacteremia: at least 10 days
    b. Uncomplicated meningitis: at least 14–21 days
  3. Treat the twin of an index case

From Committee on Infectious Diseases. 1994 Red Book (Elk Grove: American Academy of Pediatrics, 1994), pp. 439–442

VII. **RHEUMATIC FEVER**
A. **Jones criteria:** If supported by evidence of preceding group A streptococcal infection, the presence of two major manifestations or of one major and two minor manifestations indicates a high probability of acute rheumatic fever.

1. Major manifestations
   a. Carditis
   b. Polyarthritis
   c. Chorea
   d. Erythema marginatum
   e. Subcutaneous nodules
2. Minor manifestations
   a. Clinical findings
      1) Arthralgia
      2) Fever
   b. Laboratory findings
      1) Elevated acute-phase reactants
         a) ESR
         b) C-reactive protein
      2) Prolonged PR interval
3. Supporting evidence of antecedent group A strep infection
   a. Positive throat culture or rapid strep antigen test
   b. Elevated or rising streptococcal antibody titer

From Dajani et al: Guidelines for the diagnosis of rheumatic fever, 87:302, 1993.

B.   Prevention of recurrence
1. Preferred regimen: Penicillin G benzathine 1.2 million units IM Q3–4 wk
2. Alternate regimens
   a. Sulfisoxazole 0.5 g PO Q24 hr if <60 lb and 1 g PO Q24 hr if >60 lb
   b. Penicillin V 250 mg PO BID
   c. Erythromycin stearate 250 mg PO BID

From Committee on Infectious Diseases. 1994 Red Book (Elk Grove: American Academy of Pediatrics, 1994), pp. 438–439. Mandell GL, Bennett JE, Dolin R: *Principles and practice of infectious disease,* New York, 1995, Churchill Livingstone.

VIII. ISOLATION TECHNIQUES FOR SELECTED ILLNESSES (Tables 18.8 and 18.9)

TABLE 18.8.

Note: Use universal precautions during all patient encounters to reduce the risk of transmission of bloodborne pathogens. Minimize contact with blood and body fluids* of all patients as follows:
Needles and sharps: Do not recap needles; dispose needles in needle containers only.
Gowns and gloves: Wear when contact with blood and body fluids is likely.
Protective eyewear and mask: Wear when splashing is likely.

Isolation precautions	
Strict	Herpes zoster, disseminated
	Herpes zoster, localized, lesions *cannot* be covered
	Meningococcal pneumonia†
	Rubella, congenital
	Rubella, primary infection
	Rubeola
	Varicella
Contact	Diarrhea, infectious (suspected or confirmed)
	Enterococci resistant to vancomycin
	Gas gangrene
	Herpes simplex, neonatal
	Herpes zoster, localized, lesions *can* be covered‡
	Staphylococcal wound or skin infection, contained by dressing
	Syphilis, congenital†
	Wound infection, other than staphylococcal, extensive
Contact with mask	Diphtheria§
	Haemophilus influenzae, invasive†
	Influenza
	Meningitis *H. influenzae* or *N. meningitidis*†
	Meningococcemia†
	Mumps
	Parainfluenza
	Pertussis§
	Rabies
	Staphylococcal pneumonia
	Staphylococcal wound or skin infection, extensive
RSV precautions	Bronchiolitis, etiology unknown in children <2 y/o
	Respiratory syncytial virus
Airborne	Tuberculosis

RSV, Respiratory syncytial virus.
*Blood; all fluids containing visible blood; cerebrospinal fluid; vaginal secretions; semen; and synovial, pericardial, amniotic, peritoneal, and pleural fluid.
†Until 24 hours after effective treatment is begun.
‡Roommates must be immune.
§Private room required.

TABLE 18.9.

	Strict	Contact	Contact with mask	RSV precautions	Airborne*
Cart	Yes	Yes	Yes	Yes	Yes
Private Room	Required	Preferred†	Preferred†	Preferred	Required
Door closed	Yes	No	No	No	Yes
Mask	To enter room	No	At patient bedside	At patient bedside	To enter room‡
Gown	To enter room	For contact with patient	For contact with patient	For contact with patient	No
Gloves	To enter room	For contact with infective material	For contact with infective material	To enter Room	No
Disposable items: red bag	All	If soiled with infective material	If soiled with infective material	If soiled with sputum	If soiled with sputum
Large reusable items: wash	All	If soiled with infective material	If soiled with infective material	If soiled with sputum	If soiled with sputum
Linen: cloth bag at bedside	Yes	If soiled with infective material	If soiled with infective material	Yes	No
Glass thermometer	Yes	No	No	No	No
B/P apparatus	Yes	No	No	No	No
Special transport	Patient in surgical face mask and clean linens	Clean linens	Patient in surgical face mask and clean linens	Clean linens	Patient in surgical face mask

Note: Antimicrobial soap required for all categories of isolation/precautions

*For room requirements, refer to Centers for Disease Control and Prevention's "Guidelines for Preventing the Transmission of *M. tuberculosis* in Health-Care Facilities," 1994.   †Required for pertussis and diphtheria.
‡Requires HEPA respirator mask to enter patient's room. This mask is not to be worn by the patient.
From The Johns Hopkins Hospital. Infection Control Department.

MICROBIOLOGY

19

I. BACTERIA

A. Staining Techniques

Allow smear to air dry before it is fixed; then fix with gentle heat by quickly passing slide through a flame (no more than 4 times). Test temperature by tapping slide on the back of your hand; it should feel warm. Allow slide to cool before staining.

1. **Gram stain**
   a. Flood slide with **gentian (Crystal) violet** for 1 minute. Wash with gently running water.
   b. Flood with **iodine solution** for 1 minute. Wash with gently running water.
   c. Decolorize with **acetone/alcohol** for 3–4 seconds. Wash with water immediately.
   d. Counterstain with **safranin** for 30 seconds. Wash with water.
   e. Alternatively, use **rapid method.** Follow same sequence as above but have each agent on smear for only 10 seconds. Acetone/alcohol still only 3–4 sec.

2. **Wright's stain**
   a. Air-dry; do not heat-fix.
   b. Stain with **Wright's stain** for 1 minute.
   c. Add an equal amount of water, and blow on the smear to mix the stain and water. Repeat by adding more water and blowing to mix. Look for formation of a shiny surface scum. Then allow the stain to set for 3–4 minutes.
   d. Rinse with gently running water for 5 seconds.

3. **Acid-fast stain**
   a. Cover with **Kinyoun stain** for 5 minutes. Wash with water.
   b. Decolorize in **acid-alcohol** until no more color leaches from the slide for 3–4 minutes. Wash with water.
   c. Counterstain with **methylene blue** for 2 minutes.
   d. Wash with water and let dry.

4. Methylene blue stain for fecal leukocytes (see Chapter 12)

From Detmer WM et al: *Pocket guide to diagnostic tests,* Norwalk 1992, Appleton & Lange.

B. Rapid Microbiologic Identification of Common Aerobic Bacteria and Yeast (numbers in parentheses are time involved for test) (Fig. 19.1)

Note: Germ tube screen of yeast (3h): Candida albicans.

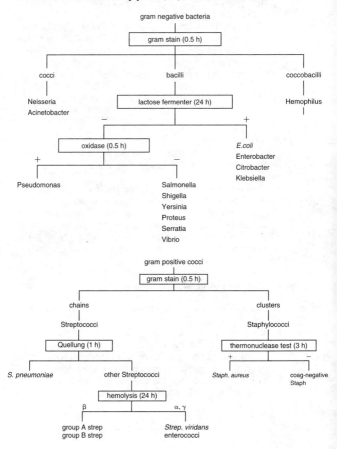

FIG. 19.1. Algorithms demonstrating identification of bacteria.

C. Antibiotic Sensitivities
1. Definitions
   a. Minimum inhibitory concentration (MIC): The lowest bacteriostatic concentration of an antimicrobial agent that prevents visible growth after an 18- to 24-hour incubation period
   b. Minimum bactericidal concentration (MBC): The lowest concentration of antimicrobial that kills > 99.9% of organisms as measured by subculturing to antibiotic-free media after 18- to 24-hour incubation
   c. Serum bactericidal test: The dilution of serum (from a patient receiving antibiotics) that kills > 99.9% of the organism grown out of the patient's original culture

From Nelson JD: *Pocket book of pediatric antimicrobial therapy,* Baltimore, 1995, Williams and Wilkins; Mandell GL, Bennett JE, Dolin R: *Principles and practice of infectious disease,* New York, 1995, Churchill Livingstone.

2. Common pitfalls: Clinically significant, common discrepancies between in vitro and in vivo antibiotic sensitivity profiles
   a. Cephalosporins vs. staphylococcus: If a staphylococcus is more than 2 dilutions more sensitive to a first generation cephalosporin than to a "staphylococcal penicillin" (e.g., oxacillin), suspect that the organism is methicillin-resistant *Staph. aureus* and consider using vancomycin rather than cephalosporins.

From Mandell GL, Bennett JE, Dolin R: *Principles and practice of infectious disease,* New York, 1995, Churchill Livingstone.

   b. Cephalosporins vs. gram-negative bacilli (nonpseudomonal): If a gram-negative rod exhibits more than a 2 dilution greater susceptibility to a first- or second-generation cephalosporin over a third-generation cephalosporin or more than a 2 dilution difference in susceptibility between two third-generation cephalosporins, it is likely to have an extended spectrum β-lactamase. Consider using a β-lactamase inhibitor-containing combination, such as ticarcillin-clavulanate or piperacillin-tazobactam.

c. Aminoglycosides vs. salmonella: Despite in vitro susceptibility to aminoglycosides, salmonella does not respond in vivo to this class of antibiotics.

From Mandell GL, Bennett JE, Dolin R: *Principles and practice of infectious disease,* New York, 1995, Churchill Livingstone.

d. The following organisms are inducibly resistant to all cephalosporins; therefore, cephalosporins should not be used as sole treatment for these organisms outside the urinary tract. β-lactamase inhibitors are potent inducers of resistance to cephalosporins in these organisms and should not be used.

- Enterobacter
- Citrobacter
- Indole-positive proteus
- *Pseudomonas aeruginosa*
- Serratia
- Providentia

From Sanders WE, Sanders CC: Inducible β-lactamases: clinical and epidemiologic implications for use of newer cephalosporins, *Rev Infect Dis* 10(4):830, 1988.

D. Bacterial Blood Cultures
Optimally, the sample volume should equal 10% of the volume of the culture medium.

II. VIRUSES
A. Staining: Tzanck smear
1. Unroof vesicle with scalpel blade, then scrape blade across vesicle base. Smear the resulting specimen on a glass slide.
2. Let smear air dry or heat-fix.
3. Stain with Wright's stain (see I.A.2.) or fresh Giemsa stain. If Giemsa stain is used, the specimen must first be fixed to the slide with methyl alcohol for 10–15 minutes.

From Detmer WM et al: *Pocket guide to diagnostic tests,* Norwalk, 1992, Appleton & Lange.

B. Serology
1. Hepatitis (Table 19.1) (From Abbott Laboratory, Chicago, Illinois.)
2. Hepatitis B (Figs. 19.2)
3. Epstein-Barr virus (Table 19.2)

TABLE 19.1. Hepatitis Panel Testing

Type	Profile name	Markers	Purpose
Diagnostic	Acute	■ HBsAg ■ Anti-HBc IgM ■ Anti-HAV IgM ■ Anti-HCV	To differentiate between HBV, HAV, and HCV acute infection. Retest for anti-HCV if negative but clinical signs/symptoms suggest hepatitis C.
Screen	Hepatitis C	■ Anti-HCV	To evaluate for late seroconversion in recent HCV infection and to identify HCV infected individuals
	Perinatal	■ HBsAg ■ HBeAg	To diagnose for HBsAg-positive pregnant women who may transmit hepatitis B to their newborn infants. If the HBsAg-positive mother is HBeAg-positive, her infant will have a 90% chance of acquiring chronic hepatitis B infection (e.g., Southeast Asians, Alaskans, health care workers).
	Immunity	■ HBsAg ■ Anti-HBc ■ Anti-HBs	1. Test blood for infection with HBsAg. 2. Test exposed person for immunity with anti-HBc and anti-HBs (in particular, dialysis patients, health care workers, recipients of frequent transfusions, and illicit drug users). 3. Test sexual partners of individuals with acute or chronic HBV in order to minimize the spread of infection by the application of prophylaxis. 4. Test to determine if an individual is currently infected or has antibodies to HBV.
Monitor	Chronic hepatitis B	■ HBsAg ■ HBeAg ■ Anti-HBe	To evaluate for late seroconversion and/or disease resolution in known HBV carrier
	Infant Follow-up	■ HBsAg ■ Anti-HBs	To monitor the success of treatment for perinatal transmission of HBV (12–15 months after birth)
	Postvaccination	■ Anti-HBs	To ensure that immunity has been achieved after vaccination

366

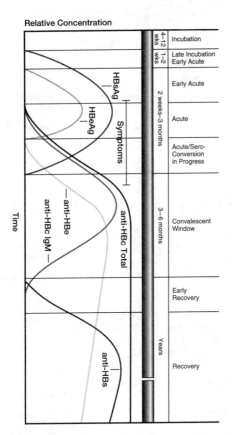

FIG. 19.2. Serologic profile in 75%–85% of patients with acute type B Hepatitis.

Note: Chronic HBV carriers will be persistently surface antigen positive.

TABLE 19.2.

Serum EBV Antibodies in EBV Infection

Antibody specificity	Time of appearance in infectious mononucleosis	Percentage of EBV-induced mononucleosis cases with antibody	Persistence	Comments
VIRAL CAPSID ANTIGENS				
IgM VCA	At clinical presentation	100	4–8 wk	Highly sensitive and specific
IgG VCA	At clinical presentation	100	Lifelong	High titer at presentation and lifelong persistence make IgG VCA more useful as epidemiologic tool than in diagnosis
EARLY ANTIGENS				
Anti-D	Peaks at 3–4 wk after onset	70	3–6 mo	Correlated with severe disease; also seen in nasopharyngeal carcinoma
Anti-R	2 wk to several mo after onset	Low	2 mo to > 3 yr	Occasionally seen with unusually severe or protracted illness; also seen in African Burkitt's lymphoma
EPSTEIN-BARR NUCLEAR ANTIGEN				
	3–4 wk after onset	100	Lifelong	Late appearance helpful in diagnosis of heterophile-negative cases
SOLUBLE COMPLEMENT-FIXING ANTIGENS (ANTI-S)				
	3–4 wk after onset	100	Lifelong	Late appearance helpful in diagnosis of heterophile-negative cases

From Mandell GL, Bennett JE, Dolin R: *Principles and practice of infectious disease,* New York, 1995, Churchill Livingstone.

NEONATOLOGY 20

I. **FETAL ASSESSMENT**
A. **Genetic Diagnosis and Fetal Anomaly Screening**
 1. Frequency of major and minor anomalies: Major malformations are structural abnormalities having surgical, medical, or cosmetic importance and occur in 2%–3% of live births.
 2. Maternal serum alpha-fetoprotein screening (MSAFP)
  a. Elevated MSAFP (> 2.5 multiples of the median (MoM)): Associated with neural tube defects (NTDs), anencephaly, multiple pregnancy, Turner syndrome, omphalocele, cystic hygroma, epidermolysis bullosa, and renal anomalies
  b. Low MSAFP (<0.75 (MoM)): Associated with underestimating gestational age, intrauterine growth retardation, and chromosomal trisomies (13, 18, and 21)
  c. Accurate gestational dating and maternal weight are critical to the interpretation of results.
 3. Amniocentesis: Performed with ultrasound guidance at 11–17 weeks gestation. Estimated fetal loss of 0.5%–1%. Indications: Women >35 years of age, previous infant with known chromosomal abnormality, suspected X-linked disorders, abnormal alphafetoprotein, and to rule out inborn errors of metabolism. Incidence of trisomy 21 in women > 35 years of age is 1/385.
 4. Chorionic villus sampling: Villi obtained by transcervical or transabdominal aspiration with ultrasound guidance between 9 and 11 weeks gestation. Complications include maternal infection, fetal demise (2.5%), limb abnormalities (1.7%), and chromosomal mosaicism (3%).
 5. Ultrasonography
  a. Routine ultrasounds: Performed on low-risk patients at 18–20 weeks gestation

    b. Amniotic fluid volume estimations (AFV): AFV is dependent upon fetal swallowing (500 ml/day at term), fetal micturition (26–43 ml/hr at term), and maternal/fetal exchange of amniotic fluid at the placenta.

    c. Oligohydramnios (<500 ml): Associated with Potter syndrome, renal or urologic abnormalities, lung hypoplasia, limb deformities, or premature rupture of membranes (PROM)

    d. Polyhydramnios (>2 L): Suggestive of gastrointestinal anomalies (gastroschisis, duodenal atresia, tracheoesophageal fistula, diaphragmatic hernia), CNS abnormalities (anencephaly, Werdnig-Hoffman), chromosomal trisomies, maternal diabetes, and cystic adenomatoid malformation of the lung

B. Fetal Maturity Assessment

1. Menstrual history: Most accurate determination of gestational age. Naegele's rule, based on a 28-day cycle, calculates EDC as 9 months (280 days) plus 7 days from the last menstrual period.

2. Ultrasound: Crown-rump length obtained between 6 and 12 weeks predicts gestational age ±3–4 days. After 12 weeks the biparietal diameter is accurate within 10 days, and beyond 26 weeks accuracy diminishes to ± 3 weeks.

3. Growth: Average fetal weight is approximately 1000 g at 25 weeks, 2500 g at 35 weeks, and 3300 g at 40 weeks.

4. Fetal lung maturity: Lecithin, the active component of surfactant, is present in amniotic fluid in increasing amounts throughout gestation compared to constant levels of sphingomyelin.

    a. The L:S ratio: L:S ratios of 2:1 or greater indicate fetal lung maturity in nondiabetic pregnancies, and ratios of 3:1 indicate lung maturity in diabetic pregnancies and with Rh isoimmunization. L/S ratio is generally 1:1 at 31–32 weeks gestation, and 2:1 by 35 weeks gestation. Ratios of 2:1 are associated with respiratory distress syndrome (RDS) in 0.5% of infants. With ratios of (1.5–1.9):1, 50% will develop RDS, and 73% with ratios of < 1.5:1.

    b. Phosphatidyl glycerol (PG): A late appearing surfactant component. The risk of RDS is < 0.5% if PG is present in amniotic fluid.

C. **Antepartum Fetal Monitoring**
 1. Non stress test (NST): Fetal heart rate is monitored with the mother at rest. In a normal, reactive NST, fetal heart rate increases >15 beats/minute for more than 15 seconds, at least twice in 20 minutes. Reactivity is absent in fetuses <30 weeks gestation because of CNS immaturity.
 2. Contraction stress test (CST): Uterine contractions are induced by parenteral oxytocin or nipple stimulation. Fetal heart rate is monitored through three successive uterine contractions during a 10 minute interval. A positive (nonreassuring) test consists of late decelerations with >50% of uterine contractions and indicates uteroplacental insufficiency. High false positive rate.
 3. Biophysical profile: Consists of a 30 minute ultrasound examination of 5 biophysical assessments. Parameters include the NST, amniotic fluid volume, fetal breathing movements, fetal movements, tone, and heart rate. Each parameter is scored 2 (if normal), or 0 (if abnormal). Total scores of 8–10 are reassuring.

D. **Intrapartum Fetal Monitoring**
 1. Fetal heart rate monitoring (Fig. 20.1)
  a. **Normal baseline FHR:** 120–160 beats/minute (BPM). Mild bradycardia: 100–120 BPM.
  b. **Normal variability:** Deviation from baseline of >6 BPM. Absence of variability is <2 BPM.
  c. **Early decelerations:** Begin with the onset of contractions, reach the nadir at the peak contraction, and return to baseline as the contraction ends. Occur secondary to changes in vagal tone after brief hypoxic episodes or head compressions and are benign.
  d. **Variable decelerations:** No uniform temporal relationship to the onset of the contraction. Represent umbilical cord compression. Variable decelerations are considered severe when the heart rate drops below 60 BPM for 60 seconds or more with slow recovery to baseline.
  e. **Late decelerations:** Occur after the peak of contraction, persist after the contraction stops, and show a slow return to baseline. Result from uteroplacental insufficiency. Normal variability indicates a physiologically compensated fetus.

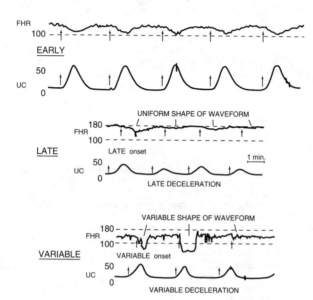

FIG. 20.1. Fetal heart tracings. *(From Taeusch H et al: Schaffer and Avery's diseases of the newborn, ed 6, Philadelphia, 1991, WB Saunders.)*

II.   **NEWBORN ASSESSMENT**
A.   **Vital Signs**

    Average heart rate and respiratory rate are 120–160 BPM and 40–60 BPM respectively. Arterial blood pressure is related to birth weight and gestational age (see Chapter 7).

B.   **Thermoregulation (Fig. 20.2)**
C.   **Apgar Scores**

    Assessed at 1 and 5 minutes. For neonatal distress, assessment is repeated at 10 and 20 minutes (Table 20.1)

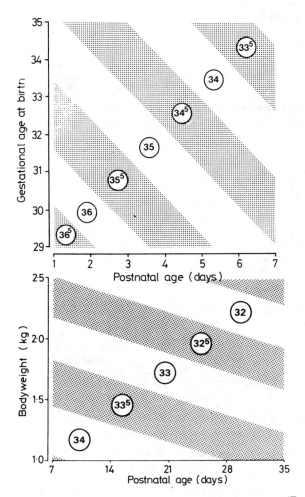

FIG. 20.2. Neutral thermal environmental temperatures. *(From Sauer PJJ, Dane HJ, Visser HKA:* Arch Dis Child *59:18, 1984.)*

TABLE 20.1

		Score	
	0	1	2
Heart rate	Absent	<100	>100
Respiratory effort	Absent, irregular	Slow, crying	Good
Muscle tone	Limp	Some flexion of extremeties	Active motion
Reflex irritability (nose suction)	No response	Grimace	Cough or sneeze
Color	Blue, pale	Extremities blue	Completely pink

Adapted from Apgar V: *Anesth Analg* 32:260, 1953.

D. Gestational Age
1. Anterior lens vessel examination (Fig. 20.3)

| Grade 4 | Grade 3 | Grade 2 | Grade 1 |
| 27 to 28 weeks | 29 to 30 weeks | 31 to 32 weeks | 33 to 34 weeks |

FIG. 20.3. Anterior Lens Vessels. *(From Hittner H et al: J Pediatr 91:455, 1977.)*

2. Neuromuscular and physical maturity (Ballard score) The Ballard is most accurate when performed between 12–20 hours or as soon as possible after stabilization.
   a. Neuromuscular maturity (Fig. 20.4)
      1) Posture: Observe infant quiet, supine. Score 0: arm, legs extended; 1: beginning flexion of hips and knees, arms extended; 2: stronger flexion of legs, arms extended; 3: arms slightly flexed, legs flexed and abducted; 4: full flexion of arms, legs.
      2) Square window: Flex hand on forearm enough to obtain fullest possible flexion without wrist rotation. Measure angle between the hypothenar eminence and the ventral aspect of the forearm.
      3) Arm recoil: With infant supine, flex forearms for 5 seconds, then fully extend by pulling on hands,

then release. Measure the angle of elbow flexion
to which the arms recoil.
4) Popliteal angle: Hold infant supine with pelvis
flat, thigh held in the knee-chest position. Extend
leg by gentle pressure and measure the popliteal
angle.
5) Scarf sign: With baby supine, pull infant's hand
across the neck toward the opposite shoulder.
Determine how far the elbow will go across.
Score 0: Elbow reaches opposite axillary line; 1:
past midaxillary line; 2: past midline; 3: elbow
unable to reach midline.
6) Heel-to-ear maneuver: With baby supine, draw
foot as near to the head as possible without
forcing it. Observe distance between foot and
head, and degree of extension at the knee. Knee
is free and may be down alongside abdomen.

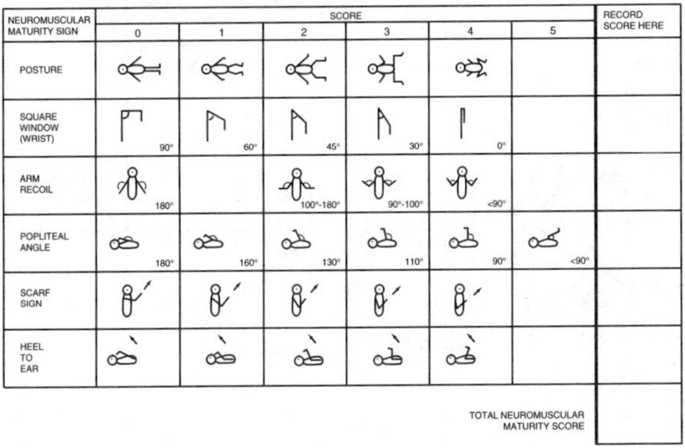

NEUROMUSCULAR MATURITY SIGN	SCORE						RECORD SCORE HERE
	0	1	2	3	4	5	
POSTURE							
SQUARE WINDOW (WRIST)	90°	60°	45°	30°	0°		
ARM RECOIL	180°		100°-180°	90°-100°	<90°		
POPLITEAL ANGLE	180°	160°	130°	110°	90°	<90°	
SCARF SIGN							
HEEL TO EAR							
					TOTAL NEUROMUSCULAR MATURITY SCORE		

FIG. 20.4. Neuromuscular maturity (Ballard). *(From Ballard J et al: J Pediatr 95:769, 1979.)*

b. Physical maturity (Table 20.2)
c. Maturity rating: Add scores for neuromuscular maturity and physical maturity assessment (Table 20.3).

TABLE 20.2

Physical maturity sign	Score						Record score here
	0	1	2	3	4	5	
Skin	Gelatinous, red, transparent	Smooth, pink, visible veins	Superficial peeling, and/or rash, few veins	Cracking; pale area; rare veins	Parchment; deep cracking; no vessels	Leathery, cracked, wrinkled	
Lanugo	None	Abundant	Thinning	Bald areas	Mostly bald		
Plantar creases	No crease	Faint red marks	Anterior transverse crease only	Creases anterior 2/3	Creases cover entire sole		
Breast	Barely perceptible	Flat areola, no bud	Stippled areola, 1–2 mm bud	Raised areola, 3–4 mm bud	Full areola, 5–10 mm bud		
Ear	Pinna flat, stays folded	Slightly curved pinna; soft with slow recoil	Well-curved, pinna; soft but ready recoil	Formed and firm with instant recoil	Thick cartilage; ear stiff		
Genitals (male)	Scrotum empty; no rugae		Testes descending; few rugae	Testes down; good rugae	Testes pendulous; deep rugae		
Genitals (female)	Prominent clitoris and labia minora		Majora and minora equally prominent	Majora large, minora small	Clitoris and minora completely covered		
						Total physical maturity score	

TABLE 20.3

Score	5	10	15	20	25	30	35	40	45	50
Weeks	26	28	30	32	34	36	38	40	42	44

III. MANAGEMENT OF THE PRETERM INFANT
A. Fluid Management (see also Chapter 11)
1. Insensible water loss: Preterm infants experience increased insensible losses through the skin because of increased surface area per unit body mass and immaturity of the skin (Table 20.4).

TABLE 20.4

Estimates of Insensible Water Loss at Different Body Weights*

Body Weight (g)	Insensible Water Loss (ml/kg/day)
<1,000	60–70
1,000–1,250	60–65
1,251–1,500	30–45
1,501–1,750	15–30
1,751–2,000	15–20

*AGA infants in a thermoneutral environment during the first week of life.
From Veille JC: *Clin Perinatol* 15(4):863, 1988.

2. Water requirements (ml/kg/24 hr) of newborns (Table 20.5)

TABLE 20.5

Water Requirements (ml/kg/24h) of Newborns

Birthweight (g)	1–2 days	Age 3–7 days	7–30 days
<750	100–250	150–300	120–180
750–1000	80–150	100–150	120–180
1000–1500	60–100	80–150	120–180
>1500	60–80	100–150	120–180

Adapted from Schaffer and Avery, editors: *Diseases of the newborn*, ed 6, Philadelphia, 1991, WB Saunders.

3. Electrolyte requirements: Common electrolyte abnormalities include hyponatremia, hypernatremia, hypokalemia, hyperkalemia, and hypocalcemia
   a. **Sodium:** None required in the first 72 hours of life, unless serum Na <135 mEq/dl, and no evidence of volume overload. After 72 hours, the sodium requirement is generally 2–3 mEq/kg/24 hr for term, and 3–5 mEq/kg/24 hr for preterm infants.
   b. **Potassium:** Added to fluids after adequate urinary output established and serum level <4.5. K requirements are generally 1–2.5 mEq/kg/day.
4. Glucose requirements: Premature neonates require approximately 5–6 mg/kg/min of glucose to maintain euglycemia (40–100 mg/dl). Term neonates require about 3–5 mg/kg/min of glucose to maintain euglycemia.

   Formula to calculate rate of glucose infusion:

$$\text{mg/kg/min glucose} = \frac{(\% \text{ of glucose in solution} \times 10) \times (\text{rate of infusion})}{(60 \times \text{wt(kg)})}.$$

From Cornblath M, Schwartz R: *Disorders of carbohydrate metabolism in infancy,* ed 3, 1991, Blackwell Scientific Publications.

IV. NUTRITION AND GROWTH OF THE NEONATE
A. Growth Rates
Expected weight gain is 20–30 g/kg/day for premature infants and 10 g/kg/day for full term infants.
B. Caloric Requirements
To maintain weight, 50–75 kcal/kg/day. Adequate growth requires 100–120 kcal/kg/day in term, 115–130 kcal/kg/day for preterm, and up to 150 kcal/kg/day for very low birth weight infants.
C. Mineral Requirements
1. Calcium: Premature infants have high calcium and phosphorus requirements and require special premature formulas or human milk fortifier. Fortifier should be added to breast milk only after the second week of life. Supplementation is recommended for infants weighing <1,000 g to provide 150–200 mg/kg/day Ca until 1,500–2,000 g weight is achieved.

2. Iron: Enterally fed premature infants require elemental iron supplementation of 2 mg/kg/day after 6–8 weeks of age.

D.   Total Parenteral Nutrition (see Chapter 23)

V.   RESPIRATORY DISEASES

A.   Surfactant Production

Type II cells synthesize and secrete pulmonary surfactant, a phospholipid protein mixture, which increases surface tension and prevents alveolar collapse. Acute asphyxia with hypoxia and acidosis inhibits surfactant production.

B.   Respiratory Distress Syndrome

1. Incidence: In general, the incidence is 60% in infants <30 weeks gestation without antenatal glucocorticoids and 35% for those with antenatal steroid exposure. Between 30 and 34 weeks gestation, the incidence is 25% in untreated or inadequately treated infants and 10% in those who have received full steroid treatment. For infants <34 weeks gestation, the incidence is 5%.

2. Risk factors: Prematurity, maternal diabetes, c-section without antecedent labor, perinatal asphyxia, second twin, previous infant with RDS. Decreased incidence occurs in long-term maternal stress (e.g., toxemia, hypertension), IUGR, maternal infection, maternal heroin exposure, and glucocorticoid treatment.

3. Clinical presentation: Respiratory distress worsens during the first few hours of life, progresses over 48 to 72 hours, and subsequently improves. Recovery is accompanied by brisk diuresis. Lung fields have a "ground glass" or "reticulogranular" pattern obscuring the heart border on chest x-ray exam.

4. Management

   a. Support ventilation and oxygenation

   b. Surfactant therapy (see Formulary for dosing)

   1) "Rescue" therapy: Administration of surfactant to infants with diagnosed RDS within the first 8 hours of birth

   2) "Prophylactic" therapy: Administration of surfactant immediately after delivery. May be more effective than rescue therapy in infants <26 weeks gestation.

C.   **Intrauterine Acceleration of Fetal Lung Maturation**
   1. Indications
      a. Threatened premature labor before 33–34 weeks gestation if pulmonary maturity is unknown
      b. Documented pulmonary immaturity, and delivery not anticipated for at least 12 hours
   2. Steroid efficacy: Maximum benefit if administered at least 24 hours before delivery. Efficacy subsides after 7 days and is not beneficial in infants > 34 weeks gestation. Incidence of RDS is decreased by about 50% in most studies.
   3. Dosing: Administer betamethasone or dexamethasone over a period of 48 hours. If the infant is not delivered in 7 days, another course of glucocorticoids may be considered.

VI.   **APNEA**
A.   **Definition**
   Respiratory pause >20 seconds or a shorter pause associated with cyanosis, pallor, hypotonia, or bradycardia <100 BPM. In premature infants apneic episodes may be central (no diaphragmatic activity), obstructive (upper airway obstruction), or mixed.
B.   **Incidence**
   Apnea occurs in the majority of infants <28 weeks gestation, approximately 50% of infants 30–32 weeks, and $<7\%$ of infants 34–35 weeks gestation.
C.   **Management**
   1. Consider a pathologic cause for apnea.
   2. Pharmacotherapy with theophylline, aminophylline, caffeine, or doxapram (see Formulary for dosing)
   3. CPAP or mechanical ventilation (see Chapter 24 for details)

VII.   **NEONATAL HYPERBILIRUBINEMIA**
A.   **Physiologic Increases in Bilirubin**
   During the first 3–4 postnatal days infants serum bilirubin increases from cord bilirubin levels of 1.5 mg/dl to $6.5+/-2.5$ mg/dl. The maximum rate of increase in bilirubin for otherwise normal infants with nonhemolytic hyperbilirubinemia is 5 mg/dl/24 hr or 0.2 mg/dl/hr. Visible jaundice on the first day of life or a bilirubin concentration

>10 mg/dl is outside the normal range for rate of increase and suggests a potentially pathologic cause.

B. **Hyperbilirubinemia in Prematurity**

Infants <37 weeks gestation tend to have maximum serum bilirubin levels 30%–50% higher compared with term infants.

C. **Evaluation of Hyperbilirubinemia in the Healthy Newborn**

1. Maternal prenatal testing: ABO and Rh(D) typing and serum screen for isoimmune antibodies
2. Infant or cord blood: Evaluation of blood smear, direct Coombs' test, blood type, and Rh(D) typing if mother has not had prenatal blood typing, is blood type O, or is Rh negative.

D. **Management of Hyperbilirubinemia in the Healthy Term Newborn**

The institution of phototherapy and exchange transfusion remains quite controversial (Table 20.6)

TABLE 20.6

Management of Hyperbilirubinemia in the Healthy Term Newborn*

Age (hr)	TSB Level, mg/dl (mcmol/L)			
	Consider† photo-therapy	Phototherapy	Exchange transfusion if intensive phototherapy fails‡	Exchange transfusion and intensive phototherapy
≤24§	. . .	. . .	. . .	. . .
25–48	≥12 (170)	≥15 (260)	≥20 (340)	≥25 (430)
49–72	≥15 (260)	≥18 (310)	≥25 (430)	≥30 (510)
>72	≥17 (290)	≥20 (340)	≥25 (430)	≥30 (510)

*TSB indicates total serum bilirubin.
†Phototherapy at these TSB levels is a clinical option, meaning that the intervention is available and may be used *on the basis of clinical judgment.*
‡Intensive phototherapy should produce a decline of TSB of 1 to 2 mg/dl within 4 to 6 hours and the TSB level should continue to fall and remain below the threshold level for exchange transfusion. If this does not occur, it is considered a failure of phototherapy.
§Term infants who are clinically jaundiced at ≤24 hours old are not considered healthy and require further evaluation.
From AAP Practice Parameter, *Pediatrics* 94(4): 558, 1994.

E.   **Management of Hyperbilirubinemia in the Preterm Newborn (Table 20.7)**

TABLE 20.7

Guidelines for the Use of Phototherapy in Infants <1 Week of Age (Bilirubin values in mg/dl)

Weight	Phototherapy	Consider exchange transfusion
500–1,000 g	5–7	12–15
1,000–1,500 g	7–10	15–18
1,500–2,500 g	10–15	18–20
>2,500 g	>15	>20

Guidelines do not apply to infants with specific, identified pathologic situations, such as hemolysis, extensive bruising, and those infants who are exceptionally ill or unstable.

F.   **Neonatal Exchange Transfusion**
     (see Chapter 15 for volume calculations)

Note: CBC, reticulocyte count, peripheral smear, bilirubin, Ca, glucose, total protein, infant blood type, and Coombs test should be performed on preexchange sample of blood since they are of no diagnostic value on postexchange blood. If indicated, save preexchange blood for serologic or chromosome studies.

1. Sensitized cells or hyperbilirubinemia
   a. Cross match donor blood against maternal serum for first exchange and against postexchange blood for subsequent exchanges.
   b. Use Type O-negative (low titer), irradiated blood; may use infant's type if no chance of maternal-infant incompatibility. Blood should be stored at room temperature, either fresh or up to 48 hours old, and anticoagulated with ACD or CPD unless infant is acidotic or hypocalcemic.
   c. Make infant NPO during and at least 4 hours after exchange. Empty stomach if infant was fed within 4 hours of procedure.
   d. Follow vital signs, blood sugar, and temperature closely; have resuscitation equipment ready.
   e. Prepare and drape patient for sterile procedure.

    f. Insert umbilical artery and vein catheters as per Chapter 3. During the exchange, blood is removed through the umbilical artery catheter and infused through the venous catheter. If unable to pass an arterial catheter, use a single venous catheter.

    g. Prewarm blood in quality-controlled blood warmer if available; do not improvise with a water bath!

    h. Exchange 15 ml increments in vigorous full-term infants, smaller volumes for smaller, less stable infants. Do not allow cells in donor unit to form sediment.

    i. Withdraw and infuse blood 2–3 ml/kg/min to avoid mechanical trauma to patient and donor cells.

    j. Give 1–2 ml of 10% calcium gluconate solution IV slowly for ECG evidence of hypocalcemia (prolonged Q-Tc intervals). Flush tubing with NaCl before and after calcium infusion. Observe for bradycardia during infusion.

    k. To complete double volume exchange, transfuse 160 ml/kg for full-term infant and 160–200 ml/kg for preterm infant.

    l. Send last aliquot withdrawn for Hct, smear, glucose, bilirubin, potassium, Ca^{2+}, and type and match.

From Kitterman JA et al *Pediatr Clin North Am* 17:895, 1970.

  2. Complications

    a. Cardiovascular: Thromboemboli or air emboli, thromboses, dysrhythmias, volume overload, and cardiorespiratory arrest

    b. Metabolic: Hyperkalemia, hypernatremia, hypocalcemia, hypoglycemia, and acidosis

    c. Hematologic: Thrombocytopenia, DIC, overheparinization, and transfusion reaction

    d. Infectious: Hepatitis, HIV, and bacteremia

    e. Mechanical: Injury to donor cells (especially from overheating), vascular or cardiac perforation, and blood loss

VII. **POLYCYTHEMIA**
A.   **Venous Hematocrit** >65% confirmed on two consecutive samples
B.   **Etiology**
     Delayed cord clamping or intrauterine hypoxia. Fetal hypoxia stimulates erythropoietin resulting in polycythemia.
C.   **Clinical Signs**
     Plethora, respiratory distress, cardiac failure, and neurologic signs including irritability tremors and seizures. Laboratory studies include hypoglycemia, thrombocytopenia, and hyperbilirubinemia
D.   **Complications**
     Hyperviscosity predisposes to venous thrombosis and CNS injury. Hypoglycemia may result from increased erythrocyte utilization of glucose.
E.   **Management**
     Partial exchange transfusion for symptomatic infants with isovolemic replacement of blood with normal saline, lactated Ringer's solution, or 5% salt poor albumin. Blood is exchanged in 10–20 ml increments to reduce HCT to <55. Volume of blood to be withdrawn (V):

$$V(ml) = EBV(ml) \times ([\text{act. HCT} - \text{desired HCT}] / \text{act. HCT})$$

(Note: EBV, Estimated blood volume; *act. HCT,* actual hematocrit.)

VIII. **NECROTIZING ENTEROCOLITIS (NEC)**
      Intestinal inflammation primarily affecting the terminal ileum and colon
A.   **Incidence**
      Approximately 2% of all NICU admissions. 3%–4% of infants with birth weight <2000 g, and <1% infants >2000 g. 75% of infants with NEC are born < 37 weeks gestation and birth weight <2000 g.
B.   **Possible Associated Factors**
      1. Prenatal factors: Maternal age > 35 years, maternal infection requiring antibiotic administration, PROM, cocaine exposure.

2. Perinatal factors: Maternal anesthesia, depressed Apgar scores at 5 minutes, birth asphyxia, respiratory distress syndrome, hypotension
3. Postnatal factors: Patent ductus arteriosus, congestive heart failure, umbilical vessel catheterization, polycythemia, and exchange transfusion
4. Staging criteria (Table 20.8)

TABLE 20.8

Clinical Staging System for NEC

Stage	Clinical findings	Radiographic findings	Treatment	Survival (%)
I (suspected NEC)	Mild abdominal distention; poor feeding; vomiting	Mild ileus	Medical, including workup for sepsis	100
II (definite NEC)	The above, plus marked abdominal distention and GI bleeding	Significant ileus; pneumatosis intestinalis; portal vein gas (9% of cases)	Medical	96
III (advanced NEC)	The above, plus deterioration of vital signs; septic shock	The above, plus pneumoperitoneum (60% of cases)	Surgical	50

From Kosloske A, Musemeche CA; *Clin Perinatol* 16(1): 103, 1989.

IX. **INTRAVENTRICULAR HEMORRHAGE (GMH/IVH)**
A. **Incidence**
   Highest in the first 72 hours of life with overall incidence of 40%–50% of low birth weight infants. Incidence of GMH/IVH increases as gestational age decreases, affecting 20%–40% of infants <25–26 weeks. Approximately 50% of hemorrhages occur on the first postnatal day and <5% after the fourth postnatal day.
B. **Diagnosis and Classification**
   1. Grade I: Hemorrhage in germinal matrix only
   2. Grade II: IVH without ventricular dilitation
   3. Grade III: IVH with ventricular dilitation (30%–45% incidence of motor/intellectual impairment)
   4. Grade IV: IVH with parenchymal extension (60%–80% incidence of motor/intellectual impairment)

From Papile L et al: *J Pediatr* 92:529, 1978; Personal communication, Marilee Allen, M.D., Johns Hopkins Hospital, 1993.

X. RETINOPATHY OF PREMATURITY
A. **Zones of the Retina (Fig. 20.5)**
B. **Stages of Retinopathy of Prematurity (Table 20.9)**

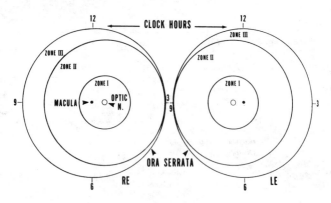

FIG. 20.5. Zones of the retina.

TABLE 20.9

Stage 1	Demarcation line separates avascular from vascularized retina.
Stage 2	Ridge forms along demarcation line.
Stage 3	Extraretinal, fibrovascular proliferation tissue forms on ridge.
Stage 4	Retinal detachment
Plus disease	Posterior tortuosity and engorgement of blood vessels that may be present at any stage
Prethreshold	Zone 1, any stage
	Zone 2, stage 2 and plus disease
	Zone 2, stage 3
Threshold	A level of severity at which the risk of blindness predicted approaches 50%; 5 contiguous or 8 total 30° sectors of stage 3 in zone 1, or zone 2 with plus disease

From Ben-Sira I et al: *Pediatrics* 74:127, 1984.

NEPHROLOGY 21

I. URINALYSIS

A "liquid biopsy of the urinary tract." Evaluate specimen within 1 hour after void, ideally collecting the first morning void.

A. Color (Table 21.1)

TABLE 21.1.

Red	Adriamycin, beets, blackberries, desferoxamine (with elevated serum iron), food-coloring, hemoglobin, phenazopyridine (acid urine), phenolphtalein (laxatives, alkaline urine), phenothiazines, phenytoin, porphyrins, Povan, pyridium, red blood cells, red diaper syndrome (nonpathogenic *Serratia marcescens*), urates (brick dust syndrome)
Yellow-brown	Antimalarials (pamaquine, primaquine, quinicrine), azulfidine (alkaline urine), B-complex vitamins, bilirubin, carotene, cascara, metronidazole, nitrofurantoin, sulfonamides
Brown-black	Hemosiderin, homogentisic urine (alkaptonuria), melanin (especially in alkaline urine), myoglobin, old blood, quinine, rhubarb
Burgundy	Porphyrins (old urine)
Deep yellow	Riboflavin
Orange	Phenazopyridine, rifampin, urates, warfarin
Blue-green	Adriamycin, amitriptyline, biliverdin (obstructive jaundice), blue diaper syndrome (familial disorder characterized by hypercalcemica, nephrocalcinosis, and indicanuria), indomethicin, methylene blue, *Pseudomonas,* UTI (rare), riboflavin

B. Turbidity

Can be normal; most often due to crystal formation at room temperature. Uric acid crystals form in acidic urine, phosphate crystals in alkaline urine. Cellular material and bacteria can also cause turbidity.

C. Specific Gravity

1. Hydrometer/urinometer: Requires at least 15 ml of urine at room temperature. Device must be free-floating in the sample.
2. Refractometer: Requires only one drop of urine. Based on the principle that the refractive index (RI) of a solution is related to the content of dissolved solids

present. The RI varies with but is not identical to specific gravity. The refractometer measures RI but is calibrated for specific gravity. Glucose, abundant protein, and iodine-containing contrast materials can give falsely high readings.

D. pH

Estimated using indicator paper or dipstick. To improve accuracy, use freshly voided specimen and pH meter.

E. Protein

1. Tests for protein: Significant proteinuria as determined by the following tests should be confirmed by a 24-hour collection:

   a. Dipstick: Easiest method. Significant if ≥ 1+ (30 mg/dl) on 2 of 3 random samples 1 week apart, if urine specific gravity is <1.015 or ≥2+ (100 mg/dl) on similarly collected urine, if specific gravity is >1.015. False positives can occur with highly concentrated alkaline urine (pH>8), gross hematuria, pyuria, bacteriuria, quaternary ammonium cleansers (e.g., antiseptics, chlorhexidine, or benzalkonium). False negatives can occur with very dilute or acidic urine (pH 4.5) and nonalbumin proteinuria.

   b. Sulfosalicylic acid (SSA) test: Add 0.5–0.8 ml (5–8 drops) of 20% SSA to 5 ml of urine (pH 4.5–6.5) and examine for turbidity. Barely evident turbidity is graded ±; increasing amounts of turbidity are graded 1–4+. False positives result from cephalosporins, concentrated urine, gross hematuria, IV contrast, TPN, penicillins, phosphates, sulfonamides, tolbutamide.

   c. Protein/creatinine ratio: Determine ratio of protein (mg/dl) and creatinine (mg/dl) concentrations in a randomly collected spot urine during normal ambulation. A ratio ≥ 0.2 suggests significant proteinuria, which should be confirmed with a 24-hour urine collection.

From Ginsberg JM et al: *N Engl J Med* 309:1543, 1983.

   d. 24-hour urine collection (see Section II.A.1.a under timed urine specimen for creatinine clearance): Most accurate method.

   Normal: ≤4 mg/m^2/hr; Abnormal: 4–40 mg/m^2/hr; Nephrotic range: ≥40 mg/m^2/hr.

From Norman ME: *Ped Clin of North Am* 34:553, 1987.

2. Types of proteinuria
   a. Glomerular proteinuria: Occurs when alterations in the charge or size barrier result in increased permeability of the glomerular capillary walls to large plasma proteins.
      1) Transient proteinuria: Most common in children. Associated with exercise, postural changes, cold exposure, fever, emotional stress, dehydration, seizure, congestive heart failure, and epinephrine infusion. Serial urines should be negative for protein.
      2) Orthostatic proteinuria: Common, not associated with renal pathology. For diagnosis, obtain a fractionated 24 hour urine collection:
         a) Have patient wake up at 8 AM, void completely, and discard the urine.
         b) Begin collecting all voided urine from this point into container #1. The patient should attempt to void at 4 PM and add the urine to container #1.
         c) All urine voided from 4 PM until bedtime should be collected in container #2. The patient should void completely before retiring and add the urine to container #2.
         d) Collect the remainder of the urine from bedtime until 8 AM in container #3. The patient should void at 8 AM since this may be the only urine in container #3. It is important that the patient does not ambulate before this void.
         e) Record the specific gravity and measure protein concentration for the urine in each container. The diagnosis of orthostatic proteinuria is confirmed if samples #1 and/or #2 have significant proteinuria, whereas the urine in container #3 yields no significant protein.
      3) Proteinuria secondary to glomerulopathies: Occurs in the presence of disorders of glomerular structure and function
   b. Tubular proteinuria: Documented by the presence of low molecular weight proteins in the urine
      1) Overload proteinuria: Occurs when excessive amounts of low molecular weight proteins over-

whelm the tubular resorptive capacity (e.g., light chains [multiple myeloma], lysozyme [monocytic and myelocytic leukemias], myoglobin [rhabdomyolysis], and hemoglobin [hemolysis])

2) Tubular proteinuria associated with tubular dysfunction or disorders (such as Fanconi's syndrome): Occurs when normal amounts of low molecular weight proteins (e.g., amino acids) are not adequately resorbed because of damaged tubular cells

3. Suggested work-up of proteinuria includes the following:

   a. Blood electrolytes, BUN, serum creatinine, protein, cholesterol, hepatitis serologies, and immunoglobulins

   b. C3, C4, ASO, ANA

   c. Renal ultrasound (and other radiologic studies as indicated)

   d. Referral to a pediatric nephrologist

   e. Consider obtaining tests for HIV

From Norman ME: *Ped Clin North Am* 34:556, 1987.

F. Sugars

Normally, urine does not contain sugars. Glucosuria is suggestive but not diagnostic of diabetes mellitus or proximal renal tubular disease (see Section II.B.1.b). The presence of other reducing sugars can be confirmed by chromatography.

1. Dipstick: Easiest method but specific for glucose. False negatives occur with high levels of ascorbic acid (used as preservative in antibiotics) in urine.

2. Clinitest tablets (Ames Co): Identifies all reducing substances in urine including reducing sugars (glucose, fructose, galactose, pentoses, lactose), amino acids, ascorbic acid, chloral hydrate, chloramphenicol, creatinine, cysteine, glucuronates, hippurate, homogentisic acid, isoniazid, ketone bodies, nitrofurantoin, oxalate, TPN, penicillin, salicylates, streptomycin, sulfonamides, tetracycline, and uric acid. Since sucrose is not a reducing sugar it is not detected by Clinitest.

   a. Method: Mix 5 drops of urine, 10 drops of water, and 1 tablet. Compare color with standard scale. (Table 21.2)

TABLE 21.2

Color	% Reducing substance
Blue	Negative
Greenish blue	Trace
Green	0.5
Greenish brown	1.0
Yellow	1.5
Brick red	2.0

G. Ketones

Except for trace amounts, ketonuria suggests ketoacidosis, usually from either diabetes mellitus or catabolism induced by inadequate intake. Neonatal ketoacidosis may occur with a metabolic defect, such as propionic acidemia, methylmalonic aciduria, or a glycogen storage disease.

1. Dipstick: Detects acetoacetic acid best, acetone less well; does not detect beta-hydroxybutyrate. False positives may occur after phthalein administration or with PKU.
2. Acetest tablets (Ames Co): Detects only acetoacetic acid and acetone

H. Hemoglobin/Myoglobin/RBCs

Centrifuged urine usually contains fewer than 5 RBCs/hpf. Significant hematuria is 5–10 RBCs/hpf and corresponds to a Chemstrip reading of 50 RBCs/hpf or Labstix reading "trace hemolyzed" or "small."

1. Dipstick: Positive with intact RBCs, hemoglobin, and myoglobin; can detect as few as 3–4 RBCs/hpf. False positives can occur with the presence of bacterial peroxidases, high ascorbic acid concentrations, and Betadine (i.e., from fingers of medical staff).
2. Microscopy: Used to differentiate hemoglobinuria or myoglobinuria from hematuria (intact RBCs). In addition, examination of RBC morphology by phase contrast microscopy may help localize the source of bleeding. Dysmorphic small RBCs suggests a glomerular origin, whereas normal RBCs suggests lower tract bleeding.
3. Differentiation of hemoglobinuria and myoglobinuria
   a. History: Hemoglobinuria is seen with intravascular hemolysis or in hematuric urine that has stood for an

extended period. Myoglobinuria is seen in crush injuries, vigorous exercise, major motor seizures, fever and malignant hyperthermia, electrocution, snakebite, ischemia, and some muscle and metabolic disorders.

   b. Lab studies: Clinical laboratories may use many techniques to directly measure hemoglobin or myoglobin. Other laboratory data may also be used to indirectly identify the source of urinary pigment. For example, in nephropathy from myoglobinuria, the BUN/creatinine ratio is low (creatinine is released from damaged muscles) and CPK is high.

4. Suggested work-up of persistent hematuria

   a. Examination of urine sediment, urine culture, sickle cell screen, urine calcium:creatinine ratio

   b. Serum electrolytes, BUN, serum creatinine, serum total protein and albumin, immunoglobulins, hepatitis serologies, and consider testing for HIV

   c. ASO titers, C3, C4, ANA

   d. Renal ultrasound and other indicated radiologic studies

   e. Referral to a pediatric nephrologist

From Norman ME: *Pediatr Clin North Am* 34:550, 1987.

I.   Bilirubin/Urobilingen

1. Dipstick: Measures each individually. Both are normally present in the urine in only very small amounts.

2. Correlating the results of both tests can provide helpful diagnostic information (Table 21.3)

TABLE 21.3

	Normal	Hemolytic disease	Hepatic disease	Biliary obstruction
Urine urobilogen	Normal	Increased	Increased	Decreased
Urine bilirubin	Negative	Negative	±	Positive

From Modern urinalysis, 1974:51.

J.   Sediment

Using light microscopy, unstained, centrifuged urine can be examined for formed elements, including casts, cells, and crystals. Centrifuge 10 ml for 5 minutes, then decant 9 ml of supernatant. Resuspend sediment in remaining 1 ml of urine. Place drop on glass slide; use coverslip. Best results with subdued light. Focus particularly on edge of coverslip since formed elements collect there. See color plates for illustration of urine sediment.

From Henry JB: *Clinical diagnosis and management by laboratory methods,* Philadelphia, 1984, WB Saunders; Greenhill A et al: *Pediatr Clin North Am* 23:661, 1976.

Urine microscopy

	Color Plate
Red blood cells and white blood cells	1
White blood cells with bacteria in an infected urine specimen	2
Fine granular cast	3
White blood cell cast (seen in intrinsic renal diseases such as pyelonephritis and glomerulonephritis; note the discernible nuclei and cell boundaries)	4
Red blood cell cast (the distinct and uniformly spherical shape of the erythrocyte is visible)	5
Epithelial cast (present in tubular disease)	6
Trichomonas vaginalis	7
Budding yeast forms	8
Calcium oxalate crystals	9
Phosphate crystals	10
Urate crystals	11
Cystine crystal (indicative of cystinuria)	12

Color Plates 1, 3–9, and 12: Urine under the microscope, 1975, ROCOM.
Color Plate 2: Birch DF et al: *A color atlas of urine microscopy,* 1994, Chapman & Hall Medical.
Color Plates 10 and 11: Netter FH, Shapter RK, Yonkman FF: The CIBA collection of medical illustrations, 6:80, 1973.

K. Screening Tests for Urinary Tract Infections (UTIs)

Note: All tests must be confirmed with a urine culture.

1. Dipstick
   a. Nitrite test: Detects nitrites produced by the reduction of dietary nitrates by urinary bacteria (especially *E. coli, Klebsiella,* and *Proteus*). A positive test is virtually diagnostic of bacteriuria. False negatives can occur with inadequate dietary nitrates, insufficient time for bacterial proliferation or conversion of nitrates to nitrites, inability of bacteria to reduce nitrates to nitrites (many gram positive organisms as

well as *Enterococcus, Mycobacterium,* and fungi), and large volumes of dilute urine.
   b. Leukocyte esterase test: Detects esterases released from broken-down leukocytes. This is therefore an indirect test for WBCs that may or may not be present with a UTI.
2. Urine gram stain: Used to screen for UTIs. One organism/hpf in uncentrifuged urine represents at least 10^5 colonies/ml.

From Feigin RD, Cherry JD: *Pediatr Infect Dis,* 483, 1992.

II. RENAL FUNCTION TESTS
A. Tests of Glomerular Function
May be determined by the following methods:
1. Creatinine clearance (Ccr)
   a. Timed urine specimen: Standard measure of glomerular filtration rate (GFR); closely approximates inulin clearance in the normal range of GFR. When GFR is low, Ccr is greater than inulin clearance. Inaccurate in children with obstructive uropathy.
      Method: Collect urine over any time period; record interval to the nearest minute. Have patient empty bladder (discard specimen) before beginning the collection. Collect all urine during the time interval, including urine voided at the end of the collection period. If the patient's renal function is stable, draw blood sample for serum creatinine once during the test period. (If function is changing rapidly, draw the blood sample at the beginning and end of the period and use the average.)

$$\text{Ccr (ml/min/1.73m}^2) = (U \times V/P) \times 1.73/SA$$

Note: U (mg/dl), Urinary creatinine concentration; V (ml/min), total urine volume (ml) divided by the duration of the collection (min) (24 hrs = 1440 min); P (mg/dl), serum creatinine concentration (may average two levels); SA (m²), surface area.

   b. Estimated creatinine clearance from plasma creatinine: Useful when a timed specimen cannot be collected; correlates well with standard creatinine clearance for children with relatively normal body habitus. If habitus is markedly abnormal, then more standard methods of measuring Ccr must be used.

Estimated Ccr (ml/min/1.73m^2) = **k×L/Pcr**

Note: k, Proportionality constant, L; height (cm); Pcr = plasma creatinine (mg/dl).

k Values

LBW during first year of life	0.33
Term AGA during first year of life	0.45
Children and adolescent girls	0.55
Adolescent boys	0.70

From Schwartz GJ et al: *Pediatr Clin North Am* 34:571, 1987.

    2. Glomerular function as determined by nuclear medicine scans (see Chapter 25)
    3. Normal values of GFR (measured by inulin clearance) (Table 21.4)

TABLE 21.4

Age	GFR - Mean (ml/min/1.73 m^2)	Range (ml/min/1.73 m^2)
Neonates <34 weeks gestational age		
2–8 days	11	11–15
4–28 days	20	15–28
30–90 days	50	40–65
Neonates >34 weeks gestational age		
2–8 days	39	17–60
4–28 days	47	26–68
30–90 days	58	30–86
1–6 months	77	39–114
6–12 months	103	49–157
12–19 months	127	62–191
2–12 years	127	89–165

From Holliday MA et al: *Pediatric nephrology*, Baltimore, 1994, Williams & Wilkins.

B. Tests of Tubular Function
    1. Proximal tubule
      a. Proximal tubule reabsorption: The proximal tubule is responsible for the resorption of electrolytes, glucose, and amino acids. Studies to determine proximal tubular function compare urine and blood levels of specific compounds arriving at a percent tubular resorption (Tx):

$$Tx = 1 - \frac{Ux/Px}{Ucr/Pcr} \times 100\%$$

(Note: Ux, Concentration of compound in urine; Px, concentration of compound in plasma; Ucr, concentration creatinine in urine; Pcr, concentration of creatinine in plasma.) This formula is also used for amino acids, electrolytes, calcium and phosphorus.

   b. Glucose reabsorption: The glucose threshold is the plasma glucose concentration at which significant amounts of glucose appear in the urine. The presence of glucosuria must be interpreted in relation to simultaneously determined plasma glucose concentration. If the plasma glucose concentration is <120 mg/dl, and glucose is present in the urine, this implies incompetent tubular reabsorption of glucose and proximal renal tubular disease. (For discussion of normal values and further studies of proximal tubule function consult Holliday MA et al: *Pediatric nephrology,* Baltimore, 1994, Williams & Wilkins.)

   c. Urine calcium: Hypercalciuria is seen with RTA, vitamin D intoxication, hyperparathyroidism, steroids, immobilization, excessive calcium intake, and loop diuretics. It may be idiopathic (associated with hematuria and renal calculi). Diagnosis is as follows:
      1) 24-hour urine: Calcium >4 mg/kg/24 hr
      2) Spot urine: Determine Ca/Cr ratio. It is recommended that an abnormal spot urine Ca/Cr ratio be followed-up with a 24-hour urine calcium determination (Table 21.5).

TABLE 21.5

Age	Ca/Cr ratio (mg/mg ratio) (95th percentile for age)
<7 months	0.86
7–18 months	0.6
19 month–6 years	0.42
Adults	0.22

From Sargent JD et al: *J Pediatr* 123: 393, 1993.

d. Bicarbonate reabsorption (proximal RTA): The majority of bicarbonate reabsorption occurs in the proximal tubule. Abnormalities in reabsorption lead to type II RTA. These patients have high fractional excretion of bicarbonate in their urine at normal serum bicarbonate levels. However, they can acidify their urine when in the face of metabolic acidosis.

2. Distal tubule

a. Urine acidification (distal RTA): A urine acidification defect should be suspected when random urine pH values are >6 in the presence of moderate systemic metabolic acidosis. Acidification defects should be confirmed by simultaneous venous or arterial pH, plasma bicarbonate concentration, and pH meter (not dipstick) determination of the pH of fresh urine.

1) Ammonium chloride test: Seldom performed since the diagnosis can usually be established by the tests above repeated at different points in time

a) Perform test in consultation with a nephrologist.

b) Proceed only if the child is well hydrated.

c) Administer 75 mEq/m^2 ammonium chloride PO over 1 hour

d) Measure urine pH (pH meter) every hour for 5 hours.

e) Measure plasma bicarbonate concentration 3 hours after administration of ammonium chloride. Normally, the plasma bicarbonate concentration should fall 4–5 mEq/L, and the urine pH should fall below 5.5. If the urine pH does not fall as the plasma bicarbonate falls, then one would suspect type I RTA. If the plasma bicarbonate concentration is not below 20 mEq/L (18 for infants), larger doses of ammonium chloride may be necessary to produce plasma bicarbonate concentrations below an abnormal renal bicarbonate reabsorption threshold. Extreme care should be taken when using larger doses of ammonium chloride.

From Edelmann CM et al: *Pediatr Res* 1452, 1967.

2) Types of RTA (Table 21.6)

TABLE 21.6

	Type I (distal)	Type II (proximal)	Type III*	Type IV†
Growth failure	+++	++	+++	+++
Nephrocalcinosis	++	Rare	±	Rare
Fractional excretion of HCO_3 at normal serum HCO_3 levels	<5	>15	5–15	<15
Plasma K^+	Low	Low	Low	High
Urine pH with acidosis (acidosis may be induced by ammonium chloride)	>5.5	<5.5	>5.5	Variable

*Defect in distal tubular hydrogen ion excretion plus bicarbonaturia.
†Associated with hyperchloremic acidosis and hyperkalemia. Seen with adrenal insufficiency, obstructive uropathy, diabetic nephropathy, pyelonephritis, and other disorders.
Modified from Kher KW, Makker SP: *Clinical pediatric nephrology,* 672; McSherry E: *Kidney Int* 20:799, 1981.

b. Urine concentration: A random urine specific gravity of 1.023 or more indicates intact concentrating ability within the limits of clinical testing; no further tests are indicated. A first-voided specimen following an overnight fast is adequate to test concentrating ability. For more formal testing, see water deprivation test (Chapter 10).

From Edelmann CM et al: *Am J Dis Child* 114:639, 1967.

III. OLIGURIA

Urine output <300 ml/m^2/24 hr; or <0.5 ml/kg/hr in children, and <1.0 ml/kg/hr in infants

A. BUN/Cr Ratio (both in mg/dl)

1. Normal: 10–20; suggests intrinsic renal disease in the setting of oliguria
2. >20: suggests dehydration, prerenal azotemia, or GI bleeding
3. <5: liver disease, starvation, inborn error of metabolism

From Greenhill A et al: *Pediatr Clin North Am* 23:661, 1976.

B. Laboratory Differentiation (Table 21.7)

TABLE 21.7

Test	Prerenal oliguria		Low output failure		ADH secretion
Urine sodium	<20	(<40)	(>40)	(>40)	>40
Specific gravity	<1.020	(1.015)	<1.010	(<1.015)	>1.020
Osmolality (mOsm/L)	>500	(>400)	<350	(<400)	>500
Urine/plasma osmolality ratio	>1.3		<1.3		>2
Urea nitrogen	>20		<10		>15
Creatinine	>40	(>20)	<20	(<15)	>30
RFI*	<1	(<3)	>1	(>3.0)	>1
FE (Na)†	<1	(<2.5)	>1	(>3.0)	Close to 1

Numbers in parenthesis are for neonates.
*RFI (renal failure index) = (UNa × 100)/UCrPCr.
†FE (Na) (fractional excretion of sodium) = (UNa/PNa)/(UCr/PCr) × 100.
Adapted from Rogers et al: *Textbook of pediatric intensive care,* Baltimore, 1992, Williams and Wilkins.

IV. ACUTE DIALYSIS
A. Indications
1. Metabolic or fluid derangements not controlled by aggressive medical management alone. Generally accepted criteria include the following, however a nephrologist should be always be consulted:
   a. Volume overload with evidence of pulmonary edema or hypertension, which is refractory to therapy
   b. Hyperkalemia >6.0 mEq/L if hypercatabolic or >6.5 mEq/L despite conservative measures
   c. Metabolic acidosis with pH <7.2 or HCO_3 <10
   d. BUN >150; lower if rising rapidly
   e. Neurologic symptoms secondary to uremia or electrolyte imbalance
   f. Calcium/phosphorus imbalance (e.g., hypocalcemia with tetany or seizures in the presence of a very high serum phosphate)
2. Dialyzable toxin or poison (i.e., lactate, ammonia)
B. Techniques
1. Peritoneal dialysis (PD): Requires catheter to access the peritoneal cavity. May be used acutely as well as chronically as in continuous ambulatory or continuous cycling peritoneal dialysis.

a. Available fluids and additives
   1) A commonly used commercial dialysate (Baxter) contains 132 mEq Na, 3.5 mEq Ca, 0.5 mEq Mg, 96 mEq Cl, and 40 mEq lactate in each liter.
   2) This solution is available with 1.5%, 2.5%, or 4.25% dextrose. Dextrose content is selected depending on the amount of ultrafiltrate desired. Fluid is removed more rapidly with higher dextrose concentrations. Excessive use of higher osmolar solutions may result in hypovolemia and hypotension.
   3) Heparin may be added (100–500 U/L) to the initial dialysate to prevent clots from forming; this can be discontinued when the outflow is clear.
   4) Cephalothin (250–500 mg/L) or other antibiotics may be added to the dialysate as the situation warrants. A nephrologist should be consulted.
   5) If the serum K is <3.5 mEq/L, then K may be given IV or added to the dialysate (3–4 mEq/L).
2. Hemodialysis (HD): Requires placement of special vascular access devices. May be the method of choice for certain toxins (e.g., ammonia, uric acid, or poisons) or when there are contraindications to peritoneal dialysis.

From Rogers MC: *Textbook of pediatric intensive care,* Baltimore, 1992, Williams and Wilkins.

3. Continuous arteriovenous hemofiltration/hemodialysis (CAVH(-D)) and continuous venovenous hemofiltration/hemodialysis (CVVH(-D)): CAVH and CVVH are therapies whose primary goal is the continuous generation of a plasma ultrafiltrate. Indications include fluid management, renal failure with profound hemodynamic instability, electrolyte disturbance(s), intoxications of substances that are freely filtered across particular ultrafiltration membrane utilized. CAVH and CVVH can be helpful in the management of oliguric patients in need of better nutritional support, postoperative cardiac patients, and patients with septicemia. CAVH-D and CVVH-D offer added dimensions to these therapies. With these procedures, the standard circuit is initiated, and dialysate is introduced into the hemofiltration car-

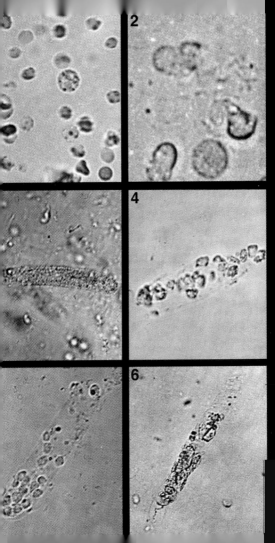

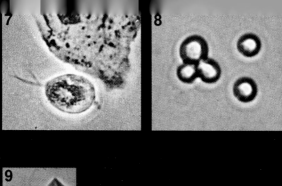

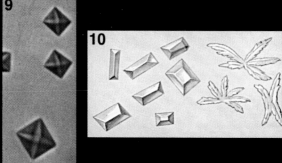

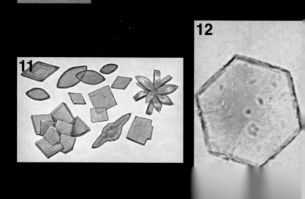

tridge, where it surrounds the blood filled capillary lumen. The exposure of the dialysate as it traverses the cartridge enhances diffusion, dramatically increasing the clearance of electrolytes. A standard PD solution can be used. These therapies also require special vascular access devices.

C. **Peritoneal Dialysis (PD) vs. Hemodialysis (HD) vs CAVH/CVVH (Table 21.8)**

TABLE 21.8

	PD	HD	CAVH/CVVH
BENEFITS			
Fluid removal	+	++	++
Urea and creatinine clearance	+	++	+
Potassium clearance	++	++	+
Toxin clearance	+	++	+
COMPLICATIONS			
Abdominal pain	+	–	–
Bleeding	–	+	+
Decreased cardiac output	+	+	+
Disequilibrium	–	+	–
Electrolyte imbalance	+	+	+
Need for heparinization	–	+	+
Hyperglycemia	+	–	–
Hypotension	+	++	+
Hypothermia	–	–	+
Infection (other than peritonitis)	–	+	+
Inguinal hernia	+	–	–
Lactic acidosis	Possible	–	Possible
Neutropenia	–	+	–
Pancreatitis	+	–	–
Peritonitis	+	–	–
Protein loss	++	–	–
Respiratory compromise	+	Possible	–
Thrombocytopenia	–	+	–
Vessel thrombosis	–	+	+

Adapted from Rogers MC: *Textbook of pediatric intensive care*, Baltimore, 1992, Williams and Wilkins.

NEUROLOGY

22

I. NEUROLOGIC EXAM
A complete neurologic exam is rarely productive in the absence of specific concerns raised by the history.

A. Mental Status
Alertness, attention, behavior, language, orientation, memory, abstraction, judgment

B. Cranial Nerves (Table 22.1)

C. Motor
1. Muscle bulk
2. Tone: High, low
   a. Least resistance to passive movement
   b. Stiffness with active skills
   c. Regional increases in tone suggesting cortical dysfunction: adducted thumbs, limited hand supination, equinus of feet

TABLE 22.1.

Function/region	Cranial nerve	Test, observation
Vision	II	Acuity, fields, color
Pupils	II, III, sympathetics	Shape, size, reaction to light, accommodation
Eye movements and eyelids	III, IV, VI	Range and quality of eye movements, saccades, pursuits, nystagmus, ptosis
Sensation	V	Corneals
Facial strength	VII	Observe degree of expression of emotions, eye or lip closure strength
Mouth, pharynx	VII, IX, X, XII	Swallowing, speech quality (nasal, deficits in labial, lingual, or palatal sound production), symmetric palatal elevation, tongue protrusion
Head control	XI	Head position and movement

3. Strength: Observe, describe activity such as arising from the floor. Quantify (e.g., distance of broad jump, time to run 30 feet, time to climb stairs)
4. Medical Research Council (MRC) Strength Rating Scale
   a. 0/5: No movement
   b. 1/5: Palpable tightening only
   c. 2/5: Movement in a gravity neutral plane
   d. 3/5: Full range of movement against gravity
   e. 4/5: Subnormal strength
   f. 5/5: Normal strength

D. **Muscle Stretch (Deep Tendon) Reflexes**
   Important for determining CNS involvement with weakness or to discern asymmetries. Less important in setting of normal strength and coordination (Table 22.2)

TABLE 22.2.

Reflex	Biceps	Brachio-radialis	Triceps	Knee	Ankle
Site	C5,6	C5,6	C7,8	L(2,3)4	S1

E. **Sensory**
   Primary disorders of sensation are rare in children, but the following tests may be useful in anatomic localization:
   1. Spinal cord dysfunction of discrete pathways
      a. Anterior cord: Test pin, temperature sensation
      b. Posterior cord: Test Romberg, position sense
   2. Transverse spinal cord dysfunction, especially of concern if bowel or bladder abnormal; use pinprick to identify level of impairment.
   3. Syringomyelia: Look for decreased pain or temperature sensibility bilaterally, with preserved proprioception, at the level of the syrinx, with preserved function below.
   4. Polyneuropathy: Look for proximal/distal gradient of loss of sensations, especially vibratory, pin.
   5. Mononeuropathies: Pinprick to localize area of anesthesia. (Figs. 22.1 and 22.2)

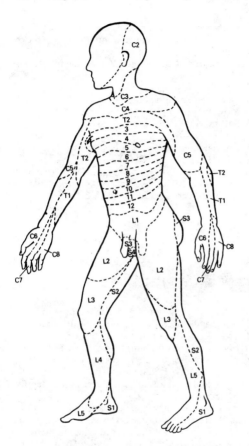

FIG. 22.1. Spinal dermatome. *(From Devinsky O, Feldman E: Examination of the cranial and peripheral nerves, New York, 1988, Churchill Livingstone.)*

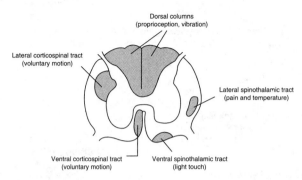

FIG. 22.2. Spinal pathways.

F. Coordination

Evaluate general coordination while watching activities like throwing a ball, dressing, playing video games. Test rapid alternation and repetitive movements, finger to nose, heel to shin, walking, and running.

G. Development

Refer to Chapter 9.

II. HEADACHES

A. Differential Diagnosis of Acute or Progressive Headache

1. Increased intracranial pressure (ICP): Trauma, hemorrhage, tumor, hydrocephalus, pseudotumor cerebri, abscess
2. Decreased ICP: After VP shunt or lumbar puncture (LP), cerebrospinal fluid (CSF) leak from basilar skull fracture
3. Meningeal pain: Meningitis, leukemia, blood
4. Vascular: Vasculitis, AVM, hypertension
5. Bone, soft tissue. Referred pain: Scalp, eyes, ears, sinuses, nose, teeth, pharynx, cervical spine

B. Differential Diagnosis of Chronic Recurrent Headache

1. Migraine (with or without aura)
2. Nonspecific ("tension" or "muscular")
3. Psychogenic: Depression, anxiety, conversion
4. Secondary to sleep deprivation (e.g., in overweight children with sleep apnea)

C. **Evaluation**
 1. History and physical: Differentiate acute or chronic progressive from stable (duration 6 months or longer), chronic recurrent headaches. Careful general neurologic and fundoscopic exams.
 2. Studies as indicated (e.g., CT/MRI for focal neurologic findings, increased ICP, atypical headache pattern, seizures)

D. **Migraine Headache**
 1. Characteristics: Chronic recurrent, throbbing/pulsatile, relieved by sleep; triggered by stress, caffeine, diet, menses; associated symptoms: nausea, vomiting, abdominal pain, photophobia
 2. Classification
    a. With aura, "classic," often fronto-temporal, unilateral (may have associated neurologic complications)
    b. Without aura, "common," often bilateral frontal
 3. Complications (rare): Paresthesias, visual field cuts, aphasia, hemiplegia, ophthalmoplegia, basilar artery migraine, confusion
 4. Treatment
    a. Prophylaxis: Avoid triggers, improve general health with good diet, aerobic exercise, regular sleep; explore issues of secondary gain/role of pain in the family's relationships; consider medications such as propranolol, cyproheptadine, verapamil, valproate.
    b. Acute symptomatic: Dark, quiet room, sleep, acetominophen, NSAIDs, ergotamine, antiemetics (e.g., metoclopramide), sumatriptan succinate (see Formulary)

From Singer H, Rowe S: *Pediatr Ann* 21:6, 369.

III. **PAROXYSMAL EVENTS**
 Transient alterations in neurologic function, which may or may not be seizures

A. **Differential Diagnosis of Recurrent Events that Mimic Epilepsy in Childhood (Table 22.3)**

B. **Evaluation of Paroxysmal Events**
 1. History: Description, time course, and setting of event; history of illness, trauma, medication, toxins, fever; presence of postictal period, past history, or family history of similar events

TABLE 22.3.

Differential Diagnosis of Recurrent Events that Mimic Epilepsy in Childhood

Event	Differentiation from epilepsy
Pseudoseizure (psychogenic seizure)	No EEG changes except movement artifact during event. Movements are thrashing rather than clonic.
Paroxysmal vertigo	Patient is frightened and crying, no loss of awareness.
GE reflux in infancy, childhood (Sandifer's syndrome)	Paroxysmal dystonic posturing associated with meals
Breath-holding spells	Loss of consciousness and convulsion are always provoked by an event that makes the child cry.
Syncope	Loss of consciousness with onset of vertigo, clouded or tunnel vision. Slow collapse to floor. Triggered by postural change, heat, emotion, etc.
Cardiogenic syncope	Abnormal ECG (e.g., prolonged QT, AV block, other arrhythmia). Exercise may trigger. Patient has episodic loss of consciousness without consistent convulsive movement.
Paroxysmal kinesigenic choreoathetosis	Event generally occurs on arising. Movements are not accompanied by change in alertness.
Shuddering attacks	Brief shivering spells with continued awareness
Night terrors	Brief nocturnal episodes of terror without typical convulsive movements
Rages	Provoked and goal-directed

Modified from Murphy JV, Dehkharghani F: Diagnosis of childhood seizure disorders, *Epilepsia* 35(Suppl 2):S7–S17, 1994.

2. Physical examination; Mental status, behavior, asymmetry, paralysis, trauma, cardiac abnormalities, phakomatosis
3. Studies: Depends on clinical setting. Consider glucose, sodium, calcium, magnesium, BUN, creatinine, CBC, toxicology screen, blood pressure (supine and upright), EEG ± video monitoring, ECG, head CT, MRI, lumbar puncture.

Note: Epilepsy is not a diagnosis of exclusion and should not be treated in the absence of strong suspicion.

C. **Seizure Disorders**
1. Seizure: Paroxysmal discharge of cortical neurons resulting in alteration of function (motor, sensory, cognitive)
2. Epilepsy: Two or more seizures not precipitated by a known cause
3. Status epilepticus: Prolonged or recurrent seizures lasting over 30 minutes without the patient regaining consciousness
4. Etiology: Idiopathic, hypoxic insult, congenital defect, acquired cortical defect (stroke, neoplasm, infection), genetic disorder, inborn error of metabolism, congenital brain malformation
5. Diagnosis: Two elements, etiology and seizure type; the seizure type (e.g., primary generalized or primary partial) generally determines treatment
6. Treatment: Individualize. Weigh the risk of further seizures without therapy against the risk of treatment side effects plus further seizures despite therapy. Monotherapy may reduce complications (Table 22.4).

D. **Special Seizure Syndromes**
1. Febrile seizure: Brief generalized seizure associated with a febrile illness but without any CNS infection or neurologic cause. Etiology seems to be lowered seizure threshold in immature brain in association with febrile illness.
   a. Incidence: 3%–5% of children, 6 months to 5 years old.
   b. Evaluation: History of event and physical examination to look for high risk, "complex" features: onset more than 24 hours after onset of illness, duration longer than 15 minutes, focality, 2 discrete episodes within 24 hours, abnormal neurologic exam. Consider further evaluation if any one of these are present.
   c. Treatment: None indicated for simple febrile seizures unless frequent recurrence disrupts normal functioning. Educate parents about benign nature of events and antipyretics.
   d. Outcome
      1) Risk of recurrence is 30% for second episode, 17% for third, 9% for greater than three.

TABLE 22.4.

Seizure type		Anticonvulsant medications*
Primary partial (focal EEG changes at onset of seizure)	Partial-simple (conscious) motor, sensory, autonomic. Partial-complex (consciousness impaired). Partial with secondary generalization: "Grand mal," tonic clonic.	CBZ, PHT, PB, VPA, (Primidone)
Primary generalized (generalized EEG spikes at outset of seizure)	Febrile	Generally not indicated
	Tonic clonic	VPA
	Absence, "Petit mal"	ES, VPA
	Juvenile myoclonic	VPA
Others	Neonatal	PB, PHT, Acetazolamide
	Infantile spasms (West syndrome)	ACTH, Corticosteroids, VPA, Benzodiazepines
	Mixed axial tonic, atypical absence, tonic clonic, myoclonic (Lennox Gastaut)	VPA

*See Formulary for doses and side effects. *CBZ,* Carbamazepine; *PHT,* phenytoin; *VPA,* valproic acid; *PB,* phenobarbital; *ES,* ethosuximide.
The Ketogenic Diet may be helpful in the management of intractable tonic and or clonic and myoclonic seizures.
Modified from Dodson WE, Bourgeois BFD: Pharmacology and therapeutic aspects of antiepileptic drugs in pediatrics, *Journal of Child Neurology* 9, Suppl. 2, 2S1–2S7, 1994.

    2) Risk of epilepsy: 2%. Increased in children with 2 or more of the following: complex febrile seizures, previously abnormal development, family history of nonfebrile seizures.

From Freeman J: *Pediatr Ann* 21:6, 355.

  2. Neonatal Seizure: Various paroxysmal behaviors or electrical events. May be tonic, myoclonic, clonic, or subtle (blinking, chewing, pedaling, apnea) because of CNS immaturity.

    a. Etiologies of neonatal seizure: Hypoxic ischemic encephalopathy (35%–42%); intracranial hemorrhage/infarction (15%–20%); CNS infection (12%–17%); CNS malformation (5%); metabolic (e.g., hypoglycemia, hypocalcemia, pyridoxine deficiency, toxins [3%–5%], other [5%–20%]).

b. Evaluation: Clinical criteria. 50% may have no EEG changes.

c. Treatment: Efficacy of standard anticonvulsants is poor (Table 22.5).

d. Outcome: Variable, depends on etiology

From Ichord R: *Pediatr Ann* 21:6, 339.

TABLE 22.5.

Treatment of Neonatal Seizures

ESTABLISH AIRWAY, ENSURE OXYGENATION AND CIRCULATION.

TREAT METABOLIC ABNORMALITIES

Hypoglycemia	0.25–0.5 g/kg IV bolus (10% dextrose) followed by a 8mg/kg/min IV drip as required
Hypocalcemia	10mg/kg elemental calcium given as calcium gluconate by slow IV infusion

TREAT WITH MEDICATIONS

Phenobarbital	15–20 mg/kg loading dose IV. Additional boluses of 5–10 mg/kg IV up to 30–50 mg/kg. If this fails, then add phenytoin and/or benzodiazepine.
Phenytoin	15–20 mg/kg IV at 1 mg/kg/min with cardiac monitoring
Diazepam	0.3 mg/kg IV; may give 0.3–0.8 mg/kg/hr IV
Lorazepam	0.05–0.1 mg/kg IV over 2–5 min
Pyridoxine	50–100 mg IV during seizure with concurrent EEG monitoring in patients with refractory neonatal seizures

Modified from Snead O: and Horton EJ: Treatment of neonatal seizures, *Semin Neurol* 13:54, 1993.

3. Infantile spasms: Head nodding with flexion or extension of the trunk and extremities, often in clusters during drowsiness or awakening. Unexpected stimuli may trigger. EEG may show hypsarrhythmia. Usual onset after 2 months, peak onset 4–6 months.

a. Etiologies: Symptomatic (67%) CNS malformation, asphyxia, tuberous sclerosis; cryptogenic (33%), associated with better outcome, less mental retardation.

b. Treatment: Controversial. ACTH 100 units/m^2/day IM divided BID for 2 to 3 weeks, then slow taper, repeat PRN. May add VPA, benzodiazepine, or use ketogenic diet.

c. Outcome: Often poor, correlates best with underlying brain pathology. Of cryptogenic cases, 30%–70% may have good outcome with treatment.

From Swaiman KF: *Principles and practice of pediatric neurology,* St Louis, 1995, Mosby.

IV. HYDROCEPHALUS

A. Diagnosis

Look for increasing head circumference, misshapen skull, bulging large anterior fontanelle, separated sutures with cracked pot sign, increased ICP, and developmental delay. Obtain head CT if increase in head circumference crosses percentiles or if patient is symptomatic. Differentiate hydrocephalus from megalencephaly or hydrocephalus ex vacuo.

B. Treatment

1. Medical
   a. Acute increase of ICP (see Chapter 1 for ICP emergencies)
   b. Slowly progressive hydrocephalus: The following medications may be effective in children 2 weeks to 10 months of age with slowly progressive hydrocephalus:
      1) Acetazolamide: PO or IV: 20 mg/kg/24 hr to maximum 100 mg/kg/24 hr divided TID. Maximum 2 g/24 hr.
      2) Furosemide: 1 mg/kg/24 hr PO or IV divided TID.
      3) Polycitra: Titrate to maintain bicarbonate > 18 mEq/L and normal Na and K. Usual dose is 2–4 mEq/kg/24 hr.
      4) Side effects: Mild lethargy, poor feeding, occasional tachypnea, transient diarrhea, increased susceptibility to dehydration (unable to concentrate urine)

From Shinnar S et al: J *Pediatr* 107:31, 1987.

2. Surgical: Have shunt placed to drain CSF from cranium.
   a. Shunt types: Ventriculoperitoneal shunts are used most commonly. Ventriculoatrial/pleural shunts are associated with cardiac arrhythmias, pleural effusions, and higher rates of infection.

    b. Shunt components: Typically a shunt is composed of three parts
      1) Proximal tubing
      2) A flushing device with a one-way valve
      3) Distal tubing
    c. Shunt complications: Shunt dysfunction may be caused by infection, obstruction (clogging or kinking), disconnection, and migration of proximal and distal tips.

C. Management of Acute Shunt Obstruction or Infection

1. Test shunt function: Depress bulb and allow it to refill. Decreased bulb depression phase may be caused by distal shunt obstruction or a stiffened bulb. Poor refill suggests obstruction at the ventricular end, or excessive ventricular decompression.
2. Evaluate shunt integrity: Obtain shunt series (skull, neck, chest, and abdominal films) to look for kinking or disconnection. Obtain head CT to evaluate shunt position, ventricular size, and evidence of increased ICP.
3. Tap shunt: This procedure should be performed by a neurosurgeon; however, if a neurosurgeon is unavailable or the patient is rapidly deteriorating, a shunt tap may be performed by any physician familiar with the procedure.
    a. Cleanse the area over the shunt bulb using aseptic technique.
    b. Insert a long-nose, 25-gauge butterfly needle into the flushing device, through the bulb diaphragm, into the proximal chamber. A stopcock attached to the butterfly tubing may help prevent air from entering the ventricular system. Measure the fluid pressure, and remove the minimum amount of fluid needed to achieve symptomatic relief.
    c. If blockage at the ventricular end is suspected and the patient continues to deteriorate, insert a spinal needle (up to 18-gauge) through the burr hole through which the shunt was placed, and direct it toward the lateral ventricles. Measure the pressure and remove the minimal amount of fluid necessary for decompression.
    d. Send CSF for culture, cell count, and differential, glucose, and protein.
4. Further management: Pursue medical and surgical management of hydrocephalus as outlined above.

NUTRITION **23**

I. ASSESSMENT OF NUTRITIONAL STATUS

Before nutritional therapy is initiated an evaluation of the child's nutritional status should be completed based on the child's needs. A complete assessment consists of the following:

- Medical history and physical exam (medical diagnosis, clinical symptoms of nutritional deficiencies)
- Dietary evaluation (feeding history, current intake)
- Lab findings (comparison to age based norms)
- Anthropometric measurements (weight, length/height, head circumference, skinfolds); data is plotted on growth charts according to age and compared with a reference population

A. Classification of Protein Energy Malnutrition (PEM) (Table 23.1)

TABLE 23.1.

$\text{Acute PEM} = \dfrac{\text{Child's actual weight (kg)}}{\text{50th percentile weight/height (kg)}}$	90%–100% normal 80%–90% mild 70%–80% moderate < 70% severe
$\text{Chronic PEM} = \dfrac{\text{Child's actual height (cm)}}{\text{50th percentile height for age (cm)}}$	95%–100% normal 90%–95% mild 85%–90% moderate < 85% severe

B. Evaluation for Obesity

1. Children ≤ 10 years old
   >120% of 50th percentile wt/ht (kg) and/or triceps skinfold >85th percentile
2. Children > 10 years old

3. Recommended cutoff values for body mass index (BMI) in kg/m^2 for adolescents who are overweight or at risk of overweight during adolescence (Table 23.2).

$$BMI = \frac{(Wt \text{ in kg})}{(Ht \text{ in meters})^2}$$

TABLE 23.2.

Age (yr)	At risk of overweight		Overweight	
	Males	Females	Males	Females
10	20	20	23	23
11	20	21	24	25
12	21	22	25	26
13	22	23	26	27
14	23	24	27	28
15	24	24	28	29
16	24	25	29	29
17	25	25	29	30
18	26	26	30	30
19	26	26	30	30
20–24	27	26	30	30

II. ESTIMATING ENERGY NEEDS
Several methods are used for estimating energy needs. Most methods are based on calculating basal metabolic rate (BMR) with adjustments made to account for activity and disease or injury factors. The RDA tables are the most frequently used.
A. Median Heights and Weights and Recommended Energy Intake (Table 23.3)
B. Seashore Formula
Used to estimate energy needs for critically ill children
1. Step 1 - Calculate BMR:

BMR (kcal/day) = (55- 2x age in years) × (weight (kg))

TABLE 23.3.

Median Heights and Weights and Recommended Energy Intake

Category	Age (yr) or condition	Weight (kg)	Weight (lb)	Height (cm)	Height (in)	REE* (kcal/day)	Multiples of REE	Average energy allowance (kcal)† Per kg	Average energy allowance (kcal)† Per day‡
Infants	0.0–0.5	6	13	60	24	320		108	650
	0.5–1.0	9	20	71	28	500		98	850
Children	1–3	13	29	90	35	740		102	1,300
	4–6	20	44	112	44	950		90	1,800
	7–10	28	62	132	52	1,130		70	2,000
Males	11–14	45	99	157	62	1,440	1.70	55	2,500
	15–18	66	145	176	69	1,760	1.67	45	3,000
	19–24	72	160	177	70	1,780	1.67	40	2,900
	25–50	79	174	176	70	1,800	1.60	37	2,900
	51 +	77	170	173	68	1,530	1.50	30	2,300
Females	11–14	46	101	157	62	1,310	1.67	47	2,200
	15–18	55	120	163	64	1,370	1.60	40	2,200
	19–24	58	128	164	65	1,350	1.60	38	2,200
	25–50	63	138	163	64	1,380	1.55	36	2,200
	51 +	65	143	160	63	1,280	1.50	30	1,900
Pregnant	1st trimester								+0
	2nd trimester								+300
	3rd trimester								+300
Lactating	1st 6 months								+500
	2nd 6 months								+500

*Calculation based on FAO equations, then rounded.
†In the range of light to moderate activity, the coefficient of variation is ±20%.
‡Figure is rounded.

2. Step 2 - Calculate total daily energy needs:

Total daily energy needs (kcal/day) =
BMR + BMR (maintenance + injury + activity factors)

- Maintenance: 0.2
- Activity: 0.1–0.25
- Sepsis: 0.13 ° C
- Simple trauma: 0.2
- Multiple injuries: 0.4
- Burns: 0.5–1
- Growth: 0.5

C. **Harris-Benedict Equation**
   Can be used to estimate BEE (basal energy expenditure) of adolescents and adults (See ref. 6)
   1. Step 1 - Calculate BEE in kcal/day

Men:

$$66+[13.7 \times weight(kg)]+[5 \times height(cm)]-[6.8 \times age (yr)]$$

Women:

$$655+[9.6 \times weight(kg)]+[1.7 \times height(cm)]-[4.7 \times age(yr)]$$

   2. Step 2 - Calculate total daily energy needs:

$$\text{Total daily energy needs (kcal/day)} = BEE + BEE (\text{activity} + \text{disease/injury factors})$$

   a. Activity factors:
   - Bed rest: 0.2
   - Ambulatory: 0.3

   b. Disease/injury factors:
   - Long bone fractures: 0.15–0.3
   - Severe infection/multiple trauma: 0.3–0.75
   - Burns: 0.25 for ~ 10% BSA to 1.15 for ~ 70% BSA

D. **Catch up Growth Requirement**
   This formula can be used to calculate the energy needs for a malnourished child to catch up to his expected growth parameters (see ref. 8):

$$\text{Kcal/kg} = \frac{\text{RDA for chronological age (kcal/kg)} \times \text{50th percentile wt/ht (kg)}}{\text{actual wt (kg)}}$$

III. RECOMMENDED DIETARY ALLOWANCES (Table 23.4)

TABLE 23.4.

Recommended Dietary Allowances*—Vitamins

Category	Age (years) or Condition	Weight (kg)	Weight (lb)	Height (cm)	Height (in)	Protein (g)	Fat-Soluble Vitamins				Water-Soluble Vitamins						
							Vitamin A (mcg RE)‡	Vitamin D (mcg)§	Vitamin E (mg α-TE)‖	Vitamin K (mcg)	Vitamin C (mg)	Thiamin (mg)	Riboflavin (mg)	Niacin (mg NE)¶	Vitamin B6 (mg)	Folate (mcg)	Vitamin B12 (mcg)
Infants	0.0–0.5	6	13	60	24	13	375	7.5	3	5	30	0.3	0.4	5	0.3	25	0.3
	0.5–1.0	9	20	71	28	14	375	10	4	10	35	0.4	0.5	6	0.6	35	0.5
Children	1–3	13	29	90	35	16	400	10	6	15	40	0.7	0.8	9	1.0	50	0.7
	4–6	20	44	112	44	24	500	10	7	20	45	0.9	1.1	12	1.1	75	1.0
	7–10	28	62	132	52	28	700	10	7	30	45	1.0	1.2	13	1.4	100	1.4
Males	11–14	45	99	157	62	45	1,000	10	10	45	50	1.3	1.5	17	1.7	150	2.0
	15–18	66	145	176	69	59	1,000	10	10	65	60	1.5	1.8	20	2.0	200	2.0
	19–24	72	160	177	70	58	1,000	10	10	70	60	1.5	1.7	19	2.0	200	2.0
	25–50	79	174	176	70	63	1,000	5	10	80	60	1.5	1.7	19	2.0	200	2.0
	51+	77	170	173	68	63	1,000	5	10	80	60	1.2	1.4	15	2.0	200	2.0
Females	11–14	46	101	157	62	46	800	10	8	45	50	1.1	1.3	15	1.4	150	2.0
	15–18	55	120	163	64	44	800	10	8	55	60	1.1	1.3	15	1.5	180	2.0
	19–24	58	128	164	65	46	800	10	8	60	60	1.1	1.3	15	1.6	180	2.0
	25–50	63	138	163	64	50	800	5	8	65	60	1.1	1.3	15	1.6	180	2.0
	51+	65	143	160	63	50	800	5	8	65	60	1.0	1.2	13	1.6	180	2.0
Pregnant						60	800	10	10	65	70	1.5	1.6	17	2.2	400	2.2
Lactating	1st 6 months					65	1,300	10	12	65	95	1.6	1.8	20	2.1	280	2.6
	2nd 6 months					62	1,200	10	11	65	90	1.6	1.7	20	2.1	260	2.6

See footnotes on p. 439.

(Continued.)

417

TABLE 23.4. (cont.)
Recommended Dietary Allowances*–Minerals

Category	Age (years) or Condition	Weight (kg)	Weight (lb)	Height (cm)	Height (in)	Minerals Calcium (mg)	Phosphorus (mg)	Magnesium (mg)	Iron (mg)	Zinc (mg)	Iodine (mcg)	Selenium (mcg)
Infants	0.0–0.5	6	13	60	24	400	300	40	6	5	40	10
	0.5–1.0	9	20	71	28	600	500	60	10	5	50	15
Children	1–3	13	29	90	35	800	800	80	10	10	70	20
	4–6	20	44	112	44	800	800	120	10	10	90	20
	7–10	28	62	132	52	800	800	170	10	10	120	30
Males	11–14	45	99	157	62	1,200	1,200	270	12	15	150	40
	15–18	66	145	176	69	1,200	1,200	400	12	15	150	50
	19–24	72	160	177	70	1,200	1,200	350	10	15	150	70
	25–50	79	174	176	70	800	800	350	10	15	150	70
	51+	77	170	173	68	800	800	350	10	15	150	70
Females	11–14	46	101	157	62	1,200	1,200	280	15	12	150	45
	15–18	55	120	163	64	1,200	1,200	300	15	12	150	50
	19–24	58	128	164	65	1,200	1,200	280	15	12	150	55
	25–50	63	138	163	64	800	800	280	15	12	150	55
	51+	65	143	160	63	800	800	280	10	12	150	55
Pregnant						1,200	1,200	320	30	15	175	65
Lactating	1st 6 months					1,200	1,200	355	15	19	200	75
	2nd 6 months					1,200	1,200	340	15	16	200	75

Table 23.4 (cont.)

Recommended Dietary Allowances

*The allowances, expressed as average daily intakes over time, are intended to provide for individual variations among most normal persons as they live in the United States under usual environmental stresses. Diets should be based on a variety of common foods in order to provide other nutrients for which human requirements have been less well defined.

†Weights and heights of Reference Adults are actual medians for the United States population of the designated age, as reported by NHANES II. The median weights and heights of those under 19 years of age were taken from Hamill et al. (1979). The use of these figures does not imply that the height-to-weight ratios are ideal.

‡Retinol equivalents. 1 retinol equivalent = 1 mcg retinol or 6 mcg β-carotene.

§As cholecalciferol. 10 mcg cholecalciferol = 400 IU of vitamin D.

‖α-Tocopherol equivalents. 1 mg d-α tocopherol = 1 α-TE.

¶1 NE (niacin equivalent) is equal to 1 mg of niacin or 60 mg of dietary tryptophan.

IV. ENTERAL NUTRITION

A. **Formula Comparison by Macronutrients (Tables 23.5 to 23.7, pp. 440–445)**
B. **Infant Formula Analysis (Table 23.8, p. 446)**
C. **Toddler and Young Children Formula Analysis (Table 23.9, p. 452)**
D. **Older Children to Adult Formula Analysis (Table 23.10, p. 454)**
E. **Single Component Enteral Nutritional Supplements (Table 23.11, p. 459)**
F. **Concentration of Infant Formulas (Table 23.12, p. 459)**
G. **Infant Multivitamin Drops Analysis (Table 23.13, p. 460)**

TABLE 23.5

Classification of Formulas by Carbohydrate

	Comments	Infant	Toddler and young child	Older child and adolescent
Lactose	Requires lactase	Enfamil Carnation Follow-Up Gerber Good Start Neocare Premature Enfamil Similac Similac Special Care Similac PM 60/40	Next Step* Toddler's Best	Carnation Instant Breakfast Scandi Shake
Sucrose & glucose polymers		Alimentum Alsoy Isomil Isomil DF (Fiber) Portagen	Kindercal (Fiber) Neocate One Plus Next Step Soy Nutren Junior PediaSure (also w/Fiber) Peptamen Junior	All other formulas

Glucose polymers		Isomil SF Lactofree Neocate Nutramigen Pregestimil ProSobee	Vivonex Pediatric	Criticare HN Deliver 2.0 Glucerna Isocal Jevity (Fiber) Peptamen Tolerex Vivonex TEN Vivonex Plus
Minimal carbohydrate	For severe carbohydrate intolerance	MJ3232A RCF		

*Also contains glucose polymers

TABLE 23.6

Classification of Formulas by Protein

	Infant	Toddler and young child	Older child and adolescent
Cow's milk protein	Requires normal GI tract	Carnation Follow-Up Enfamil Gerber Lactofree Neocare Portagen Premature Enfamil Similac Similac PM 60/40 Similac Special Care	Kindercal Next Step Nutren Junior PediaSure Toddler's Best	All other formulas
Soy protein	For cow's milk allergy if exclusively soy	Alsoy Follow Up Soy Gerber Soy Isomil Isomil DF Isomil SF ProSobee RCF	Next Step Soy	Ensure* Ensure with fiber* Isocal* Osmolite* Promote* Sustacal* Sustacal with fiber*

Nutrition **423**

Hydrolysate	Malabsorption or food allergy	Alimentum Good Start Nutramigen Pregestimil MJ3232A	Peptamen Junior	Criticare HN Peptamen Vital HN
Free amino acids	Malabsorption or food allergy	Neocate	Vivonex Pediatric Neocate One Plus	Tolerex Vivonex TEN Vivonex Plus

*Also contains cow's milk protein.

TABLE 23.7

Classification of Formulas by Fat

	Comments	Infant	Toddler and young child	Older child and adolescent
Long chain triglycerides	Requires normal fat absorption	Alsoy Enfamil Carnation Follow-Up Follow-Up Soy Gerber Gerber's Soy Good Start Isomil (all) Lactofree Neocate Nutramigen ProSobee RCF Similac Similac PM 60/40	Next Step Toddler's Best	Carnation Instant Breakfast Ensure Ensure with Fiber Ensure Plus Glucerna Magnacal Nepro Pulmocare Scandishake Suplena Sustacal Sustacal HC Sustacal with Fiber

Medium chain triglycerides and long chain triglycerides	Fat malabsorption	Alimentum Enfamil Premature MJ3232A Pregestimil Portagen Similac Neocare Similac Special Care	Kindercal Neocate One Plus Nutren Junior PediaSure Peptamen Junior Vivonex Pediatric	Deliver 2.0 Isocal Jevity Lipisorb Nutren 2.0 Nutrivent Osmolite Promote Respalor Traumacal Ultracal

TABLE 23.8

Infant Formula Analysis/100 ml

Formula	Kcal/ml (oz)	Protein g (% Cal)	Carbohydrate g (% Cal)	Fat g (% Cal)	Na (mEq)	K (mEq)	Ca (mg)	P (mg)	Fe (mg)	Osmolality mOsm/kg water	Suggested uses
Alimentum (Ross)	0.67 (20)	Casein hydrolysate, Cystine, Tyrosine Tryptophan 1.9 (11)	Sucrose 67% Modified Tapioca starch 6.9 (41)	MCT oil (50%) Safflower oil (40%) Soy oil (10%) 3.8 (48)	1.3	2	71	51	1.2	370	Infants w/food allergies, protein or fat malabsorption
Alsoy (Carnation)	0.67 (20)	Soy Isolate 2 (12)	Sucrose Maltodextrin 6.6 (39)	Soy oil 3.6 (48)	1.2	2	68	42	1.3	270	Infants with allergy to cow's milk, lactose malabsorption, galactosemia
Enfamil [w/Fe] (Mead Johnson)	0.67 (20)	Nonfat milk, Demineralized Whey 1.5 (9)	Lactose 7.0 (41)	Palm olein (45%) Soy oil (20%) Coconut oil (20%) HO Sun oil (15%) 3.8 (50)	0.8	1.9	53	36	0.3 [1.25]	300	Infants with normal GI tract
Enfamil 24 [w/Fe] (Mead Johnson)	0.8 (20)	Nonfat milk, Whey 1.8 (9)	Lactose 8.3 (41)	Palm olein (45%) Soy oil (20%) Coconut oil (20%) HO Sun oil (15%) 4.5 (50)	1	2.2	63	43	0.5 [1.5]	360	Infants with normal GI tract requiring additional calories
Enfamil Human Milk Fortifier (per packet) (Mead Johnson)	3.5 (—)	Reduced mineral Whey Caseinate 0.2 (12)	Corn syrup solids Lactose 0.7 (77)	0.033 (3)	0.08	0.1	22.5	11.5	—	120	To be mixed with human milk for the preterm infant

426

Product	Protein source (g)	Carbohydrate source (g)	Fat source (g)							Indications
Enfamil Premature 20 Formula [w/Fe] (Mead Johnson) 0.67 (20)	Demineralized whey Cow's milk solids 2 (12)	Corn syrup solids Lactose 7.4 (44)	MCT oil (40%) Soy oil Coconut oil 3.4 (44)	1.1	1.9	110	55	0.17 [1.3]	260	Preterm infants
Enfamil Premature 24 Formula [w/Fe] (Mead Johnson) 0.8 (24)	Demineralized whey Cow's milk solids 2.4 (12)	Corn syrup solids Lactose 9 (44)	MCT oil (40%) Soy oil Coconut oil 4.1 (44)	1.4	2.1	134	68	0.2 [1.5]	310	Preterm infants
Evaporated milk Formula* 0.69 (21)	Cow's milk 2.8 (16)	Lactose Corn syrup 7.5 (43)	Butterfat 3.3 (43)	2	3.3	113	87	0.2	N/A	Infants with normal GI tract; Need vitamin C and iron supplement
Follow-Up Formula (Carnation) 0.67 (20)	Nonfat milk 1.7 (10)	Corn syrup (43%) Lactose (37%) 8.8 (53)	Palm olein (47%) Soy oil (26%) Coconut oil (21%) HO saff oil (6%) 2.7 (36)	1.1	2.3	90	60	1.3	300	Infants 4-12 months with normal GI tract
Follow-Up Soy (Carnation) 0.67 (20)	Soy 2.1 (12)	Maltodextrin 6.8 (40)	Soy oil 3.7 (49)	1.2	2	90	60	1.3	270	Infants 4-12 months with allergy to cow's milk, lactose malapsorbtion, glactomsemia
Gerber [w/Fe] (Gerber) 0.67 (20)	Nonfat milk 1.5 (9)	Lactose 7.1 (42)	Palm olein Soy oil Coconut oil 3.6 (48)	0.9	1.8	50	39	0.3 [1.2]	300	Infants with normal GI tract
Gerber Soy [w/Fe] (Gerber) 0.67 (20)	Soy Isolate Methionine 2 (12)	Corn syrup Sucrose 6.7 (40)	Soy oil Coconut oil 3.5 (47%)	0.8	1.5	63	49	0.3 [1.2]	270	Infants with allergy to cow's milk, lactose malabsorption, galactosemia

*13 ounces evaporated whole milk + 19 ounces water + 2 Tbsp corn syrup.

(Continued.)

TABLE 23.8 (cont.)

Formula	Kcal/ml (oz)	Protein g (% Cal)	Carbohydrate g (% Cal)	Fat g (% Cal)	Na (mEq)	K (mEq)	Ca (mg)	P (mg)	Fe (mg)	Osmolality mOsm/kg water	Suggested uses
Good Start (Carnation)	0.67 (20)	Hydrolyzed Whey 1.6 (9.6)	Lactose Maltodextrins 7.4 (44)	Palm olein (47%) Soy oil (26%) Coconut oil (21%) HO saff oil (6%) 3.5 (4.6)	0.7	1.7	43	24	1	265	Infants with normal GI tract
Human milk Mature	0.67 (20)	Human milk 1.1 (6)	Lactose 7.2 (39)	Human milk 3.9 (55)	0.8	1.1	29	14	0.03	300	Infants
Human milk Preterm	0.67 (20)	Human milk 1.6 (9.5)	Lactose 7.3 (43.5)	Human milk 3.5 (47)	1.2	1.5	29	15	0.03	300	Infants
Isomil (Ross)	0.67 (20)	Soy isolate Methionine 1.8 (11)	Corn syrup Sucrose 6.8 (40)	Soy oil Coconut oil 3.7 (49)	1.3	1.9	71	51	1.2	240	Infants with allergy to cow's milk, lactose malabsorption, galactosemia
Isomil DF (Ross)	0.67 (20)	Soy isolate Methionine 1.8 (11)	Corn syrup Sucrose Soy fiber 6.7 (40)	Soy oil Coconut oil 3.6 (48)	1.3	1.8	70	50	1.2	240	Short term management of diarrhea; contains fiber
Isomil SF (Ross)	0.67 (20)	Soy isolate Methionine 1.8 (11)	Glucose polymers 6.7 (40)	Soy oil Coconut oil 3.6 (48)	1.3	1.8	70	50	1.2	180	Infants with allergy to cow's milk, lactose malabsorption, galactosemia
Lactofree (Mead Johnson)	0.67 (20)	Nonfat milk 1.5 (9)	Corn syrup Solids 7 (42)	Palm olein (45%) Soy oil (20%) Coconut oil (20%) HO sun oil (15%) 3.7 (49)	0.9	1.9	55	36	1.2	200	Infants with lactose malabsorption
MJ3232A (Mead Johnson)	0.42 (12.6)	Casein hydrolysate Cystine, Tyrosine Tryptophan 1.9 (17)	Tapioca starch Carbohydrate must be added 2.8 (25)	MCT oil (85%) Corn oil (15%) 2.8 (57)	1.3	1.9	63	42	1.3	250	Infants with severe CHO intolerance. (CHO must be added)

Neocate (Scientific Hospital Supply)	0.69 (21)	Free amino acids 2 (12)	Corn syrup solids 8.1 (47)	Safflower oil Coconut oil Soy oil 3.2 (41)	0.8	1.6	49	35	1.1	342	Infants with severe food allergies
Nutramigen (Mead Johnson)	0.67 (20)	Casein hydrolysate Cystine, Tyrosine Tryptophan 1.9 (11)	Corn syrup solids Corn starch 7.3 (44)	Palm olein (45%) Soy oil (20%) Coconut oil (20%) HO sun oil (15%) 3.3 (45)	1.4	1.9	63	42	1.3	320	Infants with food allergies
Portagen (Mead Johnson)	0.67 (20)	Na caseinate 2.3 (14)	Corn syrup solids Sucrose 7.7 (46)	MCT oil (85%) Corn oil (15%) 3.1 (40)	1.6	2.1	63	47	1.3	220	Infants with fat malabsorption
Pregestimil (Mead Johnson)	0.67 (20)	Caein hydrolysate Cystine, Tyrosine Tryptophan 1.9 (11)	Corn syrup solids (60%) Modified tapioca Starch (20%) Dextrose (20%) 6.9 (41)	MCT oil (55%) Corn oil (20%) HO saff oil (12.5%) Soy oil (12.5%) 3.8 (48)	1.1	1.9	63	42	1.3	320	Infants with food allergies, protein or fat malabsorption
ProSobee (Mead Johnson)	0.67 (20)	Soy isolate Methionine 2 (12)	Corn syrup solids 6.7 (40)	Palm olein (45%) Soy oil (20%) Coconut oil (20%) HO Sun oil (15%) 3.5 (48)	1	2.1	63	49	1.3	200	Infants with allergy to cow's milk, lactose malabsorption, galactosemia
RCF (Ross)	0.4 (12)	Soy isolate 2 (20)	Carbohydrate must be added —	Soy oil Coconut oil 3.5 (80)	1.3	1.9	70	50	0.15	74	Infants with severe CHO intolerance. (CHO must be added)

(Continued.)

TABLE 23.8 (cont.)

Formula	Kcal/ml (oz)	Protein g (% Cal)	Carbohydrate g (% Cal)	Fat g (% Cal)	Na (mEq)	K (mEq)	Ca (mg)	P (mg)	Fe (mg)	Osmolality mOsm/kg water	Suggested uses
Similac [w/Fe] (Ross)	0.67 (20)	Nonfat milk 1.5 (9)	Lactose 7.2 (43)	Soy oil Coconut oil 3.6 (48)	0.8	1.8	50	38	0.3 [1.2]	300	Infants with normal GI tract
Similac 24 [w/Fe] (Ross)	0.8 (24)	Nonfat milk 2.2 (11)	Lactose 8.5 (42)	Soy oil Coconut oil 4.3 (47)	1.2	2.7	73	57	0.18 [1.5]	380	Infants with normal GI tract requiring additional calories
Similac Natural Care (Ross)	0.8 (24)	Nonfat milk Whey 2.2 (11)	Lactose Glucose polymers 8.5 (42)	MCT oil (50%) Soy oil Coconut oil 4.3 (47)	1.4	2.6	168	84	0.3	280	To be mixed with human milk for the preterm infant
Similac Neocare (Ross)	0.73 (22)	Nonfat milk Whey 2.0 (11)	Glucose polymers (50%) Lactose (50%) 7.5 (41)	MCT oil (25%) Soy oil (45%) Coconut oil (30%) 4 (49)	1	2.6	77	46	1.3	290	Preterm infants, after hospital discharge, for the first year of life
Similac PM 60/40 (Ross)	0.67 (20)	Whey Na caseinate 1.6 (9)	Lactose 6.9 (41)	Soy oil Coconut oil 3.8 (50)	0.7	1.5	38	19	0.15	280	Infants who require lowered calcium and phosphorus levels
Similac Special Care 20 (Ross)	0.67 (20)	Nonfat milk Whey 1.8 (11)	Glucose polymers Lactose 7.2 (42)	MCT oil (50%) Soy oil Coconut oil 3.7 (47)	1.3	2.2	122	61	0.3	235	Preterm infants
Similac Special Care 24 (Ross)	0.8 (24)	Nonfat milk Whey 2.2 (11)	Glucose polymers Lactose 8.6 (42)	MCT oil (50%) Soy oil Coconut oil 4.4 (47)	1.5	2.7	146	73	0.3 [1.5]	280	Preterm infants

TABLE 23.9

Toddler & Young Child Formula Analysis / Liter

Formula	Kcal/ml (oz)	Protein g (% Cal)	Carbohydrate g (% Cal)	Fat g (% Cal)	Na (mEq)	K (mEq)	Ca (mg)	P (mg)	Fe (mg)	Osmolality mOsm/Kg water	Suggested uses
Cow's milk Whole	0.63 (19)	Cow's milk 34 (21)	Lactose 48 (30)	Butterfat 34 (49)	21	39	1190	930	0.5	288	Children > 1 year of age with normal GI tract
Kindercal (contains fiber) (Mead Johnson)	1.06 (32)	Sodium caseinate 34 (13)	Maltodextrins (83%) Sucrose (17%) 135 (50)	Canola oil (50%) HO sun oil (15%) Corn oil (15%) MCT oil (20%) 44 (37%)	16	33.6	850	850	10.6	310	Tube feeding and oral supplement for children with normal GI tract
Neocate One Plus (Scientific Hospital Supply)	1 (30)	Free amino acids 25 (10)	Maltodextrins Sucrose 146 (58)	MCT oil (35%) Safflower oil Canola oil 35 (32)	9	24	620	620	8	835	Children with malabsorption and protein allergy
Next Step (Mead Johnson)	0.67 (20)	Nonfat milk 17 (10)	Lactose Corn syrup solids 74 (44)	Palm olein (45%) Soy oil (20%) Coconut oil (20%) HO sun oil (15%) 33 (45)	12	22	800	550	12	270	Toddlers with normal GI tract
Next Step Soy (Mead Johnson)	0.67 (20)	Soy protein 22 (13)	Corn syrup solids Sucrose 78 (47)	Palm olein (45%) Soy oil (20%) Coconut oil (20%) HO sun oil (15%) 29 (40)	13	22	760	600	12	260	Toddlers with allergy to cow's milk, galactosemia

(Continued.)

431

TABLE 23.9 (cont.)

Formula	Kcal/ml (oz)	Protein g (% Cal)	Carbohydrate g (% Cal)	Fat g (% Cal)	Na (mEq)	K (mEq)	Ca (mg)	P (mg)	Fe (mg)	Osmolality mOsm/kg water	Suggested uses
Nutren Junior (Clintec)	1 (30)	Casein Whey 30 (12)	Maltodextrins Sucrose 128 (51)	Soy oil Canola oil MCT oil 42 (38)	20	34	1000	800	14	350	Tube feeding and oral supplement for children with normal GI tract
PediaSure (also with fiber) (Ross)	1 (30)	Sodium caseinate Whey protein 30 (12)	Hydrolyzed corn starch (70%) Sucrose (30%) (Soy fiber) 110 (44)	HO saff oil (50%) Soy oil (30%) MCT oil (20%) 50 (44)	16.5	33.5	970	800	14	310	Tube feeding and oral supplement for children with normal GI tract
Peptamen Junior (Clintec)	1 (30)	Hydrolyzed whey 30 (12)	Maltodextrin Sucrose Starch 138 (55)	MCT oil (60%) Soy oil Canola oil Lecithin 38.5 (33)	20	34	1000	800	14	260 (unflavored) 365 (flavored)	Children with malabsorption
Toddler's Best (Ross)	0.67 (20)	Nonfat milk 24 (14)	Lactose Sucrose 74 (44)	HO saff oil Coconut oil Soy oil 32 (42)	12	26	1055	642	12	357	Toddlers with normal GI tract
Vivonex Pediatric (Sandoz)	0.8 (24)	Free amino acids Glutamine 24 (12)	Maltodextrins Modified starch 130 (63)	MCT oil (68%) Soy oil (32%) 24 (25)	17	31	970	800	10	360	Children with malabsorption, protein allergy

432

TABLE 23.10

Older Child to Adult Formula Analysis / Liter

Formula	Kcal/ml (oz)	Protein g (% Cal)	Carbohydrate g (% Cal)	Fat g (% Cal)	Na (mEq)	K (mEq)	Ca (mg)	P (mg)	Fe (mg)	Osmolality mOsm/kg water	Suggested uses
Carnation Instant Breakfast w/whole milk (Clintec)	1.2 (36)	Cow's milk 53 (18)	Lactose Maltodextrin Sucrose 161 (54)	Butterfat 34 (26)	42	67	1632	1400	17	590	High calorie supplement for patients with normal GI tract
Criticare HN (Mead Johnson)	1.06 (32)	Hydrolyzed casein Amino acids 38 (14)	Maltodextrin Modified corn starch 220 (81.5)	Safflower oil 53 (4.5)	27	34	530	530	9.5	650	Patients with malabsorption
Deliver 2.0 (Mead Johnson)	2 (60)	Ca caseinate Na caseinate 75 (15)	Corn syrup 200 (40)	Soy oil (70%) MCT oil (30%) 102 (45)	35	43	1000	1000	18	640	Oral supplement or tube feeding for patients with fluid restriction or increased calorie needs
Ensure (Ross)	1.06 (32)	Na caseinate Ca caseinate Soy protein 37 (14)	Corn syrup (70%) Sucrose (30%) 145 (55)	Corn oil 37 (32)	36	40	521	521	9.4	470	Oral supplement or tube feeding for patients with normal GI tract
Ensure Plus (Ross)	1.5 (45)	Na caseinate Ca caseinate Soy protein 55 (15)	Corn syrup Sucrose 200 (53)	Corn oil 53 (32)	46	50	705	705	13	690	Oral supplement or tube feeding for patients with higher calorie needs, normal GI tract

(Continued.)

433

TABLE 23.10 (cont.)

Formula	Kcal/ml (oz)	Protein g (% Cal)	Carbohydrate g (% Cal)	Fat g (% Cal)	Na (mEq)	K (mEq)	Ca (mg)	P (mg)	Fe (mg)	Osmolality mOsm/kg water	Suggested uses
Ensure with Fiber (Ross)	1.1 (33)	Na caseinate Ca caseinate Soy protein 40 (15)	Hydrolyzed corn starch (58%) Sucrose (32%) Soy polysaccharide (10%) 162 (55)	Corn oil 37 (31)	37	43	719	719	13	480	Oral supplement or tube feeding with fiber, normal GI tract
Glucerna (Ross)	1 (30)	Na caseinate Ca caseinate 42 (17)	Glucose polymers (53%) Soy polysaccharide (25%) Fructose (21%), 94 (33)	Ho saff oil (85%) Soy oil (15%) 56 (50)	40	40	704	704	13	375	Patients with impaired glucose tolerance, also contains fiber
Isocal (Mead Johnson)	1.06 (32)	Na caseinate Ca caseinate Soy protein 34 (13)	Maltodextrin 135 (50)	MCT oil (20%) Soy oil (80%) 44 (37)	23	34	630	530	10	270	Tube feeding for patients with normal GI tract
Jevity (Ross)	1.06 (32)	Na caseinate Ca caseinate 44 (17)	Hydrolyzed corn starch Soy polysaccharide 152 (53)	Ho saff oil (50%) Canola oil (30%) MCT oil (20%) 36 (30)	40	40	909	758	14	300	Tube feeding with fiber, normal GI tract
Lipisorb (Mead Johnson)	1.35 (40)	Na caseinate Ca caseinate 57 (17)	Maltodextrin Sucrose 161 (48)	MCT oil (85%) Soy oil (15%) 57 (35)	59	43	850	850	15	630	Patients with fat malabsorption

434

Magnacal (Sherwood)	2 (60)	Na caseinate Ca caseinate 70 (14)	Maltodextrin Sucrose 250 (50)	Soy oil 80 (36)	44	32	1000	1000	18	590	Oral supplement or tube feedings for patients with fluid restriction or increased calorie needs
Nepro (Ross)	2 (60)	Ca caseinate Mg caseinate Na caseinate 70 (14)	Hydrolyzed corn starch (88%) Sucrose (12%) 215 (43)	HO saff oil (90%) Soy oil (10%) 96 (43)	36	27	1373	686	19	635	Patients with renal failure undergoing dialysis
Nutren 2.0 (Clintec)	2 (60)	K caseinate Ca caseinate 80 (16)	Sucrose Corn syrup solids Maltodextrin 196 (39)	MCT oil (73%) Canola oil Corn oil Soy Lecithin 106 (45)	57	49	1050	1050	24	710	Oral supplement or tube feedings for patients with fluid restriction or increased calorie needs
Nutrivent (Clintec)	1.5 (45)	Maltodextrin Sucrose 68 (18)	Ca caseinate K caseinate 101 (27)	MCT oil (40%) Canola oil (43%) Corn oil (13%) Lecithin (4%) 95 (55)	33	57	1200	1200	18	420	Patients requiring higher percentage of calories from fat
Osmolite (Ross)	1.06 (32)	Na caseinate Ca caseinate Soy protein 37 (14)	Hydrolyzed corn starch 145 (55)	HO saff oil (50%) Canola oil (30%) MCT oil (20%) 38 (31)	28	26	530	530	9.5	300	Tube feeding for patients with normal GI tract
Peptamen (Clintec)	1 (30)	Hydrolyzed whey 40 (16)	Maltodextrin (88%) Hydrolyzed corn starch (12%) 127 (51)	MCT oil (67%) Sunflower oil (18%) Lecithin (6%) Milk fat (9%) 39 (33)	22	32	600	500	9	270	Patients with malabsorption
Promote (Ross)	1 (30)	Na caseinate Ca caseinate Soy protein 63 (25)	Hydrolyzed corn starch (91%) Sucrose (9%) 130 (52)	HO saff oil (50%) Canola oil (30%) MCT oil (20%) 26 (23)	40	51	960	960	14	330	Oral supplement or tube feeding for patients with increased protein needs

(Continued.)

TABLE 23.10 (cont.)

Formula	Kcal/ml (oz)	Protein g (% Cal)	Carbohydrate g (% Cal)	Fat g (% Cal)	Na (mEq)	K (mEq)	Ca (mg)	P (mg)	Fe (mg)	Osmolality mOsm/kg water	Suggested uses
Pulmocare (Ross)	1.5 (45)	Na caseinate Ca caseinate 63 (17)	Hydrolyzed corn starch (46%) Sucrose (54%) 106 (28)	Corn oil 92 (55)	57	44	1056	1056	19	465	Patient's requiring higher percentage of calories from fat
Respalor (Mead Johnson)	1.5 (45)	Ca caseinate Na caseinate 76 (20)	Corn syrup Sucrose 148 (37)	Canola oil (70%) MCT oil (30%) 71 (43)	55	38	710	710	13	580	Patients requiring higher percentage of calories from fat
Scandi Shake with whole milk (Scandipharm)	2.5 (75)	Cow's milk 50 (8)	Lactose Maltodextrin 292 (47)	Coconut oil Safflower oil Soy oil Palm oil 125 (45)	240	103	391	478	trace	1094	High calorie supplement and for fat malabsorption
Suplena (Ross)	2 (60)	Na caseinate Ca caseinate 30 (6)	Hydrolyzed corn starch (90%) Sucrose (10%) 255 (51)	HO saff oil (90%) Soy oil (10%) 96 (43)	34	29	1385	728	19	600	Patients with renal failure not undergoing dialysis
Sustacal (Mead Johnson)	1 (30)	Na caseinate Ca caseinate Soy protein 61 (24)	Corn syrup Sucrose 140 (55)	Partially hydrogenated soy oil 23 (21)	40	54	1010	930	17	650	Oral supplement or tube feeding for patients with increased protein needs
Sustacal HC (Mead Johnson)	1.5 (45)	Na caseinate Ca caseinate 61 (16)	Corn syrup solids Sucrose 190 (50)	Corn oil 58 (34)	37	38	850	850	15	670	Oral supplement or tube feeding for patients with high calorie needs, normal GI tract

Product (Manufacturer)	kcal/mL (kcal)	Protein source, g/L (%)	Carbohydrate source, g/L (%)	Fat source, g/L (%)						Osmolality	Indications
Sustacal with Fiber (Mead Johnson)	1.06 (30)	Na caseinate, Ca caseinate, Soy protein 46 (17)	Maltodextrin, Sucrose 140 (53)	Corn oil 35 (30)	31	36	840	70	13	480	Oral supplement or tube feeding with fiber, normal GI tract
Tolerex (Sandoz)	1 (30)	Free amino acids 21 (8)	Maltodextrin 230 (91)	Safflower oil 1.5 (1)	20	31	560	560	10	550	Patients with malabsorption or severe food allergy
Traumacal (Mead Johnson)	1.5 (45)	Na caseinate, Ca caseinate 83 (22)	Corn syrup, Sucrose 145 (38)	Soy oil (70%), MCT oil (30%) 68 (40)	52	36	750	750	9	490	Patients with increased protein and calorie needs
Ultracal (Mead Johnson)	1.06 (30)	Na caseinate, Ca caseinate 44 (17)	Maltodextrin, Soy fiber, Oat fiber 123 (46)	MCT oil (40%), Canola oil (60%) 45 (37)	40	41	850	850	15	310	Oral supplement or tube feeding with fiber, normal GI tract
Vital HN (Ross)	1 (30)	Hydrolyzed whey, meat, and soy (87%), Free amino acids (13%) 41.7 (17)	Hydrolyzed corn starch (83%), Sucrose (17%) Lactose (<0.5%) 185 (74)	Safflower oil (55%), MCT oil (45%) 11 (9)	25	36	667	667	12	500	Patients with malabsorption
Vivonex Plus (Sandoz)	1 (30)	Free amino acids BCCA (30%) Glutamine (22%) Arginine (1%) 45 (18)	Maltodextrin 190 (76)	Soybean oil 6.7 (6)	27	28	560	560	10	650	Patients with malabsorption or severe food allergy
Vivonex TEN (Sandoz)	1 (30)	Free amino acids [BCCA (33%)] 38 (15)	Maltodextrin 210 (82)	Safflower oil 2.8 (3)	20	20	500	500	9	630	Patients with malabsorption or severe food allergy

437

TABLE 23.11.

Single Component Enteral Nutrition Supplements

Component	Source	Content	Calories
Protein			
Casec	Calcium caseinate	88 g/100 g powder	3.7 kcal/g
Promod	Whey protein	75 g/100 g powder	4.2 kcal/g
Propac	Whey protein	75 g/100 g powder	3.95 kcal/g
Carbohydrate			
Moducal	Corn starch hydrolysate	95 g/100 g powder	3.8 kcal/g
Polycose	Corn starch hydrolysate	50 g/100 ml liquid	2 kcal/ml
		94 g/100 g powder	3.8 kcal/g
Fat			
MCT oil	Fractionated coconut oil, 90%; C8 and C10 TGs	93 g/100 ml	7.7 kcal/ml
Micro lipid	Safflower oil, 50% emulsion	50 g/100 ml	4.5 kcal/ml

TABLE 23.12.

Concentration of Infant Formulas

Concentrates (40 cal/oz)

Caloric concentration (cal/oz)	Concentrate (oz)	Water (oz)
20	13	13
24	13	8.5
26	13	7
28	13	5.5
30	13	4.3

Powder (40 cal/tbsp)

Caloric concentration (cal/oz)	Powder (scoop/Tbsp)	Water (oz)
20	1	2
24	3	5
26	2	3
28	7	10
30	3	4

TABLE 23.13.

Infant Multivitamin Drops Analysis (per ml)

	Poly-Vi-Flor [with Iron] Mead Johnson	Poly-Vi-Sol [with Iron] Mead Johnson	Tri-Vi-Flor [with Iron] Mead Johnson	Tri-Vi-Sol [with Iron] Mead Johnson	Vi-Daylin ADC [with Iron] Ross	Vi-Daylin/F ADC [with Iron] Ross	Vi-Daylin Multivitamin [with Iron] Ross	Vi-Daylin/F Multivitamin [with Iron] Ross
Vitamin A, IU	1500	1500	1500	1500	1500	1500	1500	1500
Vitamin D, IU	400	400	400	400	400	400	400	400
Vitamin E, IU	5	5					5	5
Vitamin C, mg	35	35	35	35	35	35	35	35
Thiamin, mg	0.5	0.5					0.5	0.5
Riboflavin, mg	0.6	0.6					0.5	0.6
Niacin, mg	8	8					8	8
Vitamin B6, mg	0.4	0.4					0.4	0.4
Vitamin B12, mg	2	2						
Iron, mg	[10]	[10]	[10]	[10]	[10]	[10]	[10]	[10]
Fluoride, mg	0.25		0.25			0.25		0.25

V. PARENTERAL NUTRITION
A. **Initiation and Advancement of Parenteral Nutrition (Table 23.14)**
B. **Daily Parenteral Nutrient Recommendations (Table 23.15)**
C. **Parenteral MVI Formulation (Table 23.16)**
D. **Monitoring Schedule (Table 23.17)**

TABLE 23.14.

Initiation & Advancement of Parenteral Nutrition

Nutrient	Initial Dose	Advancement	Maximum
Glucose	5%–10%	2.5%–5%/day	12.5% peripheral 18 mg/kg/min (maximum rate of infusion)
Protein	0.5–1 g/kg/day	0.5–1 g/kg/day	3 g/kg/day 10%–16% of calories
Fat	0.5–1 g/kg/day	0.5–1 g/kg/day	4 g/kg/day 0.17 g/kg/hr (maximum rate of infusion)

TABLE 23.15.

Daily Parenteral Nutrient Recommendations

Component	0–1 yr	1–7 yr	> 7 yr
Energy (Kcal/kg)	80–120	55–90	55–75
Protein (g/kg)	2–3	1.5–2.5	1.5–2.5
Sodium (mEq/kg)	3–4	2–4	2–4
Potassium (mEq/kg)	2–3	2–3	2–3
Magnesium (mEq/kg)	0.25–1	0.25–1	0.25–1
Calcium (mg/kg)	40–60	10–50	10–50
Phosphorus (mg/kg)	20–45	15–40	15–40
Zinc (mcg/kg)	400 (preterm) 100	100	100 max 4 mg/day
Copper (mcg/kg)	20	20	20 max 1.5 mg/day
Chromium (mcg/kg)	0.2	0.2	0.2 max 15 mg/day
Manganese (mcg/kg)	2–10	2–10	2–10 max 0.8 mg/day
Selenium (mcg/kg)	3	3	3 max 40 mg/day

References: 9, 10, 11, 12

TABLE 23.16.

Parenteral MVI Formulation

MVI Pediatric
Each 5 ml of reconstituted product provides:

Ascorbic acid	80 mg
Vitamin A (retinol)	0.7 mg*
Ergocalciferol	10 mcg†
Thiamine	1.2 mg
Riboflavin	1.4 mg
Pyridoxine	1 mg
Niacinamide	17 mg
Dexpanthenaol	5 mg
Vitamin E	7 mg‡
Biotin	20 mcg
Folic acid	140 mcg
Cyanocobalamin	1 mcg
Phytonadione	200 mcg

*0.7 mg vitamin A equals 2300 USP units
†10 mcg ergocalciferol equals 400 USP units
‡7 mg vitamin E equals 7 USP units

TABLE 23.17.

Monitoring Schedule

Variable	Initial period*	Later period†
GROWTH		
Weight	Daily	2 times/wk
Height	Weekly (infants) Monthly	Monthly
Head circumference (infants)	Weekly	Monthly
Arm circumference	Monthly	Monthly
Skinfold thickness	Monthly	Monthly
LABORATORY STUDIES		
Electrolytes & glucose	Daily until stable	Weekly
BUN/creatinine	2 times/wk	Weekly
Albumin or prealbumin	Weekly	Weekly
Ca, Mg, P	2 times/wk	Weekly
ALT, AST, Alk P	Weekly	Weekly
Total & direct bilirubin	Weekly	Weekly
CBC	Weekly	Weekly
Triglycerides	With each increase	Weekly
Vitamins	—	As indicated
Trace minerals	—	As indicated

*The period before nutritional goals are reached or during any period of instability.
†When stability is reached, no changes in nutrient composition.

REFERENCES

Waterlow JC: Classification and definition of protein calorie malnutrition, *Br Med J* 3:565, 1972.

Dietz WH: Obesity in infants, children and adolescents in the United States I: identification, natural history and after effects, *Nutr Res* 3:43, 1983.

Himes JH, Dietz WH: Guidelines for overweight in adolescent preventive services: recommendations from an expert committee, *Am J Clin Nutr* 59:307, 1994.

Food and Nutrition Board, National Academy of Sciences National Research Council. Recommended Dietary Allowances. 1989.

Seashore JH: Nutritional support of children in the intensive care unit, *Yal J Biol Med* 57:111, 1984.

Harris JA, Benedict FG: *A biometric study of basal metabolism in man,* Washington, DC, 1919, Carnegie Institute.

Wilmore D: *The metabolic management of the critically ill,* New York, 1977, Plenum.

MacLean WC et al: Nutritional management of chronic diarrhea and malnutrition: primary reliance on oral feeding, *J Pediatr* 97:316, 1980.

Committee on Nutrition of the AAP. Commentary on parenteral nutrition. *Pediatr* 73:547, 1983.

Kerner JA: *Manual of pediatric nutrition,* New York, 1983, John Wiley & Sons.

Collier SB: Parenteral nutrition. In Hendricks KM, Walker WA, editors: *Manual of pediatric nutrition,* Toronto, BC, 1990, Decker.

Cox JH, Cooning SW: Parenteral nutrition. In Queen PM, Lang CE, editors: *Handbook of pediatric nutrition,* Gaithersburg, 1993, Aspen Publishers.

PULMONOLOGY 24

I. NORMAL RESPIRATORY RATES (Table 24.1)

TABLE 24.1.

Age (yr)	Boys	Girls	Age (yr)	Boys	Girls
0–1	31 ± 8	30 ± 6	9–10	19 ± 2	19 ± 2
1–2	26 ± 4	27 ± 4	10–11	19 ± 2	19 ± 2
2–3	25 ± 4	25 ± 3	11–12	19 ± 3	19 ± 3
3–4	24 ± 3	24 ± 3	12–13	19 ± 3	19 ± 2
4–5	23 ± 2	22 ± 2	13–14	19 ± 2	18 ± 2
5–6	22 ± 2	21 ± 2	14–15	18 ± 2	18 ± 3
6–7	21 ± 3	21 ± 3	15–16	17 ± 3	18 ± 3
7–8	20 ± 3	20 ± 2	16–17	17 ± 2	17 ± 3
8–9	20 ± 2	20 ± 2	17–18	16 ± 3	17 ± 3

Mean respiratory rates ± 1 standard deviation.
From Illif A, Lee V: *Child Development,* 23:240, 1952.

II. PULMONARY FUNCTION TESTS (PFTs)
Pulmonary function testing provides objective and reproducible measurements of airway function and lung volumes, which can be used to characterize disease, assess severity, and follow response to therapy.

A. Peak Expiratory Flow Rate (PEFR)
The maximum flow rate that can be generated during a forced expiratory maneuver. Provides a simple, quantitative, reproducible measure of airway obstruction that can be obtained using inexpensive, portable, hand-held peak flow meters. Effort dependent, insensitive to small airway function. PEFRs may be useful in following both the course of asthma and a patient's response to therapy. If possible, it is ideal to compare a patient's PEFR to previous "personal best" rather than normal predicted value (Table 24.2).

TABLE 24.2.

Predicted Average Peak Expiratory Flow Rates for Normal Children

Height (in)	PEFR (L/min)	Height (in)	PEFR (L/min)
43	147	56	320
44	160	57	334
45	173	58	347
46	187	59	360
47	200	60	373
48	214	61	387
49	227	62	400
50	240	63	413
51	254	64	427
52	267	65	440
53	280	66	454
54	293	67	467
55	307		

From Polger G, Promedhat V: *Pulmonary function testing in children: techniques and standards,* Philadelphia, 1971, WB Saunders.

B. Spirometry

A rapid, forceful, and complete expiration from total lung capacity to residual volume (FVC maneuver) is used to measure forced vital capacity (FVC), forced expiratory volume in one second (FEV_1), and forced expiratory flow between 25% and 75% of vital capacity (FEF_{25-75}). Can also be used to obtain measurements of tidal volume (TV), minute ventilation (VE), maximal voluntary ventilation (MVV), expiratory reserve volume, inspiratory capacity, and inspiratory reserve volume. May be done before and after bronchodilators to assess response to therapy or after bronchial challenge to assess for airway hyperreactivity. Can reliably be performed by most children 6 years and older.

1. FVC: The maximum volume of air that can be exhaled from the lungs after a maximum inspiration. Bedside measurement of vital capacity with a hand-held spirometer can be useful in confirming or predicting hypoventilation. An FVC<15 ml/kg is an indication for ventilatory support.

2. FEV_1: The volume exhaled during the first second of a FVC maneuver. Single best measure of airway function.

3. FEF$_{25-75}$: The mean rate of airflow over the middle half of the FVC—between 25% and 75% of FVC. Sensitive to small airway obstruction.
4. MVV: Patient breathes as hard and as fast as possible for 12–15 seconds (sprint maneuver), and minute ventilation is calculated. Good measure of overall pulmonary function. Useful in assessing respiratory muscle function.

C. **Flow-Volume Curves**
   Plot of air flow versus lung volume. Useful in characterizing different patterns of airway obstruction (Fig. 24.1).

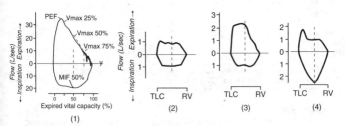

FIG. 24.1. Flow-volume loops.

1. Normal flow/volume curve
2. Fixed upper airway obstruction (tracheal stenosis): Flattening of both inspiratory and expiratory phases
3. Variable extrathoracic obstruction (obstructive apnea, tracheomalacia, paralyzed vocal cords): Flattened **inspiratory** phase as negative inspiratory pressure favors extrathoracic airway collapse
4. Variable intrathoracic obstruction (tumor): Flattened **expiratory** phase as positive pleural pressure compresses trachea and increases resistance

D. **Maximal Inspiratory and Expiratory Pressures**
   Obtained by having patient inhale/exhale against fixed obstruction. Low pressures suggest neuromuscular problem or submaximal effort. A negative inspiratory pressure < 20–25 is an indication for ventilatory support.

E. **Lung Volumes**

Total lung capacity (TLC), functional residual capacity (FRC), and residual volume (RV) cannot be determined by spirometry and require determination by helium dilution, nitrogen washout, or body plethysmography (Fig. 24.2).

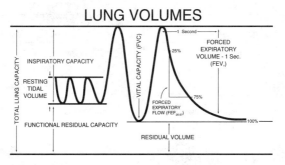

FIG. 24.2. Lung volumes.

D. **Interpretation (Table 24.3)**

TABLE 24.3.

	Obstructive disease (asthma, cystic fibrosis)	Restrictive disease (interstitial fibrosis, scoliosis)
SPIROMETRY		
FVC*	Normal or reduced	Reduced
FEV$_1$*	Reduced	Reduced§
FEV$_1$/FVC†	Reduced	Normal
FEF$_{25-75}$	Reduced	Normal or reduced§
PEFR*	Normal or reduced	Normal or reduced§
LUNG VOLUMES		
Total lung capacity (TLC)*	Normal or increased	Reduced
Residual volume (RV)*	Increased	Reduced
RV/TLC‡	Increased	Unchanged
Functional residual Capacity (FRC)	Increased	Reduced

*Normal range: ± 20% of predicted.	†Normal range: > 85%.
‡Normal range: 20 ± 10%.	§Reduced proportional to FVC.

III. PULMONARY GAS EXCHANGE
A. Arterial Blood Gas (ABG)
Used to assess oxygenation (PaO_2), ventilation ($PaCO_2$), and acid/base status (pH and HCO_3).
1. Normal mean ABG values (Table 24.4)

TABLE 24.4.

	pH	PaO_2 (mm Hg)	$PaCO_2$ (mm Hg)	HCO_3 (mEq/L)
Newborn (birth)	7.26–7.29		55	
Newborn (24 hr)	7.37	70	33	20
Infant (1–24 mo)	7.40	90	34	20
Child (7–19 yr)	7.39	96	37	22
Normal range (adult)	7.35–7.45	90–110	35–45	22–26

Adapted from Rogers M: *Textbook of pediatric intensive care,* ed 2, Baltimore, 1992, Williams and Wilkins.

2. Analysis of acid/base disturbances
Henderson-Hasselbach Equation:

$$pH = pK + \log\left(\frac{[HCO_3]}{a \times [PaCO_2]}\right)$$

where $pK = 6.10$ and $a = 0.0301$
   a. Approximate changes in pure acid/base disturbances
      1) Pure respiratory acidosis or alkalosis: 10 mm Hg rise (fall) in $PaCO_2$ accompanies a 0.08 fall (rise) in pH.
      2) Pure metabolic acidosis or alkalosis: 0.15 fall (rise) in pH accompanies a 10 mEq/L fall (rise) in HCO_3.
   b. Determine primary disturbance and then assess for mixed disorder by calculating expected compensatory response (Table 24.5).
B. Venous Blood Gas (VBG)
Peripheral venous samples are strongly affected by the local circulatory or metabolic environment and have limited usefulness, especially in assessing oxygenation. Can be used to assess acid-base status. Sampling from central venous catheters is preferred. A mixed-venous sample from the pulmonary artery may be used to evaluate the shunt fraction as well as total body oxygen consumption (see Reference Data).

TABLE 24.5.

Disturbance	Primary change	pH	Expected compensatory response
Acute respiratory acidosis	↑ $PaCO_2$	↓ pH	↑ **HCO_3^-** by 1 mEq/L for each 10 mm Hg rise in $PaCO_2$
Acute respiratory alkalosis	↓ $PaCO_2$	↑ pH	↓ **HCO_3^-** by 1–3 mEq/L for each 10 mm Hg fall in $PaCO_2$
Chronic respiratory acidosis	↑ $PaCO_2$	↓ pH	↑ **HCO_3^-** by 4 mEq/L for each 10 mm Hg rise in $PaCO_2$
Chronic respiratory alkalosis	↓ $PaCO_2$	↑ pH	↓ **HCO_3^-** by 2–5 mEq/L for each 10 mm Hg fall in $PaCO_2$
Metabolic acidosis	↓ HCO_3^-	↓ pH	↓ **$PaCO_2$** by 1–1.5 × fall in HCO_3
Metabolic alkalosis	↑ HCO_3^-	↑ pH	↑ **$PaCO_2$** by 0.25–1 × rise in HCO_3

Adapted from Schrier RW: *Renal and electrolyte disorders,* ed 3, Boston, 1986, Little, Brown and Company.

C. **Capillary Blood Gas (CBG)**
   Correlation with arterial sampling is generally best for pH, moderate for PCO_2, and worst for PO_2.
D. **Pulse Oximetry**
   1. Noninvasive method of indirectly measuring arterial oxygen saturation. Uses light absorption characteristics of oxygenated and deoxygenated hemoglobin to estimate oxygen saturation based on empirically derived algorithm. The oxyhemoglobin dissociation curve (see Fig. 24.4) relates O_2 saturation to PaO_2.
   2. Important uses
      a. Rapid and continuous assessment of oxygenation in acutely ill patients
      b. Monitoring of patients requiring oxygen therapy
      c. Assessment of oxygen requirements during feeding, sleep, and exercise
      d. Home monitoring of physiologic effects of apnea/bradycardia
   3. Technique limitations
      a. Measures **saturation** (SaO_2) and **not O_2 delivery** to tissues. A marginally low saturation may be clinically significant in an anemic patient.
      b. Unreliable if poor detection of pulse signal due to physiologic conditions (hypothermia, hypovolemia, shock) or movement artifact. The oximeter's pulse rate should match the patient's heart rate.

    c. Insensitive to hyperoxia ($PaO_2 > 100$ mm Hg) because of the sigmoid shape of the oxyhemoglobin curve. This limits its usefulness in premature infants.

    d. SaO_2 artificially **increased** by carboxyhemoglobin levels >1%–2% (chronic smokers, smoke inhalation)

    e. SaO_2 artificially **decreased** by intravenous dyes, like methylene blue or indocyanine green, and opaque nail polish

    f. SaO_2 artificially **increased or decreased** by methemoglobin levels >1%–2% (nitroglycerin ingestion), patient motion, electrosurgical interference, or xenon arc surgical lamps

From Murray CB, Loughlin GM: *Contemp Pediatr* 12:45, 1995.

  F. **Capnography**

    Measures CO_2 concentration of expired gas by infrared spectroscopy or mass spectroscopy. End-tidal CO_2 ($ETCO_2$) is the highest CO_2 during the expiratory phase. $ETCO_2$ correlates with $PaCO_2$ (usually within 5 mm Hg of $PaCO_2$ in healthy subjects). Can be used for demonstrating proper placement of endotracheal tube, for continuous monitoring of CO_2 trends in ventilated patients, and for monitoring ventilation during polysomnography.

IV. OXYGEN DELIVERY SYSTEMS

A. Nasal Cannula (nasal prongs)

    1. Provides low to moderate O_2 concentrations (22%–40%) at flow rates of 1/8 to 4 liters per minute (lpm).

    2. High flow rates may be uncomfortable, dry mucous membranes, and cause gastric distention or headaches.

    3. FIO_2 delivered is somewhat unpredictable depending on how much ambient air is entrained (influenced by age, inspiratory flow rate, and minute ventilation) during inspiration.

    4. Mouth breathing is usually not a factor since O_2 can be entrained from nasopharynx.

    5. Use appropriate size cannula for age.

B. Masks (see Fig. 24.3)

    Should be soft and pliable. Should be clear so that regurgitation can be detected. Will increase dead space. CO_2 retention may occur if O_2 flow rate is not sufficient.

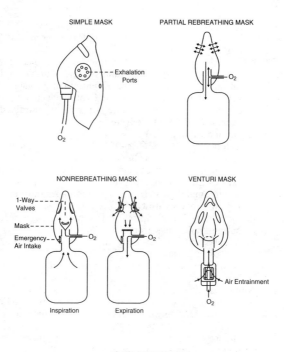

SIMPLE MASK

PARTIAL REBREATHING MASK

Exhalation Ports

O_2

O_2

NONREBREATHING MASK

VENTURI MASK

1-Way Valves

Mask

Emergency Air Intake

O_2

O_2

Inspiration

Expiration

Air Entrainment

O_2

TRACHEOSTOMY MASK

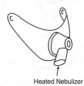

Heated Nebulizer

FIG. 24.3. Masks *(From Burgess WR, Chernick V: Respiratory therapy in newborn infants and children, New York 1982, Thieme-Stratton.)*

1. **Simple mask**
   a. Delivers FIO_2 of 35%–55% at flow rates of 6–10 lpm.
   b. FIO_2 determined by O_2 flow rate supplied relative to inspiratory flow rate and tidal volume. During inspiration, O_2 mixes with room air entrained through the vents and around mask. As tidal volume increases for a given O_2 flow rate, more air will be entrained, decreasing the FIO_2 delivered.

2. **Partial rebreathing mask**
   a. Can deliver FIO_2 of 60%–95% depending on inspiratory flow rate, tidal volume, and leaks.
   b. Has reservoir bag but no valve system to prevent expired air from entering reservoir.
   c. Approximately first 1/3 of expiration goes into reservoir and mixes with O_2.
   d. Remaining 2/3 of expiration is vented through ports on mask and leaks around mask.
   e. A collapsed reservoir bag indicates inadequate O_2 flow or huge leak.
   f. O_2 flow rates should be >6 lpm to avoid CO_2 retention.

3. **Nonrebreathing mask**
   a. Commonly used to deliver FIO_2 approaching 100%. Requires relatively tight seal with face and high rate of gas flow.
   b. Has reservoir bag and one-way valve to prevent expired air from entering reservoir.
   c. Inspired gas comes exclusively from the mask and reservoir bag. Negative inspiratory pressure closes exhalation ports and opens valve to the reservoir.
   d. Exhaled gas is vented through the exhalation ports.
   e. If the O_2 source disconnects, a safety valve permits room air to enter the system.

4. **Venturi mask**
   a. Designed to deliver specific O_2 concentrations
   b. Especially useful in chronic lung disease where control of FIO_2 is crucial.
   c. Based on Bernoulli principle. O_2 flows through a jet at a set flow rate, and room air enters through entrainment ports. FIO_2 determined by the flow rate, the size of the jet, and the entrainment ports. Allows for

predictable O_2 concentrations between 24% and 50%.
      d. If back pressure develops on the jet, less room air may be entrained, and FIO_2 may increase unpredictably.
      e. It may be useful to confirm manufacturer's specifications by analyzing FIO_2 in the mask.
   5. **Tracheostomy mask**
      a. Provides a relatively controlled O_2 and humidity source.
      b. FIO_2 not predictable unless Venturi circuit (same principle as Venturi mask) is used. FIO_2 should be analyzed for each patient individually.
      c. Should be properly positioned over tracheostomy.
C. **Oxygen Hoods/Headboxes**
   1. Useful for patients who will not tolerate masks or cannulae (i.e., infants).
   2. May achieve very high O_2 concentrations.
   3. Flow rate must be sufficient to reduce CO_2 accumulation (usually >10 lpm).
   4. Disadvantages: An O_2 gradient may develop within the hood/box, and patients must be taken out for feeding and cares.
D. **Oxygen Tents**
   1. Usually provide FIO_2 up to 50% range.
   2. Leaks are a major problem.
   3. Flow rate must be sufficient to prevent CO_2 build-up.
   4. Can be used to provide humidified air (croup or mist tent).
   5. Disadvantages: Development of O_2 gradient, decreases in FIO_2 resulting from frequently entering the tent, and claustrophobia (may become a problem for older children). Sparks in or near the tent may be hazardous. Close monitoring of patient and apparatus are required.

From Burgess WR, Chernick V: *Respiratory therapy in newborn infants and children,* New York, 1982, Thieme-Stratton.

V. MECHANICAL VENTILATION
A. **Types of Ventilatory Support**
   1. **Volume limited**
      a. Delivers a preset tidal volume to a patient regardless of pressure required

    b. Risk of barotrauma reduced by pressure alarms and pressure pop-off valves that limit peak inspiratory pressure

  2. **Pressure limited**

    a. Gas flow is delivered to the patient until a preset pressure is reached and then held for the set inspiratory time (reduces the risk of barotrauma).

    b. Useful for neonatal and infant ventilatory support (<10 kg) where the volume of gas being delivered is small in relation to the volume of compressible air in the ventilator circuit, making reliable delivery of a set tidal volume difficult.

B. Ventilator Parameters

  1. Peak inspiratory pressure **(PIP):** Maximum inspiratory pressure attained during the respiratory cycle

  2. Positive end-expiratory pressure **(PEEP):** Airway pressure maintained between inspiratory and expiratory phases (prevents alveolar collapse during expiration, decreasing work of reinflation and improving gas exchange)

  3. Rate **(IMV):** The number of mechanical breaths delivered per minute

  4. Inspired oxygen concentration **(FIO$_2$):** The fraction of oxygen present in inspired gas

  5. Inspiratory time **(Ti):** Length of time spent in the inspiratory phase of the respiratory cycle

  6. Tidal volume **(TV):** Volume of gas delivered during inspiration

C. Modes of Operation

There are several modes of operation on most volume-cycled ventilators.

  1. **IMV** (intermittent mandatory ventilation): A preset number of breaths are delivered each minute. The patient can take breaths on his own, but the ventilator may cycle on during a patient breath.

  2. **SIMV** (synchronized IMV): Similar to IMV, but the ventilator synchronizes delivered breaths with inspiratory effort, and allows the patient to finish expiration before cycling on.

  3. **AC or AMV** (assist control): Every inspiratory effort by the patient triggers a ventilator-delivered breath at the set tidal volume. Ventilator-initiated breaths are delivered

when the spontaneous rate falls below the backup rate.

4. **PSV** (pressure support ventilation): Inspiratory effort opens a valve allowing air flow at a preset positive pressure. Patient determines rate and inspiratory time. May be used in combination with other modes of operation.

5. **CPAP** (continuous positive airway pressure): Delivers air flow (with set FIO_2) such that a set pressure is maintained

D. **Initial Ventilator Settings**
   1. **Volume limited**
      a. Rate: Approximately normal range for age
      b. Tidal volume: Approximately 10–15 ml/kg
      c. Inspiratory time: Generally use I:E ratio of 1:2. More prolonged expiratory times are required for obstructive diseases to avoid air trapping.
      d. FIO_2: Selected to maintain targeted saturations and PaO_2
   2. **Pressure limited**
      a. Rate: Approximately normal range for age
      b. PEEP: Start with 3 cm H_2O and increase as clinically indicated. (Monitor for decreases in cardiac output with increasing PEEP.)
      c. PIP: Set at pressure required to produce adequate chest wall movement (approximate this using hand-bagging and manometer).
      d. FIO_2: Selected to maintain targeted saturations and PaO_2

E. **Further Ventilator Management**
   1. Follow patient closely with serial blood gas measurements and clinical assessment. Adjust ventilator parameters as indicated (Table 24.6).
   2. Parameters predictive of successful extubation
      a. Normal $PaCO_2$
      b. PIP generally <14–16 cm H_2O
      c. PEEP <2–3 cm H_2O (infants) or <5 cm H_2O (children)
      d. IMV <2–4 (infants); children may wean to CPAP
      e. FIO_2 <40% (maintaining PaO_2 > 70)
      f. Maximum negative inspiratory pressure >20–25 cm H_2O

TABLE 24.6.

Ventilator setting changes	Effects on blood gases	
	$PaCO_2$	PaO_2
↑ PIP	↓	↑
↑ PEEP	↑	↑
↑ Rate (IMV)	↓	Min ↑
↑ I:E ratio	No change	↑
↑ FIO2	No change	↑
↑ Flow	Min ↓	Min ↑

From Carlo WA, Chatburn RL: *Neonatal respiratory care*, ed 2, Chicago, 1988, Mosby.

VI. REFERENCE DATA
A. Minute Ventilation (VE)

$$VE = \text{respiratory rate} \times \text{tidal volume (TV)}$$
$$VE \times PaCO_2 = \text{constant (for volume-limited ventilation)}$$
$$\text{normal TV} = 10\text{–}15 \text{ml/kg}$$

B. Alveolar Gas Equation

$$PAO_2 = PIO_2 - (PACO_2/R)$$
$$PIO_2 = FIO_2 \times (PB - 47 \text{ mm Hg})$$

1. PIO_2 = partial pressure of inspired O_2 (150 mm Hg at sea level on room air)
2. R = respiratory exchange quotient (CO_2 produced/O_2 consumed) = 0.8
3. $PACO_2$ = partial pressure of alveolar CO_2 ≅ partial pressure of arterial CO_2 ($PaCO_2$)
4. PB = atmospheric pressure = 760 mm Hg
5. PAO_2 = partial pressure of O_2 in the alveoli

C. Alveolar-arterial Oxygen Gradient (A-a gradient)

$$\text{A-a gradient} = PAO_2 - PaO_2$$

1. Obtain ABG measuring PaO_2 and $PaCO_2$ with patient on 100% FIO_2 for at least 15 minutes.
2. Calculate the PAO_2 (as in Section B above) and then the A-a gradient.
3. The larger the gradient the more serious the respiratory

compromise. A normal gradient is 20–65 on 100% O_2 or 5–20 mm Hg on room air.

D. Oxygen Content (CaO_2)

$$O_2 \text{ content of sample (ml/dl)} = (O_2 \text{ capacity} \times O_2 \text{ saturation [as decimal]}) + \text{dissolved } O_2$$

1. O_2 capacity = hemoglobin (g/dl) $\times$ 1.34
2. Dissolved O_2 = PO_2 (of sample) $\times$ 0.003
3. Hemoglobin carries over 99% of O_2 in blood under standard conditions.

E. Arterial-venous O_2 Difference (AV DO_2)

$$AV \ DO_2 = CaO_2 - CmvO_2 = \text{arterial } O_2 \text{ content} - \text{mixed venous } O_2 \text{ content}$$

1. Usually done after placing patient on 100% FIO_2 for 15 minutes
2. Obtain ABG and mixed venous blood sample (best obtained from pulmonary artery catheter), and measure O_2 saturation.
3. Calculate arterial and mixed venous oxygen contents (see Section D above) and then AV DO_2 (normal $\cong$ 5 ml/100 dl).

F. O_2 Extraction Ratio

$$O_2 \text{ extraction} = (AV \ DO_2/CaO_2) \times 100$$
$$(\text{normal range } 28\%–33\%)$$

1. Calculate AV DO_2 and O_2 contents (see sections D and E above).
2. Extraction ratios are indicative of the adequacy of O_2 delivery to tissues, with increasing extraction ratios suggesting that metabolic needs may be outpacing the oxygen content being delivered.

From Rogers M: *Textbook of pediatric intensive care,* ed 2, Baltimore, 1992, Williams and Wilkins.

G. Oxygenation Index (OI)

$$OI = (\text{mean airway pressure (cm } H_2O) \times FIO_2 \times 100) / PaO_2$$
$$OI > 35 \text{ for 5–6 hr is one criterion for ECMO support}$$

H. Intrapulmonary Shunt Fraction (Qs/Qt)

$$\frac{Qs}{Qt} = \frac{(\text{A-a gradient}) \times 0.003}{(\text{AV DO}_2) + (\text{A-a gradient} \times 0.003)}$$

(Note: Qt, Cardiac output; Qs, flow across right-to-left shunt.)

1. Above formula assumes blood gases obtained on 100% FIO_2.
2. Represents the mismatch of ventilation and perfusion and is normally < 5%
3. A rising shunt fraction (usually >15%–20%) is indicative of progressive respiratory failure.

I. Oxyhemoglobin Dissociation Curve

1. Increased hemoglobin affinity for oxygen **(shift to the left)** occurs with alkalemia, hypothermia, hypocarbia, decreased 2, 3-diphosphoglycerate, increased fetal hemoglobin, and anemia.
2. Decreased hemoglobin affinity for oxygen **(shift to the right)** occurs with acidemia, hyperthermia, hypercarbia, and increased 2, 3-diphosphoglycerate (Fig. 24.4).

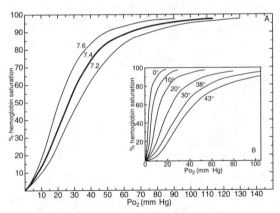

FIG. 24.4. Oxyhemoglobin dissociation curve *(From Lanbertsten CJ: Transport of oxygen, CO₂, and inert gases by the blood. In Mountcastle VB, editor:* Medical physiology, *ed 14, St Louis, 1980, Mosby.)*

RADIOLOGY

25

To avoid inadvertent irradiation of a fetus or embryo, elective diagnostic radiographs of the abdomen, pelvis, hips, and upper thighs of postmenarchal women should only be performed in the first 10 days of the menstrual cycle. If dates of menses cannot be established, a rapid sensitive urine pregnancy test should be performed. Gonadal shields should be used in all instances unless attempting to visualize the bony pelvis.

I. IMAGING MODALITIES
A. Plain Films
X-rays are produced when high-speed electrons decelerate rapidly. Structures that absorb the x-rays, such as bone, appear white on plain films. X-rays magnify the imaged object to some extent because of beam divergence and the distance between the object and the film. As this distance increases, so does the degree of magnification. Anteroposterior (AP) films of the chest, for example, magnify anterior structures such as the heart more than posteroanterior (PA) films.

1. **Chest:** Chest films are usually obtained to look for evidence of intrathoracic pathology of pulmonary, cardiac, or mediastinal origin. Also commonly obtained to check placement of endotracheal tubes and central venous catheters.

   a. **Interlobar fissures:** Visible only when tangential to the x-ray beam. Minor fissure is normally located at the level of the 6th rib at the right lateral chest wall. The major fissure is usually not visible on frontal views but runs at a 45° angle down from T_4–T_5 on lateral view.

   b. **Silhouette sign:** A term used to describe the blurring of the normally sharp borders between air-containing lung and other intrathoracic structures. Upper, lingular, and middle lobe processes silhouette anterior structures, particularly the heart border. Lower lobe processes silhouette posterior structures, such as the diaphragm and descending aorta.

c. **Air bronchograms:** Linear air shadows created by air-filled bronchi surrounded by pulmonary infiltrate, atelectasis, infarction, or edema. Helpful in distinguishing between intraparenchymal lesions and lesions in mediastinum or pleural space. Not helpful in differentiating between infection and atelectasis.

d. **Volume loss pattern**
1) Right middle lobe (RML), right upper lobe (RUL) classic locations
2) Fissure may shift toward region of volume loss (Fig. 25.1)
3) Compensatory hyperinflation may develop in remaining aerated areas.

e. **Consolidative process**
1) Any lobe may be involved.
2) Fissure is usually not displaced.
3) Air bronchograms are often visible.

f. **Central line placement:** Central venous catheters ideally placed with the catheter tip at the junction of the superior vena cava (SVC) and RA. Some extension into the RA is acceptable, but if catheter is noted to curve to the left on a PA film, or ventrally/anteriorly on a lateral film, the catheter may be positioned in the RV (Fig. 25.2)

g. **Endotracheal tube placement:** The end of the endotracheal tube (ETT) should rest approximately 2–3 cm above the carina, at the level of T_3–T_4 (this may vary somewhat depending on the size of the patient). The lung fields should show symmetric aeration; deviation of the ETT down a mainstem bronchus, obvious asymmetry in the lung fields, or atelectasis in the lung fields may indicate need for repositioning.

2. **Abdomen:** X-ray exams of the abdomen are useful in evaluating for obstruction, pneumoperitoneum, and mass effect. In the radiologic evaluation of the acute abdomen at least two films should be obtained.

a. Supine: Provides useful information concerning bowel distention
b. Either a left lateral decubitus of the abdomen or a supine cross table lateral for diagnosis of free air, necrotizing enterocolitis, or intussusception

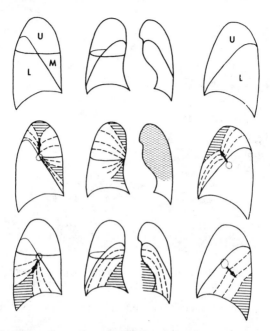

FIG. 25.1. Patterns of volume loss or consolidation. **Top panel:** Diagrammatic depiction of the three lobes of the right lung and the two lobes of the left lung. The lateral perspectives are shown for each lung from the side: right lung (left side), left lung (right side). **Middle panel:** Diagrammatic representation of typical patterns of atelectasis of the five major lobes. The upper and middle lobe patterns of atelectasis are shown separately from the lower lobes (**bottom panel**). The patterns of atelectasis reflect the manner in which the remaining aerated lung can hyperexpand to fill the space left by the atelectatic lung. The hilar structures shift accordingly. *(From Reginald E, Greene RE: Anatomical and functional basis of imaging the respiratory system. In Tavaras JM, Ferrucci JT, editors:* Radiology: diagnosis—imaging—intervention, *Philadelphia, 1990, JB Lippincott.*

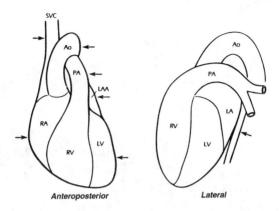

FIG. 25.2. Diagram of the heart (*Ref: Kirks DR et al: Practical pediatric imaging: diagnostic radiology of infants and children, Boston, 1991, Little, Brown, and Co.)*

   c. A chest x-ray exam should always be considered to exclude pulmonary pathology, which can mimic an abdominal process.
3. **Cervical spine:** After immobilization in a collar, lateral/AP x-ray exams of the cervical spine should be performed in all children who have sustained significant head trauma, deceleration injury, or who have undergone unwitnessed trauma for which no history can be obtained. Flexion/extension films may be helpful, especially in patients with Down's syndrome where atlantoaxial subluxation is a concern.
4. **Airway films:** The lateral view of the upper airway is the single most useful film to evaluate a child with stridor. If possible this view should be obtained on inspiration. A radiologic workup should always include AP and lateral views of the chest, with inclusion of the upper airway on the AP chest.

a. Diagnosis of diseases based upon airway x-ray exam (Table 25.1 and Fig. 25.3)

TABLE 25.1.

Diagnosis	Findings on airway films
Croup	AP and lateral films with subglottic narrowing ("steeple sign")
Epiglottitis	Enlarged, indistinct epiglottis on lateral film ("thumb sign")
Vascular ring	AP and lateral films with narrowing; double or right aortic arch
Retropharyngeal abscess or pharyngeal mass	Soft tissue air, or persistent enlargement of prevertebral soft tissues; >1/2 of a vertebral body above C_3, and 1 vertebral body below C_3
Immunodeficiency	Absence of adenoidal and tonsillar tissue after age 6 months

AP, Anteroposterior.

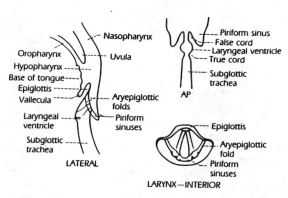

FIG. 25.3. Upper airway anatomy

  b. Foreign bodies
    1) Lower airway foreign bodies: In the absence of a radiopaque foreign body (FB), radiologic findings include air trapping, hyperinflation, atelectasis, consolidation, pneumothorax, and pneumomediastinum. If suspected clinically or on the basis of an initially abnormal CXR, further evaluative studies should include expiratory films (cooperative patient), bilateral decubitus chest films (uncooperative patient), or airway fluoroscopy.
    2) Esophageal foreign bodies (FBs): Esophageal FBs usually lodge at one of three locations: 1) at the thoracic inlet, 2) at the level of the aortic arch-left main-stem bronchus, or 3) at the gastroesophageal junction. Evaluation should include the following:
      a) Lateral airway film
      b) AP of the chest and abdomen (including the supraclavicular region)
    3) If these films are normal and the diagnosis is still suspected, a contrast study of the esophagus may reveal the foreign body. If perforation is suspected, use a nonionic, water-soluble contrast.
5. **Extremity x-ray exams:** In suspected trauma, an adequate evaluation requires at least two views, usually an AP and a lateral. Restricting the film to include only the area of interest improves the resolution (e.g., for a thumb injury, ask for an image of the thumb, not of the hand). In general, comparison films of the uninvolved extremity are not necessary, but they may be helpful in several instances, such as evaluation of joint effusions (particularly the hip), suspected osteomyelitis or pyarthrosis, and/or evaluation of subtle fractures, especially in areas of multiple ossification centers such as the elbow. Bone age determinations (traditionally using a PA view of the left hand and the wrist) may be helpful in the diagnosis and management of many endocrine, genetic, and nutritional disorders.
6. **Skeletal survey:** The skeletal survey is the appropriate radiologic series to order in cases of suspected child abuse. This survey should include a lateral skull with cervical spine, AP chest (bone technique), oblique view

of the ribs, pelvis, abdominal film (bone technique) with lateral thoracic and lumbar spine, as well as AP long bone films. Classic findings are multiple epiphyseal and metaphyseal injuries of various ages. In addition, suspicions should be raised by fracture at unusual sites or solitary spiral and transverse fractures of the long bones with a history of inadequate trauma.

B. Conventional Gray Scale Ultrasound

Images are created by echos returned from structures in the body. Measurements are based on the rate of sound wave travel and the interval between transmitted and returned signal.

1. **Applications**
   a. Pyloric stenosis
   b. Abdominal masses in young children
   c. Intussusception
   d. Tubo-Ovarian abscess
   e. Acute intracranial hemorrhage in newborns
   f. Definition of renal anatomy
   g. Congenital hip dislocation, in children <4 months of age
   h. Fluid collections (e.g., hip effusions, pleural effusions, ascites)
2. **Advantages:** No radiation exposure, painless, no sedation required, portable
3. **Disadvantages:** Gas and fat may degrade image, operator-dependent

C. Color Doppler Flow Imaging

Ultrasound frequency shifts caused by moving red blood cells are assigned color; usually, red is used for flow toward the transducer and blue is used for flow away from it. This modality (in conjunction with duplex Doppler) is used to evaluate deep vein thrombosis, vascular patency, intracranial blood flow, cardiac shunt flow, transplant vascularity, and scrotal perfusion.

D. CT Scan

1. **Applications**
   a. Modality of choice for evaluation of acute intracranial trauma, hydrocephalus, pulmonary parenchymal disease, calcifying processes, abdominal and chest trauma, and complicated inflammatory bowel disease. In children with blunt abdominal trauma, a computer-

ized tomography (CT) scan of the abdomen, including the lower portion of the chest, should be done.

b. Three-dimensional CT reconstruction is useful for evaluating complex craniofacial anomalies and injuries and other complex skeletal deformities.

2. **Advantages:** Cheaper than magnetic resonance imaging (MRI), sensitive to Ca^{++}, standardized interpretation, wide field of view

3. **Disadvantages:** Ionizing radiation exposure, not sensitive to diffuse white matter or cutaneous abnormalities, limited scanning planes, and IV contrast exposure

E. **Special CT Scans**

1. Ultrafast CT: This technique permits cine imaging, reduced radiation dosing, and takes only 50–100 ms to complete. A disadvantage is a somewhat decreased image quality compared to conventional CT.

2. Spiral CT: This technique permits continuous volume acquisition; however, the image may be degraded by motion.

3. High resolution CT: This technique permits edge enhancement and is good for imaging lung parenchyma.

F. **MRI Scans**

Radiowaves that have been altered in a stable fashion by a magnetic field stimulate atomic nuclei. Images are then created when absorbed energy is reemitted in the form of radio signals. Four parameters (proton density within a tissue, T_1 relaxation, T_2 relaxation, chemical shift) can be weighted to best evaluate dynamic physiology and tissue composition.

1. **Applications**

a. CNS: Better than CT for evaluating posterior fossa, brain stem, and spinal cord, including defects such as meningomyelocele. Excellent for evaluating demyelinating disorders because it differentiates between areas of normal and abnormal myelin content. Useful in the workup of focal seizures where a structural lesion may be involved. However, MRI may not reveal calcifications that characterize some neoplastic lesions.

b. Mediastinal lymphadenopathy

c. Cardiac: MRI provides excellent contrast between flowing blood and myocardium without the use of IV contrast agents.

  d. Abdomen: More sensitive than CT for evaluating extent of hepatic tumors before surgical resection
  e. Skeletal: Useful in detecting early signs of osteomyelitis and avascular necrosis of the femoral head. Can detect extension of bone tumors and marrow replacement by leukemic infiltrates.
 2. **Advantages:** No ionizing radiation, multiple imaging planes, sensitive to the presence of abnormal tissues
 3. **Disadvantages:** Difficult to accommodate critical care equipment, patients with implanted ferromagnetic devices cannot be scanned, sensitive to motion degradation; frequently requires sedation, poor signal from Ca^{++} and gas.
G. **Radionuclide Imaging:** Allows observation of dynamic function with a fixed amount of radiation.
 1. **Bone scan:** Useful in evaluating unexplained skeletal pain. Generally positive long before plain films for both benign conditions and malignancies such as metastatic neuroblastoma and leukemia. A three phase study should be ordered if infection is suspected. The phases are 1) blood flow scan, 2) equilibration scan at ten minutes, 3) delayed scan at 2–4 hours. Bone scanning is most commonly performed with technetium (^{99m}Tc) methylene diphosphonate (MDP).
 2. **Gallium-67 imaging:** Gallium-67 binds to transferrin, lactoferrin, and intracellular lysosomes and is useful in detecting occult abscesses and some types of tumors. Because gallium-67 is partially excreted by the colon, a standard barium enema prep (see p. 470) with a tapwater enema should be given just before sending the patient to nuclear medicine. It is not necessary to keep children NPO. Images are typically obtained at 24, 48, 72, or 96 hours after gallium-67 injection.

Note: Gallium interferes with the detection of technetium for up to 2 weeks. Thus when both technetium and gallium scans are indicated, the technetium scan should be done first. Injections for both scans can be made on the same day.

 3. **Radionuclide cystography:** Useful in the workup of urinary tract infections in children. Allows quantitative measurements and sensitive detection of vesicoureteral reflux, with approximately 1/100 the gonadal radiation

dose of voiding cystourethrogram (VCUG). The urethra is not evaluated by this technique, so it should not be used as the initial study in males who may have obstructions such as posterior urethral valves.

4. **Radionuclide renal imaging:** Tc-DTPA (^{99m}Tc diethylenetriamine pentaacetic acid) is eliminated by glomerular filtration, and is used for evaluation of renal function, glomerular filtration rate (GFR), vesicoureteral reflux, and renovascular hypertension. **Tc-DMSA** (^{99m}Tc dimercaptosuccinic acid), which selectively binds renal tubular cells, is used for evaluating renal structure and relative cortical function. Focal defects occur with pyelonephritis and scarring. **Glucoheptanate** binds to renal tubular cells and can be used as a substitute for Tc-DMSA. However, compared with DMSA, which has a 42% binding affinity, glucoheptanate has a 13% binding affinity to tubular cells. This leads to decreased cortical appearance and targeting of bladder.

5. **Gastrointestinal imaging**
   a. **Hepatobiliary scan:** Evaluates function and is often useful in diagnosing biliary atresia. Requires 5 days of preparation using phenobarbital (3-8 mg/kg/day, PO) to increase biliary excretion of the ^{99m}Tc-IDA compounds. May be useful in children with sickle cell disease for identifying biliary causes for abdominal crises.
   b. **Meckel's scan:** ^{99m}Tc-pertechnetate is trapped and secreted in the mucus-producing cells. The scan is therefore useful for detecting ectopic gastric mucosa.
   c. **Gastroesophageal reflux studies:** More information than pH probe and much less radiation exposure than with upper gastrointestinal series (UGI). Allows continuous imaging for a prolonged period with visual documentation of reflux frequency and timing, esophageal clearance of refluxed material, gastric emptying, and tracheal aspiration. Esophageal and gastric outlet anatomy is not well evaluated, so patients presenting with vomiting also require a limited UGI.

6. **Cerebral imaging:** Cerebral flow imaging may be helpful in assessing presence or absence of cerebral perfusion when brain death is at issue. Also useful in cases of early encephalitis such as herpes simplex.
7. **Nuclear cardiology:** Gated blood pool (MUGA) scanning is used to evaluate ventricular function in patients with congenital or acquired heart disease and oncology patients receiving cardiotoxic chemotherapeutic agents. Lung scanning can be used to evaluate pulmonary perfusion and patency of surgically created systemic-to-pulmonary shunts.

From Kirchner PT, editor: In *Nuclear medicine in review syllabus,* New York, 1980, Society of Nuclear Medicine; Majd M: Radionuclide imaging in pediatrics, *Pediatr Clin North Am* 32(6):1559, 1985.

8. **Ventilation/perfusion scan:** Perfusion is evaluated by labeling macroaggregated albumin (MAA) with Tc-99m. The particles become trapped in the capillary bed and are almost completely extracted during their first pass through the pulmonary circulation. Perfusion scans can be used to demonstrate congenital vascular malformations or pulmonary emboli. Ventilation scanning utilizes Xe-133 gas, Kr-81m, and Tc-DTPA aerosol in order to evaluate function in such disorders as cystic fibrosis, congenital lobar emphysema, hyperlucent lung syndrome, and postoperative diaphragmatic hernia.

From Kendig, EL, Jr, Chernick V: *Kendig's disorders of the respiratory tract in children,* ed 5, Philadelphia, 1990, WB Saunders.

II. SEDATION

Patient motion commonly degrades the quality of pediatric imaging examinations. Gentle handling and occasional physical restraints are often all that are needed for successful studies. However, sedation is often required, particularly for children under 4 years of age undergoing CT or MRI examination. See Chapter 27 for guidelines and medications.

III. CONTRAST

Plain film contrast agents are based on solutions with components of high atomic number that absorb x-rays well.

Oral contrast agents do not require consent for administration. IV contrast agents can rarely cause major adverse reactions, including anaphylaxis, upon administration. Minor reactions including hives or sneezing may also occur. Examinations usually will not be done if there is a previous history of allergy to iodine or severe reaction to a contrast agent. If there has been a previous minor reaction, steroid premedication may suffice. Most hospitals require that a parent or legal guardian read and sign a special consent form for administration of IV contrast agents.

IV. PREPARATORY PROCEDURES
A. Bisacodyl (Dulcolax)
   1. **Contraindications:** Acute surgical abdomen, acute ulcerative colitis
   2. **Tablets:** Bisacodyl acts directly on the colonic mucosa to produce peristalsis in the colon. Enteric-coated tablets must be swallowed whole; they must not be chewed or crushed. Use suppositories unless assured that child can swallow tablets whole. They should not be taken within 1 hour of antacids or milk. (See Formulary for dosage guidelines.)
   3. **Suppositories:** May be used at any age. (See Formulary for dosage guidelines.)
B. Specific Examination Requirements
   1. **Upper gastrointestinal series**
      a. Patient <18 mo: NPO for 3 hours before the study
      b. Patient >18 mo: Clear liquids after supper. No carbonated beverages on day of study. Bisacodyl pills or suppositories the evening before the examination, NPO for 4 hours before procedure.
   2. **Contrast enema**
      a. Infants <18 mo: Liquid diet starting evening before study. No carbonated beverages.
      b. Patients >18 mo: Liquid diet for 24 hours before study. No carbonated beverages. Bisacodyl pills or suppositories evening before. Bisacodyl suppository the morning of the study. If >10 years, give lukewarm tapwater enemas until clear the morning of study. Omit bisacodyl and enema when evaluation is for active colitis, acute surgical abdomen, or possible Hirschsprung disease.

   c. Air contrast barium enema (>18 mo): Clear liquid diet 24 hours before study. No carbonated beverages. Bisacodyl pills or suppositories the evening before. Lukewarm tapwater enemas until clear (i.e., no stool in the water). This usually takes 2 enemas. Bisacodyl enema (Fleet Bisacodyl Prep) will be given in radiology 1 hour before the examination.

3. **Intravenous pyelogram (IVP)** (an ultrasound exam of the kidneys frequently can substitute for an IVP): All patients should be normally hydrated but have an empty stomach. Notation must be made on requisition of previous drug reactions and allergies.

   a. Infants <18 mo: NPO before examination for same length of time as the usual interval between feedings.

   b. Patients >18 mo: Bisacodyl pills or suppositories the night before the examination. NPO 4 hours before examination.

4. **Voiding cystourethrogram:** No preparation is required.

5. **Head and body computerized tomography:** Oral and/or IV contrast agents may be necessary, depending upon the specific examination and the information required. IV contrast precautions and procedures apply as per Section III (p. 469). Patients should be NPO 4 hours before examination.

6. **Ultrasound examinations:** Because sound waves do not penetrate bone, gas, or barium, sonograms should be obtained before barium contrast studies.

   a. Pelvic and lower abdomen: Patients should be well hydrated with oral or IV fluids and, if possible, should not void for 1–3 hours before the examination. A bladder catheter may be necessary to fill the bladder.

   b. Liver, gallbladder, and biliary tree
     1) Infants: NPO 3–4 hours before examination, if possible
     2) Children: NPO 6–12 hours before examination

7. **Nuclear medicine examinations:** The general rules regarding protection from radiation as previously outlined apply to all nuclear studies. Most procedures do not require special patient preparation. Consultation with the nuclear medicine physician is encouraged before a study is performed.

PART III

Formulary

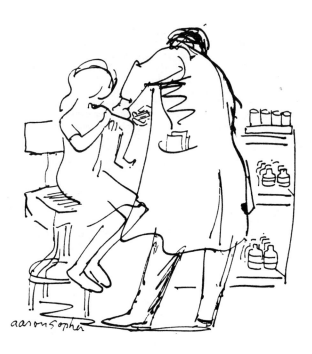

DRUG DOSES

26

The following formulary contains both generic and trade names, how drugs are supplied, and their usual dose, and routes of administration. Brief remarks about the side effects, drug interactions, precautions, and other relevant factors are included. For many generic drugs, we have provided a list of trade names. We have not attempted to make this list of trade names exhaustive: please consult books in the reference section for more detailed information.

Note: Please note in the "How Supplied" category: the unit quantity in which a drug is supplied is noted in parentheses after the drug concentration. For example, amoxicillin suspension, 125 mg/5 ml, is available in 80-, 100-, 150-, and 200-ml bottles. Suspension formulations that are footnoted are not commercially available and need to be extemporaneously compounded by a pharmacist. In addition, further dilutions of various neonatal medications may be necessary for proper dose delivery. Consult the references or a pharmacist for specific information.

Drug/How Supplied	Dose and Route	Remarks
ACETAMINOPHEN (Tylenol, Tempra, Panadol, Feverall, Anacin-3, and others) *Analgesic, antipyretic* Tabs: 325, 500, 650 mg Chewable tabs: 80, 160 mg Infant drops, solution/suspension: 80 mg/0.8 ml Child solution/suspension: 160 mg/5 ml Elixir: 80, 120, 130, 160, 325 mg/5 ml Caplet: 160, 325, 500 mg Suppositories: 80, 120, 125, 325, 650 mg (Combination product with Codeine, see Codeine)	*Pediatric:* 10–15 mg/kg/dose PO/PR Q4–6 hr; dosing by age: *0–3 mo:* 40 mg/dose *4–11 mo:* 80 mg/dose *12–24 mo:* 120 mg/dose *2–3 yr:* 160 mg/dose *4–5 yr:* 240 mg/dose *6–8 yr:* 320 mg/dose *9–10 yr:* 400 mg/dose *11–12 yr:* 480 mg/dose *Adult:* 325–650 mg/dose **Max dose:** 4 g/24 hr, 5 doses/24 hr	$T_{1/2}$: 1–3 hr, 2–5 hr in neonates; metabolized in the liver; some preparations contain alcohol (7%–10%) and/or phenylalanine; see Chapter 2 for management of overdosage; **contraindicated** in patients with known G6PD deficiency. All suspensions should be shaken before use.
ACETAZOLAMIDE (Diamox) *Carbonic anhydrase inhibitor, diuretic* Tabs: 125, 250 mg Suspension*: 30, 50 mg/ml Capsules (sustained release): 500 mg Injection (sodium): 500 mg/5 ml Contains 2.05 mEq Na/500 mg drug	*Diuretic (PO, IV)* *Child:* 5 mg/kg/dose QD-QOD *Adult:* 250–375 mg/dose QD-QOD *Glaucoma* *Child:* 20–40 mg/kg/24 hr ÷ Q6 hr IM/IV; 8–30 mg/kg/24 hr ÷ Q6–8 hr PO *Adult:* 1000 mg/24 hr ÷ Q6 hr PO; for rapid decrease in intraocular pressure, administer 500 mg/dose IV *Seizures:* 8–30 mg/kg/24 hr ÷ Q6–12 hr PO **Max dose:** 1 g/24 hr	$T_{1/2}$: 4–10 hr; possible side effects (more likely with long-term therapy) include GI irritation, paresthesias, sedation, hypokalemia, acidosis, reduced urate secretion, aplastic anemia, polyuria, and development of renal calculi; IM injection may be painful; bicarbonate replacement therapy may be required during long-term use (see Citrate or Sodium Bicarbonate) **contraindicated** in patients with hepatic failure.

*Indicates suspensions not commercially available; need to be extemporaneously compounded by a pharmacist. See references 1 and 2.

(Continued.)

Drug/How Supplied	Dose and Route	Remarks
ACETAZOLAMIDE—(cont.)	*Urine alkalinization:* 5 mg/kg/dose repeated BID-TID *Management of hydrocephalus:* see Chapter 22	
ACETYLCYSTEINE (Mucomyst) *Mucolytic, antidote for acetaminophen toxicity* Solution: 100 mg/ml (10%) or 200 mg/ml (20%) (4, 10, 30 ml)	For acetaminophen poisoning, see Chapter 2 *Meconium ileus:* 5–10 ml/kg of 10% solution PR by soft rubber catheter. This may be given up to Q6 hr. *Nebulizer:* 3–5 ml of 20% solution (diluted with equal volume of H_2O, or sterile saline to equal 10%), or 6–10 ml of 10% solution; administer TID-QID.	May induce bronchospasm, stomatitis, drowsiness, rhinorrhea, nausea, vomiting, and hemoptysis. Prior hydration is essential for meconium ileus treatment.
ACTH (Corticotropin, Acthar) *Polypeptide.* Aqueous (inj): 25, 40 U/vial Gel: 40, 80 U/ml (1, 5 ml) 1 unit = 1 mg	*Antiinflammatory:* *Aqueous:* 1.6 U/kg/24 hr IV, IM, or SC ÷ Q6–8 hr *Gel:* 0.8 U/kg/24 hr ÷ Q12–24 hr IM *Infantile spasms:* many regimens exist *Gel:* 20–40 U/24 hr IM QD or 80 U IM QOD; taper dose gradually	**Contraindicated** in acute psychoses, CHF, Cushing's disease, TB, peptic ulcer, ocular herpes, fungal infections, recent surgery, sensitivity to porcine products; IV administration for diagnostic purposes only. Can have hypersensitivity reaction. Similar adverse effects as corticosteroids.

ACYCLOVIR

(Zovirax)

Antiviral

Capsules: 200 mg

Tabs: 800 mg

Suspension: 200 mg/5 ml

Ointment: 5% (15 g)

Inj (with sodium): 500 mg/10 ml

Contains 4.2 mEq Na/1 g drug

IMMUNOCOMPETENT:

Neonatal HSV and HSV encephalitis: All ages: 30 mg/kg/24 hr or 1500 mg/m²/24 hr ÷ Q8 hr IV × 14–21 days

Mucocutaneous HSV (including genital):

Initial infection:

IV: 15 mg/kg/24 hr or 750 mg/m²/24 hr ÷ Q8 hr × 7 days

PO: 1200 mg/24 hr ÷ Q8 hr × 7–10 days

Recurrence:

PO: 1200 mg/24 hr ÷ Q8 hr × 5 days

Chronic suppressive therapy:

PO: 800–1000 mg/24 hr ÷ 2–5×/day for up to 1 year

Zoster:

IV: 30 mg/kg/24 hr or 1500 mg/m²/24 hr ÷ Q8 hr × 7–10 days

PO: 4000 mg/24 hr ÷ 5×/24 hr × 5–7 days for patients >12 yr

Varicella:

IV: 30 mg/kg/24 hr or 1500 mg/m²/24 hr ÷ Q8 hr × 7 days

PO: 80 mg/kg/24 hr ÷ QID × 5 days (begin treatment at earliest signs/symptoms)

Max dose: 3200 mg/24 hr

Can cause renal impairment; adequate hydration and slow (1 hr) IV administration is essential to prevent crystallization in renal tubules; dose alteration necessary in patients with impaired renal function; has been infrequently associated with headache, vertigo, insomnia, encephalopathy, GI tract irritation, rash, urticaria, arthralgia, fever, and adverse hematologic effects. See most recent edition of the Red Book* for further details. Oral absorption is unpredictable.

(Continued.)

Drug/How Supplied	Dose and Route	Remarks
ACYCLOVIR—(cont.)	IMMUNOCOMPROMISED: *HSV:* *IV:* 750–1500 mg/m²/24 hr ÷ Q8 hr × 7–14 days *PO:* 1000 mg/24 hr ÷ 3–5 times/24 hr × 7–14 days *Varicella or Zoster:* *IV:* Same as immunocompetent dosing × 7–10 days **Max dose** of oral acyclovir in children = 80 mg/kg/24 hr	
ADENOSINE (Adenocard) *Antiarrhythmic* Inj: 3 mg/ml (2 ml)	*Supraventricular tachycardia:* *Children:* 0.1 mg/kg rapid IV push; may increase dose by 0.05 mg/kg increments every 2 min to **max** of 0.25 mg/kg (up to 12 mg), or until termination of SVT **Max dose:** 12 mg	$T_{1/2}$: <10 sec; may precipitate bronchoconstriction. Side effects include facial flushing, headache, shortness of breath, dyspnea, nausea, chest pain, lightheadedness. **Contraindicated** in 2nd and 3rd degree AV block or sick-sinus syndrome unless pacemaker placed.
ALBUMIN, HUMAN (Albuminar, Albutein, Buminate, Plasbumin-5, Human Albumin, other) *Blood product derivative, plasma volume expander* Inj: 5% (50 mg/ml); 25% (250 mg/ml); each contains 130–160 mEq Na/L	*Hypoproteinemia:* *Children:* 1 g/kg/dose IV over 30–120 min *Adult:* 25 g/dose IV over 30–120 min; repeat Q1–2 days PRN *Hypovolemia:* *Children:* 1 g/kg/dose IV rapid infusion *Adult:* 25 g/dose IV rapid infusion; may repeat PRN **Max dose:** 6 g/kg/24 hr	**Contraindicated** in cases of CHF or severe anemia; rapid infusion may cause fluid overload; hypersensitivity reactions may occur; may cause rapid increase in serum sodium levels **Caution:** 25% concentration contraindicated in preterm infants due to risk of IVH. For infusion, use 5 micron filter or larger.

ALBUTEROL
(Proventil, Ventolin)
Beta-2-adrenergic agonist
Tabs: 2, 4 mg
Sustained release tabs: 4 mg
Oral solution: 2 mg/5 ml (473 ml)
Aerosol inhaler: 90 mcg/actuation (200 actuations/inhaler)
Rotacaps for inhalation: 200 mcg/capsule
Nebulization solution: 0.5% (5 mg/ml) (20 ml)
Prediluted nebulized solution: 2.5 mg in 3 ml NS (0.083%)

Oral:
Children <6 yr: 0.3 mg/kg/24 hr PO ÷ TID; **max dose:** 12 mg/24 hr
6–11 yr: 6 mg/24 hr PO ÷ TID; **max dose:** 24 mg/24 hr
12 yr and adults: 2–4 mg/dose PO TID-QID; **max dose:** 32 mg/24 hr
Inhalations:
Aerosol: 1–2 puffs (90–180 mcg) Q4–6 hr PRN
Rotacaps: 200 mcg Q4–6 hr
Neonate/Infant: 0.05–0.15 mg/kg/dose Q4–6 hr
1–5 yr: 1.25–2.5 mg/dose Q4–6 hr
5–12 yr: 2.5 mg/dose Q4–6 hr
>12 yr: 2.5–5 mg/dose Q6 hr

Possible side effects include tachycardia, palpitations, tremor, insomnia, nervousness, nausea, and headache. Nebulization may be given more frequently than indicated. In such cases, consider cardiac monitoring and monitoring of serum potassium. Systemic effects are dose related. **Please verify the concentration of the nebulization solution used.** The use of tube spacers or chambers may enhance efficacy of the metered dose inhalers.

ALLOPURINOL
(Lopurin, Zyloprim, and others)
Uric acid lowering agent, xanthine oxidase inhibitor
Tabs: 100, 300 mg
Suspension*: 10, 20 mg/ml

Child: 10 mg/kg/24 hr PO ÷ BID-QID;
Max dose: 600 mg/24 hr
Adult: 200–300 mg/24 hr PO ÷ BID-TID

Adjust dose in renal insufficiency. Must maintain adequate urine output and alkaline urine. Side effects include rash, neuritis, hepatotoxicity, GI disturbance, bone marrow suppression, and drowsiness. Drug interactions: increases serum theophylline level; may increase the incidence of rash with ampicillin and amoxicillin.

*Indicates suspensions not commercially available; need to be extemporaneously compounded by a pharmacist. See references 1 and 2.

(Continued.)

Drug/How Supplied	Dose and Route	Remarks
ALPROSTADIL	See Prostaglandin E₁	
ALUMINUM HYDROXIDE (Amphojel, Dialume, Nephrox, Alu-Tab, and others) *Antacid* Tabs: 300, 600 mg Caps: 475, 500 mg Suspension: 320 mg/5 ml, 450 mg/5 ml, 600 mg/5 ml, 675 mg/5 ml (150, 360 ml) Each 15 ml contains <0.3 mEq Na.	*Peptic ulcer:* *Child:* 5–15 ml PO Q3–6 hr or 1–3 hr PC and HS *Adult:* 15–45 ml PO Q3–6 hr or 1–3 hr PC and HS *Prophylaxis against GI bleeding:* *Neonates:* 1 ml/kg/dose Q4 hr PRN *Infant:* 2–5 ml PO Q1–2 hr *Child:* 5–15 ml PO Q1–2 hr *Adults:* 30–60 ml PO Q1–2 hr *Hyperphosphatemia:* 50–150 mg/kg/24 hr ÷ Q4–6 hr PO	May cause constipation, decreased bowel motility, and phosphorus depletion. Interferes with the absorption of several orally administered medications, including digoxin, indomethicin, isoniazid, tetracycline, and iron.
ALUMINUM HYDROXIDE WITH MAGNESIUM HYDROXIDE (Maalox, Mylanta, and others) *Antacid* Chewable tabs: (Al (OH)₃; Mg (OH)₂) 200 mg: 200 mg (Maalox, Mylanta) Suspension: 200 mg: 200 mg + Simethicone 20 mg/5 ml (Mylanta) 225 mg: 200 mg/5 ml (Maalox); many other combinations (contain 0.04–0.1 mEq Na/5 ml)	Same as for aluminum hydroxide preparations	May have laxative effect. May cause hypokalemia. Use with caution in patients with renal insufficiency, gastric outlet obstruction.

AMANTADINE HYDROCHLORIDE
(Symadine, Symmetrel, and others)
Antiviral agent
Capsule: 100 mg
Syrup: 50 mg/5 ml (480 ml)

Influenza A prophylaxis and treatment:
1–9 yr: 5–9 mg/kg/24 hr PO ÷ QD-BID;
    max dose: 200 mg/24 hr
>9 yr: 200 mg 24 hr ÷ QD-BID
Prophylaxis:
  Single exposure: at least 10 days
  Repeated/uncontrolled exposure: up to 90 days
  Use with influenza A vaccine when possible
Symptomatic treatment:
  Continue for 24–48 hr after disappearance of symptoms

Dose must be adjusted in patients with renal insufficiency. May cause dizziness, anxiety, depression, mental status change, rash (livedo reticularis), nausea, orthostatic hypotension, edema, CHF, and urinary retention. Use with caution in patients with liver disease, seizures, renal disease, and in those receiving CNS stimulants.

AMIKACIN SULFATE
(Amikin)
Antibiotic, aminoglycoside
Injection: 50, 250 mg/ml

Neonates: IV/IM

Post-conceptional age (wk)	Postnatal age (days)	Dose (mg/kg/dose)	Interval (hr)
≤29*	0–28	7.5	24
	>28	10	24
30–36	0–14	10	24
	>14	7.5	12
≥37	0–7	7.5	12
	>7	7.5	8

*or significant asphyxia

Adjust dose in renal failure. May cause ototoxicity, nephrotoxicity, neuromuscular blockade, and rash. Loop diuretics may potentiate the ototoxicity of all aminoglycoside antibiotics. **Therapeutic levels: peak, 20–30 mg/L; trough 5–10 mg/L.** Rapidly eliminated in patients with cystic fibrosis, burns, and in febrile neutropenic patients.

(Continued.)

Drug/How Supplied	Dose and Route	Remarks
AMIKACIN SULFATE—(cont.)	*Infants and Children:* 15–22.5 mg/kg/24 hr ÷ Q8 hr IV/IM *Adults:* 15 mg/kg/24 hr ÷ Q8–12 hr IV/IM **Initial max dose:** 1.5 g/24 hr, then monitor levels	
AMINOCAPROIC ACID (Amicar and others) *Hemostatic agent* Tabs: 500 mg Syrup: 250 mg/ml (480 ml) Injection: 250 mg/ml .	*Children:* *Loading dose:* 100–200 mg/kg IV/PO *Maintenance:* 100 mg/kg/dose Q4–6 hr **Max dose:** 30 g/24 hr	Hypercoagulation may be produced when given in conjunction with oral contraceptives. May cause nausea, diarrhea, malaise, weakness. **Contraindications:** DIC, hematuria. May cause elevation of serum potassium, especially in patients with renal impairment.
AMINOPHYLLINE (Aminophyllin, Phylocontin, and others) *Bronchodilator, methylxanthine* Tabs: 100, 200 mg (79% theophylline) Liquid (oral): 105 mg/5 ml (240 ml) (86% theophylline) Injection: 25 mg/ml (79% theophylline) Suppository: 250, 500 mg (79% theophylline) Tablet (sustained release): 225 mg (79% theophylline)	*IV loading:* 6 mg/kg IV over 20 min (each 1.2 mg/kg dose raises the serum theophylline concentration 2 mg/L) *IV maintenance:* Continuous IV drip: *Neonates:* 0.2 mg/kg/hr *6 wk–6 mo:* 0.5 mg/kg/hr *6 mo–1 yr:* 0.6–0.7 mg/kg/hr *1–9 yr:* 1–1.2 mg/kg/hr *9–12 yr and young adult smokers:* 0.9 mg/kg/hr *12 yr healthy nonsmokers:* 0.7 mg/kg/hr The above total daily doses may also be administered IV ÷ Q4–6 hr.	Consider mg of theophylline available when dosing aminophylline Monitoring serum levels is essential especially in infants and young children. Infants and children 1–5 yr may require Q4 hr dosing regimen due to enhanced metabolism. Side effects: restlessness, GI upset, arrhythmias, seizures (may occur in absence of other side effects with toxic levels). **Therapeutic level: for asthma, 10–20 mg/L; for neonatal apnea, 6–13 mg/L.**

note: Pharmacy may dilute IV and oral dosage forms to enhance accuracy of neonatal dosing.

PO:

Infants: (see Theophylline)
1–9 yr: 27 mg/kg/24 hr ÷ Q4–6 hr
9–12 yr: 20 mg/kg/24 hr ÷ Q6 hr
12–16 yr: 16 mg/kg/24 hr ÷ Q6 hr
Adults: 12.5 mg/kg/24 hr ÷ Q6 hr

Neonatal apnea:
Loading dose: 5–6 mg/kg IV or PO
Maintenance dose: 1–2 mg/kg/dose Q6–8 hr, IV or PO

Guidelines for obtaining levels:
IV bolus: 30 min after infusion
IV continuous; 12–14 hr after initiation of infusion
PO liquid, immediate-release tab:
  Peak: 1 hr post dose
  Trough: just before dose
PO sustained-release:
  Peak: 4 hr post dose
  Trough: just before dose
Ideally, obtain levels after steady state has been achieved (after at least one day of therapy). See Theophylline for drug interactions.

AMIODARONE HCl
(Cordarone)
Antiarrhythmic, Class III
Tabs: 200 mg

Children PO:
<1 yr: 600–800 mg/1.73 m²/24 hr ÷ Q12–24 then reduce to 200–400 mg/1.73 m²/24 hr
>1 yr: 10–15 mg/kg/24 hr ÷ Q12–24 hr × 7–14 days and/or until adequate control achieved then reduce to 5 mg/kg/24 hr ÷ Q12–24 hr if effective

Adults PO:
Loading dose: 800–1600 mg QD for 1–3 wk

Long elimination half-life (40–55 days). Major metabolite is active.
Asymptomatic corneal microdeposits. Alters liver enzymes, thyroid function. Pulmonary fibrosis reported in adults. May cause worsening of preexisting arrhythmias with bradycardia and AV block. May cause anorexia, nausea, vomiting, dizziness, paresthesias, ataxia, and tremor. Increases digoxin, dilantin, warfarin, and quinidine levels.
Therapeutic level: 0.5–2.5 mg/L.

(Continued.)

Drug/How Supplied	Dose and Route	Remarks
AMIODARONE HCl—(cont.)	*Maintenance:* 600–800 mg QD × 1 mo, then 200–400 mg QD Can reduce doses to lowest effective dose	
AMMONIUM CHLORIDE *Diuretic, urinary acidifying agent* Tabs: 500 mg Enteric coated tabs: 500 mg Injection: 5 mEq/ml (26.75%); 1 mEq = 53 mg	*Urinary acidification:* *Child:* 75 mg/kg/24 hr ÷ Q6 hr PO or IV **Max dose:** 6 g/24 hr *Adult:* 1.5 g/dose IV Q6 hr. **Max dose:** 6 g/24 hr IV or 8–12 g/24 hr PO ÷ Q6 hr *Injection:* Dilute to concentration not >0.4 mEq/ml. **Infusion not to exceed** 50 mg/kg/hr or 1 mEq/kg/hr.	May produce acidosis, hyperammonemia. **Contraindicated** in hepatic or renal insufficiency; **use with caution in infants.** May cause GI irritation. Monitor serum chloride level, acid/base status.
AMOXICILLIN (Amoxil, Trimox, Wymox, Polymox, and others) *Antibiotic, aminopenicillin* Drops: 50 mg/ml (15, 30 ml) Suspension: 125, 250 mg/5 ml (80, 100, 150, 200 ml) Caps: 250, 500 mg Chewable tabs: 125, 250 mg	*Child:* 20–50 mg/kg/24 hr ÷ Q8 hr PO *Adult:* 250–500 mg/dose Q8 hr PO **Max dose:** 2–3 g/24 hr *SBE prophylaxis:* See Chapter 7	Renal elimination. Serum levels about twice those achieved with equal dose of ampicillin. Less GI effects, but otherwise similar to ampicillin. Side effects: rash and diarrhea.
AMOXICILLIN-CLAVULANIC ACID (Augmentin) *Antibiotic, aminopenicillin with beta lactmase inhibitor*	**Dosage based on amoxicillin component.** *Children <3 months:* 30 mg/kg/24 hr ÷ Q12 hr PO Recommended dosage form is 125 mg/5 ml suspension	Clavulanic acid extends the activity of amoxicillin to include beta-lactamase producing strains of *H. Influenzae, M. catarrhalis,* some *S. aureus.* The BID dosing schedule is associated with

Tabs: 250, 500, 875 mg amoxicillin (all
with 125 mg clavulanate)
Chewable Tabs: 125, 200, 250, 400 mg
amoxicillin (31.25, 62.5 mg
clavulanate/5 ml)
Suspension: 125, 250 mg amoxicillin/
5 ml) (31.25, 62.5 mg clavulanate/5ml)
(75, 100, 150 ml)
200, 400 mg amoxicillin/ 5 ml (28.5, 57
mg clavulanate/ 5 ml) (50, 75, 100 ml)

Children 3 months and older:
TID dosing (see comments):
20–40 mg/kg/24 hr ÷ Q8 hr PO
BID dosing (see comments):
25–45 mg/kg/24 hr ÷ Q12 hr PO
Adult: 250–500 mg/dose Q8 hr PO
Max dose: 2 g/24 hr

less diarrhea. For BID dosing the
200mg, 400mg chewable tabs or the
200mg/5ml, 400mg/5ml suspensions
should be used. These BID dosing
forms contain phenylalanine and
should not be used by
phenylketonurics. For TID dosing, the
125mg, 250mg chewable tabs or the
125mg/5ml, 250mg/5ml suspensions
should be used.

AMPHOTERICIN B
(Fungizone)
Antifungal
Injection: 50 mg vials
Cream: 3% (20 g)
Lotion: 3% (30 ml)
Ointment, topical: 3% (20 g)

Topical: Apply BID-QID
IV: mix with D$_5$W to concentration 0.1
mg/ml (peripheral administration) or 0.2
mg/ml (central line only). pH >4.2.
Infuse over 4–6 hr.
Test dose: 0.1 mg/kg/dose IV up to **max**
1 mg (followed by remaining initial
dose)
Initial dose: 0.25 mg/kg/24 hr
Increment: Increase as tolerated by
0.25–0.5 mg/kg/24 hr QD or QOD
Maintenance: 1 mg/kg/24 hr -or- QOD:
1.5 mg/kg/dose QOD
Max dose: 1.5 mg/kg/24 hr
Intrathecal: 25–100 mcg Q48–72 hr
Increase to 500 mcg as tolerated.

Fever, chills, nausea, vomiting are
common side effects; may premedicate
with acetaminophen and
diphenhydramine 30 min before and 4
hr after infusion. Demerol (meperidine)
useful for chills. Hydrocortisone, 1
mg/mg ampho (max 25 mg) added to
bottle may help prevent immediate
adverse reactions. Monitor renal,
hepatic, electrolyte, and hematologic
status closely. Hypercalciuria,
hypokalemia, RTA, renal failure, acute
hepatic failure, and phlebitis may
occur.

(Continued.)

Drug/How Supplied	Dose and Route	Remarks
AMPICILLIN (Omnipen, Polycillin, Principen, Totacillin) *Antibiotic, aminopenicillin* Drops: 100 mg/ml (20 ml)	*Neonate IM/IV:* *<7 days:* *<2 kg:* 50–100 mg/kg/24 hr IM/IV ÷ Q12 hr *≥2 kg:* 75–150 mg/kg/24 hr IM/IV ÷ Q8 hr	Use higher doses to treat CNS disease. Produces the same side effects as penicillin, with cross-reactivity. Rash commonly seen at 5–10 days. May cause interstitial nephritis.
AMPICILLIN—(cont.) Suspension: 125, 250 mg/5 ml (80, 100, 150, 200 ml); 500 mg/5 ml (100 ml) Caps: 250, 500 mg Injection: 125, 250, 500 mg; 1, 2, 10 g Contains 3 mEq Na/1 g IV drug	*≥7 days:* *<1.2 kg:* 50–100 mg/kg/24 hr ÷ Q12 hr IM/IV *1.2–2 kg:* 75–150 mg/kg/24 hr ÷ Q8 hr IM/IV *>2 kg:* 100–200 mg/kg/24 hr ÷ Q6 hr IM/IV *Child:* *Mild-moderate infections:* 100–200 mg/kg/24 hr ÷ Q6 hr IM/IV 50–100 mg/kg/24 hr ÷ Q6 hr PO **Max PO dose:** 2–3 g/24 hr *Severe infections:* 200–400 mg/kg/24 hr ÷ Q4–6 hr IM/IV *Adult:* 500–3000 mg Q4–6 hr IM/IV 250–500 mg Q6 hr PO **Max IV dose:** 12 g/24 hr	Adjust dose in renal failure (see Chapter 29).

AMPICILLIN/SULBACTAM
(Unasyn)
Antibiotic, aminopenicillin with beta-lactamase inhibitor
Injection:
1.5 g = ampicillin 1 g + sulbactam 0.5 g
3 g = ampicillin 2 g + sulbactam 1 g
Contains 5 mEq Na per 1.5 g drug combination

Dosage based on ampicillin component
Child: 100–200 mg/kg/24 hr ÷ Q6 hr IM/IV
Adult: 1–2 g Q6–8 hr IM/IV
Max dose: 8 g ampicillin/24 hr

Similar side effects to ampicillin. Adjust in renal failure.

AMRINONE LACTATE
(Inocor)
Adrenergic agonist
Injection: 5 mg/ml (20 ml)

Neonate: 0.75 mg/kg IV bolus over 2–3 min, followed by maintenance infusion of 3–5 mcg/kg/min
Children and Adults: 0.75 mg/kg IV bolus over 2–3 min, followed by maintenance infusion of 5–10 mcg/kg/min
(IV bolus may need to be repeated in 30 min in neonates and children)
Max dose: 10 mg/kg/24 hr

Monitor for hypotension (which can be controlled with NS fluid boluses), thrombocytopenia, hepatotoxicity, and GI effects; monitor fluid and electrolytes. Diuresis may result from improvement in cardiac output and may require dosage reduction of diuretics.

ANTIPYRINE AND BENZOCAINE
(Auralgan and others)
Otic analgesic
Otic solution: Antipyrine 5.4%,
Benzocaine 1.4% (10, 15 ml)

Fill external ear canal Q1–2 hr PRN for ear pain

Benzocaine sensitivity may develop.
Contraindicated if tympanic membrane perforated.

ASCORBIC ACID
(vitamin C, others)
Tabs: 25, 50, 100, 250, 500 mg, 1 g

Scurvy PO/IM/IV/SC
Children: 100–300 mg/24 hr ÷ QD-BID for at least 2 weeks

Adverse reactions: nausea, vomiting, heartburn, flushing, headache, faintness, dizziness, hyperoxaluria.

(Continued.)

Drug/How Supplied	Dose and Route	Remarks
Chewable tabs: 100, 250, 500, 1000 mg Caps (timed release): 0.5, 1, 1.5 g Injection: 250, 500 mg/ml Syrup: 100 mg/ml (5, 10, 120, 480 ml) Lozenges: 60 mg	*Adults:* 100–250 mg QD-BID for at least 2 weeks See Chapter 23 for U.S. RDA	Oral dosing is preferred, but can give parenterally (IM preferred).
ASPIRIN (ASA, Anacin, Bufferin, and various trade names) *Nonsteroidal antiinflammatory agent, antiplatelet agent* Tabs: 325, 500, 650 mg Tabs, enteric-coated: 80, 165, 325, 500, 650, 975 mg Tabs, time-release: 650, 800 mg Tabs, buffered: 325 mg Tabs, caffeinated: 400 mg ASA + 32 mg caffeine Tabs, chewable: 81 mg Caps: 325 mg Suppository: 60, 120, 125, 130, 195, 200, 300, 325, 600, 650 mg, and 1.2 g	*Analgesic/antipyretic:* 10–15 mg/kg/dose PO Q4 hr up to total 60–80 mg/kg/24 hr **Max dose:** 4 g/24 hr *Anti-inflammatory:* 60–100 mg/kg/24 hr PO ÷ Q6–8 hr *Kawasaki disease:* 80–100 mg/kg/24 hr PO ÷ QID during febrile phase until defervesces then decrease to 3–5 mg/kg/24 hr PO QAM. Continue for at least 8 weeks or until both platelet count and ESR normal.	Do not use in children <16 yr for treatment of chicken pox or flu-like symptoms. May cause GI upset, allergic reactions, liver toxicity, and decreased platelet aggregation. See Chapter 2 for management of overdose. **Therapeutic levels:** **antipyretic/analgesic: 30–50 mg/L,** **antinflammatory: 150–300 mg/L,** Tinnitus may occur at levels of **200–400 mg/L.**
ASTEMIZOLE (Hismanal) *Antihistamine, less sedating* Tabs: 10 mg	<6 yr: 0.2 mg/kg/24 hr PO QD 6–12 yr: 5 mg/24 hr PO QD >12 yr: 10 mg/24 hr PO QD *To achieve therapeutic level faster:* >12 yr: day 1, 30 mg; day 2, 20 mg; day 3 and subsequent days, 10 mg/24 hr	Long elimination half-life. Less sedating than traditional anti-histamines. High doses may cause cardiovascular complications. **Can result in severe life-threatening cardiac arrhythmias if given with drugs that reduce hepatic**

metabolism; e.g., erythromycin, quinine, itraconazole, ketoconazole, cimetidine, ciprofloxacin, and disulfiram. Use with caution in hepatic disease.

ATENOLOL
(Tenormin)
Beta-1 selective adrenergic blocker
Injection: 0.5 mg/ml (10 ml)
Tab: 25, 50, 100 mg

Children: 1–1.2 mg/kg/dose PO QD
Max dose: 2 mg/kg 24 hr
Adults: 25–100 mg/dose PO QD
Max dose: 200 mg/24 hr

May cause bradycardia hypotension, second or third degree AV block, dizziness, fatigue, lethargy, headache. Wheezing and dyspnea have occurred when daily dosage exceeds 100 mg/24 hr. Avoid abrupt withdrawal of the drug. Crosses blood-brain barrier less than propanolol. **IV administration rate not to exceed 1 mg/min.**

ATROPINE SULFATE
Anticholinergic agent
Tabs: 0.4, 0.6 mg
Injection: 0.05, 0.1, 0.3, 0.4, 0.5, 0.8, 1 mg/ml
Ointment (ophthalmic): 0.5%, 1% (3.5 g)
Solution (ophthalmic): 0.5%, 1%, 2%, 3% (1, 2, 5 ml)

Pre-anesthesia dose:
Child: 0.01 mg/kg/dose SC/IV, **max dose:** 0.4 mg/dose; **min dose:** 0.1 mg/dose; may repeat Q4–6 hr
Adult: 0.5 mg/dose SC/IV
Cardiopulmonary Resuscitation:
Child: 0.02 mg/kg/dose IV Q5 min × 2–3 doses PRN; **min dose:** 0.1 mg; **max single dose:** 0.5 mg in children, 1 mg in adolescents; **max total dose:** 1 mg children, 2 mg adolescents

In case of bradycardia, may give via endotracheal tube (dilute with NS to volume of 1–2 ml). Side effects include: dry mouth, blurred vision, fever, tachycardia, constipation, urinary retention, CNS signs (dizziness, hallucinations, restlessness). **Contraindicated** in glaucoma, obstructive uropathy, tachycardia, thyrotoxicosis. **Caution** in patients sensitive to sulfites.

(Continued.)

Drug/How Supplied	Dose and Route	Remarks
	Adult: 0.5–1 mg/dose IV Q5 min; **max dose:** 2 mg *Bronchospasm:* 0.05 mg/kg/dose in 2.5 ml NS; **min dose** 0.25 mg; **max dose:** 1 mg Q6–8 hr via nebulizer	
ATROPINE SULFATE—(cont.)	*Ophthalmic:* *Child:* (0.5% solution) 1–2 drops in each eye QD-TID *Adult:* (1% solution) 1–2 drops in each eye QD-TID	
AZATHIOPRINE (Imuran) *Immunosuppressant* Suspension*: 2 or 50 mg/ml Tabs: 50 mg Injection: 5 mg/ml	*Immunosuppression:* *Initial:* 3–5 mg/kg/24 hr IV/PO QD *Maintenance:* 1–3 mg/kg/24 hr IV/PO QD	Toxicity: bone marrow suppression, rash, stomatitis, alopecia, arthralgias, and GI disturbances. Use 1/4–1/3 dose when given with allopurinol. Monitor CBC, platelets, total bilirubin, alkaline phosphatase, BUN, creatinine. Adjust dose in renal failure (see Chapter 29).
AZITHROMYCIN (Zithromax) *Antibiotic, macrolide* Capsules: 250 mg Suspension: 100 mg/5 ml (15 ml), 200 mg/5 ml (15, 22.5 ml)	*Children:* *Otitis Media:* 10 mg/kg PO day 1 (not to exceed 500 mg), followed by 5 mg/kg/24 hr PO QD (not to exceed 250 mg/24 hr) on days 2–5 *Pharyngitis/Tonsillitis:* 12 mg/kg/24 hr PO QD × 5 days (not to exceed 500 mg/24 hr)	Can cause increase in hepatic enzymes, cholestatic jaundice. Aluminum- and magnesium-containing antacids decrease absorption. Should be taken at least 1 hour before or two hours after meals. Contraindicated in hypersensitivity to macrolides.

Adolescents and Adults:
Respiratory tract, skin, and soft tissue infection: 500 mg PO day 1, then 250 mg/24 hr PO on days 2–5
Uncomplicated chlamydial urethritis or cervicitis: single 1 g dose PO

AZTREONAM
(Azactam)
Antibiotic, monobactam
Injection: 0.5, 1, 2 g

Neonate:
30 mg/kg/dose:
  <1.2 kg and 0–4 wk age: Q12 hr IV/IM
  1.2–2 kg and 0–7 days: Q12 hr IV/IM
  1.2–2 kg and >7 days: Q8 hr IV/IM
  >2 kg and 0–7 days: Q8 hr IV/IM
  >2 kg and >7 days: Q6 hr IV/IM
Children:
90–120 mg/kg/24 hr ÷ Q6–8 hr IV/IM
Cystic fibrosis:
150–200 mg/kg/24 hr ÷ Q6–8 hr IV/IM; **max dose:** 8 g/24 hr

Well-absorbed IM. Low cross-allergenicity between aztreonam and other beta-lactams. Adverse reactions: thrombophlebitis, eosinophilia, leukopenia, neutropenia, thrombocytopenia, elevation of liver enzymes, hypotension, seizures, confusion. Adjust dose in renal failure (see Chapter 29).

BACLOFEN
(Lioresal)
Centrally acting skeletal muscle relaxant
Tabs: 10, 20 mg
Suspension*: 10 mg/ml

Children; PO:
≥2 yr: 10–15 mg/24 hr ÷ Q8 hr
  Max dose, <8 yr: 40 mg/24 hr
  Max dose, ≥8 yr: 60 mg/24 hr
Adults; PO:
5 mg TID; **max dose:** 80 mg/24 hr

Avoid abrupt withdrawal of drug. Use with **caution** in patients with seizure disorder, impaired renal function. Adverse effects: drowsiness, fatigue, nausea, vertigo, psychiatric disturbances, rash, urinary frequency, hypotonia.

*Indicates suspensions not commercially available; need to be extemporaneously compounded by a pharmacist. See references 1 and 2 for specific formulations.

(Continued.)

rug/How Supplied	Dose and Route	Remarks
ECLOMETHASONE IPROPIONATE Beclovent, Beconase AQ, Vanceril, Vancenase AQ) *Corticosteroid* Inhalation, oral: 42 mcg/inhalation (200 inhalations) (16.8 g) Inhalation, nasal: 42 mcg/inhalation 200 inhalations (16.8 g) Spray, aqueous nasal: 42 mcg/inhalation, 200 metered doses (25 g)	*Inhalant (oral):* 6–12 yr: 1–2 inhalations TID–QID or 2–4 inhalations BID; **max** 10 inhalations/24 hr >12 yr: 2 inhalations TID–QID; **max** 20 inhalations/24 hr (1 inhalation = 42 mcg *Inhalant (nasal):* 6–12 yr: 1 spray each nostril TID >12 yr: 1 spray each nostril BID–QID or 2 sprays each nostril BID *Aqueous nasal spray:* ≥6 yr and adults: 1–2 sprays each nostril BID	Rinse mouth and gargle with water after inhalation; may cause thrush. Avoid using higher than recommended doses, since hypothalamic, pituitary, or adrenal suppression may occur. **Not recommended** for children <6 yr. Consider using with tube spacers for oral inhalation.
BERACTANT	See Surfactant, pulmonary	
BETHANECHOL CHLORIDE (Urecholine and other brand names) *Cholinergic agent* Tabs: 5, 10, 25, 50 mg Suspension*: 1 mg/ml Injection: 5 mg/ml	*Children:* *Abdominal distention/urinary retention* PO: 0.6 mg/kg/24 hr ÷ Q6–8 hr SC: 0.15–0.2 mg/kg/24 hr ÷ Q6–8 hr *Gastroesophageal reflux:* 0.1–0.2 mg/kg/dose ½–1 hr AC and HS **Max:** 4 doses/24 hr	**Contraindicated** in asthma, mechanical GI or GU obstruction, peptic ulcer disease, hyperthyroidism, seizure disorder. May cause hypotension, nausea, bronchospasm, salivation, flushing, abdominal cramps. **Warning:** severe hypotension may occur when given with ganglionic blockers (trimethaphan). **Do not give IV or IM.** Atropine is the antidote.

BISACODYL
(Dulcolax and various other names)
Laxative, stimulant
Tabs (enteric-coated): 5 mg
Suppository: 5, 10 mg
Enema: 10 mg/30 ml (37.5 ml)
Powder: 1.5 mg with tannic acid, 2.5 g/packet (25s, 50s)

Adults:
PO: 10–50 mg Q6–12 hr
SC: 2.5–5 mg TID-QID, up to 7.5–10 mg Q4 hr for neurogenic bladder

Oral:
Child: 0.3 mg/kg/24 hr or 5–10 mg to be given 6 hr before desired effect
Adult (>12 yr): 5–15 mg QD
Rectal:
<2 yr: 5 mg
2–11 yr: 5–10 mg
>11 yr: 10 mg

Do not chew or crush tablets; do not give within 1 hr of antacids or milk. **Do not** use in newborn period. May cause abdominal cramps, nausea, vomiting, rectal irritation. Oral usually effective within 6–10 hr; rectal usually effective within 15–60 min.

BRETYLIUM TOSYLATE
(Bretylol)
Antiarrhythmic, class III
Injection: 50 mg/ml (10, 20 ml)

IV: 5–10 mg/kg/dose; may repeat Q10–20 min for total dose of 30 mg/kg.
IM: 2–5 mg/kg × 1
Maintenance dose (IM, IV): 5 mg/kg/dose Q6–8 hr

May cause initial hypertension followed by hypotension. May cause PVCs and increased sensitivity to digitalis and catecholamines.

BUDESONIDE
(Rhinocort)
Corticosteroid
Nasal aerosol: 32 mcg/acuation (7 g, delivers approx 200 sprays)

>6 yr: Initial: 2 sprays *in each nostril* QAM and QHS or, 4 sprays in each nostril QAM
Max total dose 250 mcg/24 hr (8 sprays)

Reduce maintenance dose to as low as possible to control symptoms. May cause pharyngitis, cough, epistaxis, and nasal irritation. Although not yet approved in the United States at the publication of this book, nebulized budesonide has been shown effective in mild to moderate croup at doses of 2 mg × 1. Ref: *N Engl J Med* 331(5):285.

(Continued.)

*Indicates suspensions not commercially available; need to be extemporaneously compounded by a pharmacist. See references 1 and 2 for specific formulations.

Drug/How Supplied	Dose and Route	Remarks
BUMETANIDE (Bumex) *Loop diuretic* Tabs: 0.5, 1, 2 mg Injection: 0.25 mg/ml	*Children: PO, IM, IV* ≥6 mo: 0.015–0.1 mg/kg/dose QD-QOD *Adults:* 0.5–2 mg/dose PO QD-BID 0.5–1 mg IM/IV over 1–2 min. May give additional doses Q2–3 hr PRN **Usual max dose: 10 mg/24 hr or 0.1 mg/kg/24 hr**	Side effects include cramps, dizziness, hypotension, headache, electrolyte losses (hypokalemia, hypocalcemia, hyponatremia, hypochloremia), and encephalopathy. May also lead to metabolic alkalosis. Cross-allergenicity may occur in patients allergic to sulfonamides.
CAFFEINE (Caffeine base, caffeine citrate) *Methylxanthine, respiratory stimulant* Injectable and oral liquid*: 20 mg/ml (citrate salt), 10 mg/ml (caffeine base) (also available as powder for compounding)	*Neonatal apnea (caffeine base):* *Loading dose:* 10 mg/kg IV/PO × 1 *Maintenance dose:* 2.5–5 mg/kg/dose PO/IV QD, to begin 24 hr after loading dose **Note: doses for caffeine citrate are twice the doses above.**	**Therapeutic levels: 5–25 mg/L.** Cardiovascular, neurologic, or GI toxicity reported at serum levels >50 mg/L. Caffeine benzoate formulation has been associated with causation of kernicterus in neonates.
CALCITRIOL (1,25-dihydroxycholecalciferol) (Rocaltrol, Calcijex) *Active form Vitamin D, fat soluble* Caps: 0.25, 0.5 mcg Inj: (Calcijex) 1, 2 mcg/ml (1 ml)	*Renal failure:* *Children:* Oral: Suggested dose range 0.01–0.05 mcg/kg/24 hr. Titrate in 0.005–0.01 mcg/kg/24 hr increments Q4–8 wk based on clinical response. IV: 0.01–0.05 mcg/kg/dose given 3 ×/week *Adults:* Initial: 0.25 mcg/24 hr PO. Increment: 0.25 mcg/24 hr PO Q2–4 wk	Most potent vitamin D metabolite available. Monitor serum calcium and phosphorus. Avoid concomitant use of Mg++-containing antacids. Side effects include: weakness, headache, vomiting, constipation, hypotonia, polydipsia, polyuria, metastatic calcification, etc. **Contraindicated** in patients with hypercalcemia, vitamin D toxicity. IV dosing applies if patient undergoing hemodialysis.

Adult: IV: 0.5 mcg/24 hr given 3
×/week. Usual dose is 0.5–3 mcg/24
hr given 3 ×/week

Side effects: constipation, hypercalcemia,
hypophosphatemia, nausea, vomiting,
headache, confusion. May reduce
absorption of tetracycline. May
potentiate effects of digoxin. Some
products may contain trace amounts of
Na.

CALCIUM CARBONATE
(Tums, Os-Cal) (40% Ca)
Calcium supplement, antacid
Tab, chewable: 420, 500, 750, 835, 850,
1250 mg
Tab: 650, 1250, 1500 mg
Susp: 1000 mg/5 ml, 1250 mg/5 ml
Caps: 1250 mg
Powder: 6500 mg/packet
Each 1000 mg of salt contains 20 mEq
elemental Ca (400 mg elemental Ca).

**Doses expressed in mg of elemental
Calcium.** To convert to mg of salt,
divide elemental dose by 0.4.
Hypocalcemia:
  Neonates: 50–150 mg/kg/24 hr ÷
  Q4–6 hr PO
  Max dose: 1 g/24 hr
  Children: 20–65 mg/kg/24 hr PO ÷
  QID
  Adults: 1–2 g/24 hr PO

CALCIUM CHLORIDE
(27% Ca)
Calcium supplement
Injection: 100 mg/ml (10%) (1.36 mEq
Ca++/ml); each gram of salt contains
13.6 mEq (270 mg) Ca

Doses expressed in mg of CaCl
Cardiac arrest:
Infant/Child: 20 mg/kg/dose IV (0.2
ml/kg/dose) Q10 min
Adults: 250–500 mg/dose IV (2.5–5
ml/dose) Q10 min or 2–4 mg/kg/dose
Q10 min.
**Do not exceed 100 mg/min with IV
infusion.**

Use IV with extreme caution.
Extravasation may lead to necrosis.
Hyaluronidase may be helpful for
extravasation. Rapid IV infusion
associated with bradycardia,
hypotension, and peripheral
vasodilation. May cause
hyperchloremic acidosis.

§Indicates suspensions not commercially available; need to be extemporaneously compounded by a pharmacist. See references 1
and 2 for specific formulations.

(Continued.)

Drug/How Supplied	Dose and Route	Remarks
CALCIUM GLUBIONATE (Neo-Calglucon) (6.4% Ca) *Calcium supplement* Syrup: 1.8 gm/5 ml (480 ml); each gram of salt contains 3.2 mEq (64 mg) Ca.	**Doses expressed in mg Calcium glubionate** *Neonatal hypocalcemia:* 1200 mg/kg/24 hr PO ÷ Q4–6 hr *Maintenance:* *Infant/Child:* 600–2000 mg/kg/24 hr PO ÷ QID; **max dose: 9 g/24 hr** *Adult:* 6–18 g/24 hr ÷ QID	Side effects include GI irritation, dizziness, and headache. Best absorbed when given before meals. Absorption inhibited by high phosphate load. High osmotic load of syrup (20% sucrose) may cause diarrhea.
CALCIUM GLUCEPTATE (8.2% Ca) *Calcium supplement* Injection: 220 mg/ml (22%); each gram of salt contains 4.1 mEq (82 mg) Ca.	**Doses expressed in mg of Calcium gluceptate** *Hypocalcemia:* *Children:* 200–500 mg/kg/24 hr ÷ Q6 hr *Adult:* 500–1100 mg/dose as needed *Cardiac arrest:* *Children:* 110 mg/kg/dose IV Q10 min **Do not exceed 50 mg/min with IV infusion**	See calcium gluconate.
CALCIUM GLUCONATE (9% Ca) *Calcium supplement* Tabs: 500, 650, 1000 mg Injection: 100 mg/ml (10%); each gram of salt contains 4.8 mEq (90 mg) Ca	**Doses expressed in mg Calcium gluconate** *Maintenance/hypocalcemia:* *Neonates:* IV: 200–800 mg/kg/24 hr ÷ Q6 hr *Infants:* IV: 200–500 mg/kg/24 hr ÷ Q6 hr PO: 400–800 mg/kg/24 hr ÷ Q6 hr	Avoid peripheral infusion. Extravasation may cause tissue necrosis. IV infusion associated with hypotension and bradycardia. Also associated with arrythmias in digitalized patients. May precipitate when used with bicarbonate. **Do not use scalp veins! Do not administer IM or SC.**

Child: 200–500 mg/kg/24 hr IV or PO ÷ Q6 hr

Adult: 5–15 g/24 hr IV or PO ÷ Q6 hr

For cardiac arrest:

Infants and children: 100 mg/kg/dose (1 ml/kg/dose) IV Q10 min

Adults: 500–800 mg/dose (5–8 ml/dose) IV Q10 min

Do not exceed 50 mg/min with IV infusion

Give with meals. Do not dissolve tablets in milk.

CALCIUM LACTATE
(13% Ca)
Calcium supplement
Tabs: 325, 650 mg; each gram of salt contains 6.5 mEq (130 mg) Ca

Doses expressed in mg of Calcium lactate.

Infants: 400–500 mg/kg/24 hr PO ÷ Q4–8 hr

Children: 500 mg/kg/24 hr PO ÷ Q4–8 hr; **max dose:** 9 g/24 hr

Adult: 1.5–3 g PO Q8 hr; **max dose:** 9 g/24 hr

CAPTOPRIL
(Capoten)
Angiotensin converting enzyme inhibitor,
anti-hypertensive
Tabs: 12.5, 25, 50, 100 mg
Suspension*: 1 mg/ml

Neonates: 0.1–0.4 mg/kg/24 hr PO ÷ Q6–8 hr

Infants: Initially 0.15–0.3 mg/kg/dose; Titrate upward to **max dose:** 6 mg/kg/24 hr ÷ QD-QID

Children: Initially 0.5–1 mg/kg/24 hr ÷ Q8 hr; titrate to minimal effective dose; **max dose:** 6 mg/kg/24 hr ÷ QD-QID

Adolescents and adults: Initially 12.5–25 mg/dose PO TID; increase weekly if necessary by 25 mg/dose to **max dose:** 450 mg/24 hr

Onset within 15–30 min of administration. Peak effect within 1–2 hr. Adjust with renal failure. May cause rash, proteinuria, neutropenia, cough, hypotension, or diminution of taste perception. Known to decrease aldosterone and increase renin production. Should be administered 1 hr before meals. Titrate to minimal effective dose.

(Continued.)

*Indicates suspensions not commercially available; need to be extemporaneously compounded by a pharmacist. See references 1 and 2 for specific formulations.

Drug/How Supplied	Dose and Route	Remarks
CARBAMAZEPINE (Epitrol, Tegretol) *Anticonvulsant* Tabs: 200 mg Chewable tabs: 100 mg Suspension: 100 mg/5 ml (450 ml)	*<6 yr:* *Initial:* 5–10 mg/kg/24 hr PO ÷ BID-QID *Increment:* q5–7 days up to 20 mg/kg/24 hr PO *6–12 yr:* *Initial:* 10 mg/kg/24 hr PO ÷ BID up to **max dose:** 100 mg/dose BID *Increment:* 100 mg/24 hr at 1 wk intervals (÷ TID-QID) until desired response is obtained *Maintenance:* 20–30 mg/kg/24 hr PO ÷ BID-QID; **max dose:** 1000 mg/24 hr *>12 yr:* *Initial:* 200 mg PO BID *Increment:* 200 mg/24 hr at 1 wk intervals (÷ BID-QID) until desired response is obtained *Maintenance:* 600–1200 mg/24 hr PO ÷ BID-QID **Max dose:** *12–15 yr:* 1000 mg/24 hr *Adult:* 1.6–2.4 g/24 hr	**Therapeutic blood levels:** 4–12 mg/L. **Contraindicated** for patients taking MAO inhibitors. Erythromycin, verapamil, cimetidine, and INH may increase serum levels. Carbamazepine may decrease activity of warfarin, doxycycline, oral contraceptives, theophylline, phenytoin, benzodiazepines, ethosuximide, and valproic acid. Side effects include sedation, dizziness, diplopia, aplastic anemia, neutropenia, urinary retention, nausea, SIADH, and Stevens-Johnson syndrome. Pretreatment CBC is suggested. Patient should be monitored for hematologic and hepatic toxicity. $T_{1/2}$ = 10–30 hours. See Chapter 2 for management of ingestions

CARBENICILLIN
(Geocillin, Geopen, Pyopen)
Antibiotic, penicillin (extended spectrum)
Tabs (as Indanyl sodium): 382 mg; each 382 mg tab contains 1 mEq Na

Mild infection:
Children: 30–50 mg/kg/24 hr PO ÷ Q6 hr; **max dose:** 2–3 g/24 hr
Adults: 382–764 mg PO Q6 hr

Most frequent side effects are nausea, vomiting, diarrhea, abdominal cramps, and flatulence. May cause hepatotoxicity. Furry tongue is a reported side effect. Adjust dose in renal failure. Use with **caution** in penicillin allergic patients.

CEFACLOR
(Ceclor)
Antibiotic, cephalosporin (2nd generation)
Caps: 250, 500 mg
Suspension: 125, 187, 250, 375 mg/5 ml (75, 150 ml)

Infant and child: 40 mg/kg/24 hr PO ÷ Q8 hr; **max dose:** 2 g/24 hr
Adult: 250–500 mg/dose PO Q8 hr; **max dose:** 4 g/24 hr

Use with **caution** in patients with penicillin allergy or renal impairment. May cause positive Coombs or false-positive test for urinary glucose. **Serum sickness** reactions have been reported in patients receiving multiple courses of cefaclor.

CEFADROXIL
(Duricef, Ultracef)
Antibiotic, cephalosporin (1st generation)
Suspension: 125, 250, 500 mg/5 ml (50, 100 ml)
Tabs: 1 g
Caps: 500 mg

Infant and child: 30 mg/kg/24 hr PO ÷ Q12 hr
Adult: 1–2 g/24 hr PO ÷ Q12 hr; **max dose:** 2 g/24 hr

See cephalexin. Side effects include nausea, vomiting, pseudomembranous colitis, pruritus, neutropenia, vaginitis, and candidiasis.

CEFAMANDOLE
(Mandol)
Antibiotic, cephalosporin (2nd generation)
Injection: 0.5, 1, 2, 10 g (3.3 mEq Na/gm)

Child: 50–150 mg/kg/24 hr IM/IV ÷ Q4–6 hr
Adult: 4–12 g/24 hr IM/IV ÷ Q4–8 hr; **max dose:** 12 g/24 hr, 2 g/dose

See cefaclor. May cause elevated liver enzymes, coagulopathy, transient neutropenia, and disulfiram-like reaction with ethanol.

(Continued.)

Drug/How Supplied	Dose and Route	Remarks
CEFAZOLIN (Ancef, Kefzol, Zolicef, others) *Antibiotic, cephalosporin (1st generation)* Injection: 0.25, 0.5, 1, 5, 10, 20 g (2 mEq Na/g)	*Neonate IM, IV:* *Postnatal age ≤7 days:* 40 mg/kg/24 hr ÷ Q12 hr *Postnatal age >7 days:* ≤2000 g: 40 mg/kg/24 hr ÷ Q12 hr >2000 g: 60 mg/kg/24 hr ÷ Q8 hr *Infant >1 mo/children:* 50–100 mg/kg/24 hr ÷ Q8 hr IV/IM; **max dose:** 6 g/24 hr *Adult:* 2–6 g/24 hr ÷ Q6–8 hr IV/IM; **max dose:** 12 g/24 hr	See cephalexin. Use with **caution** in renal impairment or in penicillin-allergic patients. May cause phlebitis, leukopenia, thrombocytopenia, elevated liver enzymes, false-positive urine reducing substance.
CEFIXIME (Suprax) *Antibiotic, cephalosporin (3rd generation)* Tabs: 200, 400 mg Suspension: 100 mg/5 ml (50, 100 ml)	*Infant and child:* 8 mg/kg/24 hr ÷ Q12–24 hr PO; **max dose:** 400 mg/24 hr *Adolescent/Adult:* 400 mg/24 hr ÷ Q12–24 hr PO *N. gonorrhoeae infection:* 400 mg × 1 PO	Use with **caution** in patients with penicillin allergy or renal failure. Adverse reactions include diarrhea, abdominal pain, nausea, headaches. **Do not** use tablets for the treatment of otitis media due to reduced bioavailability.
CEFOPERAZONE (Cefobid) *Antibiotic, cephalosporin (3rd generation)* Injection: 1, 2 g (1.5 mEq Na/gm)	*Infant and child:* 50–200 mg/kg/24 hr ÷ Q8–12 hr IV/IM *Adult:* 2–4 g/24 hr ÷ Q12 hr IV/IM; **max dose:** 12 g/24 hr	Use with **caution** in penicillin-allergic patients or in patients with renal and hepatic failure. May cause disulfiram-like reaction with ethanol.
CEFOTAXIME (Claforan) *Antibiotic, cephalosporin (3rd generation)*	*Neonates: IV/IM:* *Postnatal age ≤7 days:* 100 mg/kg/24 hr ÷ Q12 hr	Use with **caution** in penicillin-allergic patients or in presence of renal impairment. Toxicities similar to other

Injection: 1, 2, 10 g (2.2 mEq Na/g)

Postnatal age >7 days:
  <1200 g: 100 mg/kg/24 hr ÷ Q12 hr
  ≥1200 g: 150 mg/kg/24 hr ÷ Q8 hr
Infant and child: (<50 kg): 100–200
  mg/kg/24 hr ÷ Q6–8 hr IV/IM (see
  remarks)
  Meningitis: 200 mg/kg/24 hr ÷ Q6 hr
  IV/IM (see remarks)
Adult: (≥50 kg): 2–12 g/24 hr ÷ Q4–8 hr
  IV/IM; **max dose:** 12 g/24 hr

cephalosporins: allergy, neutropenia,
thrombocytopenia, eosinophilia,
positive Coombs, elevated BUN,
creatinine, and liver enzymes. Higher
doses of 225–300 mg/kg/24 hr ÷
Q6–8 hr have been recommended for
penicillin-resistant pneumococci.

CEFOTETAN
(Cefotan)
Antibiotic, cephalosporin (2nd generation)
Injection: 1, 2 g (3.5 mEq Na/g)

Infant and child: 40–80 mg/kg/24 hr ÷
  Q12 hr IV/IM
Adult: 2–6 g/24 hr ÷ Q12 hr IV/IM;
  max dose: 6 g/24 hr

Use with **caution** in penicillin-allergic
patients or in presence of renal
impairment.

CEFOXITIN
(Mefoxin)
Antibiotic, cephalosporin (2nd generation)
Injection: 1, 2 g (2.3 mEq Na/g)

Infant and child: 80–160 mg/kg/24 hr ÷
  Q4–6 hr IM/IV
Adult: 4–12 g/24 hr ÷ Q6–8 hr IM/IV;
  max dose: 12 g/24 hr

Use with **caution** in penicillin-allergic
patients or in presence of renal
impairment.

CEFPODOXIME PROXETIL
(Vantin)
Antibiotic, cephalosporin (2nd generation)
Tabs: 100, 200 mg
Suspension: 50, 100 mg/5 ml (100 ml)

5 mo–12 yr: 10 mg/kg/24 hr PO ÷
  Q12–24 hr
  max dose: 400 mg/24 hr
≥13 yr–adult: 200–800 mg/24 hr PO ÷
  Q12 hr
Uncomplicated gonorrhea: 200 mg PO × 1

Use with **caution** in penicillin-allergic
patients or in presence of renal
impairment. Tablets should be
administered with food to enhance
absorption. Suspension may be
administered without regard to food.
High doses of antacids or H_2 blockers
may reduce absorption.

(Continued.)

Drug/How Supplied	Dose and Route	Remarks

CEFPROZIL
(Cefzil)
Antibiotic, cephalosporin (2nd generation)
Tabs: 250, 500 mg
Suspension: 125, 250 mg/5 ml (50, 75, 100 ml)
	Otitis Media:
	  6 mo–12 yr: 30 mg/kg/24 hr PO ÷ Q12 hr
	Pharyngitis/Tonsillitis:
	  2–12 yrs: 15 mg/kg/24 hr PO ÷ Q12 hr
	Other:
	  ≥12 yr: 500–1000 mg/24 hr PO ÷ Q12–24 hr
		Use with **caution** in penicillin-allergic patients or in presence of renal impairment.
		Absorption is not affected by food.

CEFTAZIDIME (Fortaz, Tazidime, Tazicef, Ceptaz [arginine salt]) *Antibiotic, cephalosporin (3rd generation)* Injection: 0.5, 1, 2, 6 g (2.3 mEq Na/g)	*Neonates: IV/IM:* *Postnatal age ≤7 days:* 100 mg/kg/24 hr ÷ Q12 hr *Postnatal age >7 days:* <1200 g: 100 mg/kg/24 hr ÷ Q12 hr ≥1200 g: 150 mg/kg/24 hr ÷ Q8 hr *Infant and child:* 90–150 mg/kg/24 hr ÷ Q8 hr IV/IM *Meningitis:* 225 mg/kg/24 hr ÷ Q8 hr IV/IM *Cystic fibrosis:* 150 mg/kg/24 hr ÷ Q8 hr IV/IM *Adult:* 2–6 g/24 hr ÷ Q8–12 hr IV/IM; **max dose:** 6 g/24 hr	Use with **caution** in penicillin-allergic patients or in presence of renal impairment.
CEFTIBUTEN (Cedax) *Antibiotic, cephalosporin (3rd generation)* Suspension: 90 mg/5 ml (30, 60, 90, 120 ml) Tabs: 400 mg	*Children:* 9 mg/kg/24 hr PO QD; **max dose:** 400 mg/24 hr	Use with caution in penicillin-allergic patients or in presence of renal impairment.

CEFTIZOXIME
(Cefizox)
Antibiotic, cephalosporin (3rd generation)
Injection: 1, 2 g (2.6 mEq Na/g)

Infant and child: 150–200 mg/kg/24 hr ÷ Q6–8 hr IV/IM
Adult: 2–12 g/24 hr ÷ Q8–12 hr IV/IM;
max dose: 12 g/24 hr

Use with **caution** in penicillin-allergic patients or in presence of renal impairment.

CEFTRIAXONE
(Rocephin)
Antibiotic, cephalosporin (3rd generation)
Injection: 0.25, 0.5, 1, 2, 10 g (3.6 mEq Na/gm)

Infant and child: 50–75 mg/kg/24 hr ÷ Q12–24 hr IM/IV
Meningitis:
100 mg/kg/24 hr IM/IV ÷ Q12–24 hr;
max dose: 4 g/24 hr
Adult: 1–4 g/24 hr ÷ Q12–24 hr IV/IM;
max dose: 4 g/24 hr
Uncomplicated gonorrhea: 125 mg IM × 1
Chancroid: 250 mg IM × 1

Use with **caution** in penicillin-allergic patients or in presence of renal impairment. May cause reversible cholelithiasis, sludging in gallbladder, and jaundice. Use with **caution** in neonates at risk for hyperbilirubinemia. For further information on STDs, see Chapter 18.

CEFUROXIME (IV, IM) /
CEFUROXIME AXETIL (PO)
(IV: Zinacef, Kefurox; PO: Ceftin)
Antibiotic, cephalosporin (2nd generation)
Injection: 0.75, 1.5, 7.5 g (2.4 mEq Na/g)
Tabs: 125, 250, 500 mg
Suspension: 125 mg/5 ml (50, 100, 200 ml)

IM/IV:
Neonates: 20–50 mg/kg/24 hr ÷ Q12 hr
Infant/Child: 75–150 mg/kg/24 hr ÷ Q8 hr;
Max dose: 6 g/24 hr
Adults: 750–1500 mg/dose Q8 hr;
Max dose: 9 g/24 hr
PO:
Children:
  Pharyngitis:
    Suspension: 20 mg/kg/24 hr ÷ Q12 hr
    Tab: 125 mg Q12 hr
  Otitis Media:
    Suspension: 30 mg/kg/24 hr ÷ Q12 hr
    Tab: 250 mg Q12 hr
Adults: 250–500 mg BID
Max dose: 1 g/24 hr

Use with **caution** in penicillin-allergic patients or in presence of renal impairment. May cause thrombophlebitis at the infusion site.
Not recommended for meningitis.

(Continued.)

Drug/How Supplied	Dose and Route	Remarks
CEPHALEXIN (Keflex, Cefanex, C-Lexin, and others) *Antibiotic, cephalosporin (1st generation)* Tabs: 250, 500 mg, 1 g Caps: 250, 500 mg Suspension: 125 mg/5 ml, 250 mg/5 ml (60, 100, 200 ml) Drops: 100 mg/ml (10 ml)	*Infant and Child: Mild/Moderate* Infections: 25–50 mg/kg/24 hr PO ÷ Q6–12 hr Severe Infections: 75–100 mg/kg/24 hr PO ÷ Q6–12 hr *Adult:* 1–4 g/24 hr PO ÷ Q6–12 hr; **max dose: 4 g/24 hr**	Some cross-reactivity with penicillins. Use with **caution** in renal insufficiency.

CEPHALOTHIN
(Keflin)
Antibiotic, cephalosporin (1st generation)
Injection: 1, 2, 4 g (2.8 mEq Na/g)
	Neonates:
	IV: <2 kg:
	  0–7 days: 40 mg/kg/24 hr ÷ Q12 hr
	  >7 days: 60 mg/kg/24 hr ÷ Q8 hr
	≥2 kg:
	  0–7 days: 60 mg/kg/24 hr ÷ Q8 hr
	  >7 days: 80 mg/kg/24 hr ÷ Q6 hr
	Infant and child: 80–160 mg/kg/24 hr ÷ Q4–6 hr IV or deep IM
	Adults: 2–12 g/24 hr ÷ Q4–6 hr IV/IM; **max dose: 12 g/24 hr**
		See cephalexin. May cause phlebitis.

CEPHRADINE (Velosef, Anspor, and others) *Antibiotic, cephalosporin (1st generation)* Suspension: 125, 250 mg/5 ml (100, 200 ml) Caps: 250, 500 mg Tabs: 1 g	*Child: PO:* 25–50 mg/kg/24 hr ÷ Q6–12 hr *Adult: PO:* 1–4 g/24 hr ÷ Q6 hr **Max dose: 4 g/24 hr**	See cephalexin.

CHARCOAL, ACTIVATED

See Chapter 2

CHLORAL HYDRATE

(Noctec, Somnos, Aquachloral)

Sedative, hypnotic

Caps: 250, 500 mg

Syrup: 250, 500 mg/5 ml

Suppository: 324, 500, 648 mg

Children:

Sedative: 25–50 mg/kg/**24 hr** PO/PR ÷ Q6–8 hr

Sedation for procedures: 25–100 mg/kg/**dose** PO/PR

Max dose: 2 gm/dose

Adult:

Sedative: 250 mg/dose TID PO/PR

Hypnotic: 500–1000 mg/dose PO/PR; **max dose:** 2 g/24 hr

Not analgesic. May cause GI irritation, paradoxical excitement, hypotension, and myocardial/respiratory depression. **Requires same monitoring as other sedatives. Contraindicated** in patients with hepatic or renal disease. Chronic administration in neonates can lead to accumulation of active metabolites. Sudden withdrawal may cause delirium tremens.

CHLORAMPHENICOL

(Chloromycetin and others)

Antibiotic

Caps: 250, 500 mg

Injection: 1 gm

Otic solution: 0.5% (7.5 ml)

Ophthalmic solution: 0.5%

Ophthalmic ointment: 1% (3.5 g)

Topical cream: 1%

Neonates IV:

Loading dose: 20 mg/kg

Maintenance dose:

≤7 days: 25 mg/kg/24 hr QD

>7 days:

≤2 kg: 25 mg/kg/24 hr QD

>2 kg: 50 mg/kg/24 hr ÷ Q12 hr

The first maintenance dose should be given 12 hours after the loading dose

Infants/children/adults: 50–100 mg/kg/24 hr IV/PO ÷ Q6 hr; **max dose:** 4 g/24 hr

Dose recommendations are just guidelines for therapy; monitoring of blood levels is essential in neonates and infants. Follow hematologic status for related or idiosyncratic marrow suppression. "Gray baby" syndrome may be seen with levels >50 mg/L. Concomitant use of phenobarbital and rifampin may lower chloramphenicol serum levels. Chloramphenicol may increase phenytoin levels. **Therapeutic levels: 15–25 mg/L for meningitis; 10–20**

(Continued.)

Drug/How Supplied	Dose and Route	Remarks
CHLORAMPHENICOL—(cont.)	*Ophthalmic:* 1–2 drops or ribbon of ointment in each eye Q3–6 hr *Topical:* apply to affected area TID-QID	mg/L for other infections. **Trough: 5–15 mg/L for meningitis; 5–10 mg/L for other infections.** Note: higher serum levels may be achieved using the oral, rather than the IV route.
CHLOROTHIAZIDE (Diuril, Diurigen) *Thiazide diuretic* Tabs: 250, 500 mg Suspension: 250 mg/5 ml (237 ml) Injection: 500 mg	*<6 mo:* 20–40 mg/kg/24 hr ÷ Q12 hr PO/IV *≥6 mo:* 20 mg/kg/24 hr ÷ Q12 hr PO/IV *Adults:* 250–1000 mg/dose QD-QID PO/IV; **max dose: 2 g/24 hr**	Use with **caution** in liver and severe renal disease. May increase serum calcium, bilirubin, glucose, uric acid. May cause alkalosis, pancreatitis, blood dyscrasias, hypokalemia, and hypomagnesemia. **Avoid IM administration.**
CHLORPHENIRAMINE MALEATE (Chlor-Trimeton and others) *Antihistamine* Tabs: 4, 8, 12 mg Caps: 12 mg	*PO, IM, IV, SC* *Children:* 0.35 mg/kg/24 hr ÷ Q4–6 hr **or** dose based on age below *2–6 yr:* 1 mg/dose PO Q4–6 hr PRN; **max dose:** 4 mg/24 hr *6–12 yr:* 2 mg/dose PO Q4–6 hr; **max dose** 12 mg/24 hr	May cause sedation, dry mouth, urinary retention, polyuria, and disturbed coordination. Young children may be paradoxically excited. Sustained release forms are **not recommended** in children less than 6 years old.

Sustained release caps and tabs: 8, 12 mg

Chewable tab: 2 mg

Syrup: 2 mg/5 ml (120, 473 ml)

Injection: 10, 100 mg/ml

Sustained release (6–12 yr): 8 mg/dose PO BID PRN

≥12 yrs/adults: 4 mg/dose Q4–6 hr PO PRN; **max dose:** 24 mg/24 hr

Sustained release: 8–12 mg PO BID PRN

CHLORPROMAZINE

(Thorazine)

Antiemetic, antipsychotic, phenothiazine derivative

Tabs: 10, 25, 50, 100, 200 mg

Extended-release caps: 30, 75, 150, 200, 300 mg

Syrup: 10 mg/5 ml (120 ml)

Suppository: 25, 100 mg

Oral concentrate: 30 mg/ml (120 ml), 100 mg/ml (60, 240 ml)

Injection: 25 mg/ml

Children >6 mo:

IM or IV: 2.5–6 mg/kg/24 hr ÷ Q6–8 hr

PO: 2.5–6 mg/kg/24 hr ÷ Q4–6 hr

PR: 1 mg/kg/dose Q6–8 hr

Max IM/IV dose:

  <5 yr: 40 mg/24 hr

  5–12 yr: 75 mg/24 hr

Adult:

Initial: 25 mg IM/IV; increase by 25–50 mg/dose Q1–4 hr up to **max** of 400 mg/dose Q4–6 hr

PO: 10–25 mg/dose Q4–6 hr;

  Max dose: 2 g/24 hr

PR: 50–100 mg/dose Q6–8 hr

Adverse effects include drowsiness, jaundice, lowered seizure threshold, extrapyramidal/anticholinergic symptoms, hypotension, arrhythmias, agranulocytosis. May potentiate effect of narcotics, sedatives, other drugs. Monitor BP closely. ECG changes include prolonged PR interval, flattened T waves and ST depression.

CHOLESTYRAMINE

(Questran, Questran Light, Cholybar)

Antilipemic, binding resin

Powder: 4 g anhydrous resin per 9 g packet; Questran Light: 4 g anhydrous resin per 5 g packet. Contains aspartame.

All doses based in terms of anhydrous resin.

Children: 240 mg/kg/24 hr ÷ TID. Give PO as slurry in water, juice, or milk before meals.

Adult: 3–4 g of cholestyramine BID-QID

May cause constipation, diarrhea, vomiting, vitamin deficiencies (A, D, E, K), and rash. Give other oral medications 4–6 hr after cholestyramine or 1 hr before dose to avoid decreased absorption.

(Continued.)

Drug/How Supplied	Dose and Route	Remarks
CHOLESTYRAMINE—(cont.) Cans: 378 g of powder (4 g resin/9 g powder) Chewable Bars: 4 g	**Max dose:** 32 g/24 hr	Hyperchloremic acidosis may occur with prolonged use.
CHOLINE MAGNESIUM TRISALICYLATE (Trilisate) *Nonsteroidal antiinflammatory agent* Tabs: 500, 750, 1000 mg Liquid: 500 mg/5 ml	**Dose based on total salicylate content.** *Children:* 30–60 mg/kg/24 hr ÷ TID-QID *Adults:* 500 mg–1.5 g QD-TID	Avoid use in patients with suspected varicella or influenza due to concerns of Reye Syndrome. Ratio of choline salicylate to magnesium salicylate in dose forms is 1:1.24. No antiplatelet effects. Less GI irritation than aspirin and other NSAIDs. Therapeutic salicylate levels, see aspirin.
CIMETIDINE (Tagamet, Tagamet HB [OTC]) *Histamine-2-antagonist* Tabs: 100 (OTC), 200, 300, 400, 800 mg Injection: 150 mg/ml Syrup: 300 mg/5 ml (237 ml)	*Neonates:* 10–20 mg/kg/24 hr IM/IV/PO ÷ Q6 hr *Infants:* 10–20 mg/kg/24 hr IM/PO/IV ÷ Q6hr *Children:* 20–40 mg/kg/24 hr IM/PO/IV ÷ Q6 hr *Adults (PO/IM/IV):* 300 mg/dose QID **or** 400 mg/dose BID **or** 800 mg/dose QHS *Ulcer prophylaxis:* 400–800 mg PO QHS: **max dose:** 2400 mg/24 hr	Diarrhea, rash, myalgia, confusion, neutropenia, gynecomastia, elevated liver function tests, or dizziness may occur. Inhibits cytochrome P-450 oxidase system, therefore increases levels of hepatically metabolized drugs (i.e., Theophylline).

CIPROFLOXACIN

(Cipro, Ciloxan ophthalmic)

Antibiotic, quinolone

Tabs: 250, 500, 750 mg

Injection: 10 mg/ml

Ophthalmic solution: 3.5 mg/ml (2.5, 5 ml)

Children:

PO: 20–30 mg/kg/24 hr ÷ Q12 hr; **max** 1.5 g/24 hr

IV: 10–20 mg/kg/24 hr ÷ Q12 hr

Adults:

PO: 250–750 mg/dose Q12 hr; **max** 2 g/24 hr

IV: 200–400 mg/dose Q12 hr

Ophthalmic: 1–2 gtts Q2 hr while awake × 2 days, then 1–2 gtts Q4 hr while awake × 5 days

Can cause GI upset, renal failure. **Do not** administer antacids or other divalent salts with or within 4 hours of ciprofloxacin dose. Like other quinolones, ciprofloxacin has caused arthropathy in immature animals; use with **caution** in children less than 18 years old.

CISAPRIDE

(Propulsid)

GI stimulant, prokinetic agent

Suspension: 1 mg/ml (450 ml)

Tabs: 10, 20 mg

Children: 0.2–0.3 mg/kg/dose TID-QID PO

Adults: 10 mg QID, administer 15 min AC and QHS PO

Contraindicated in patients taking ketoconazole, itraconazole, miconazole, fluconazole, erythromycin, clarithromycin, and troleandomycin, due to reported fatal cardiac arrhythmias. Frequent adverse reactions are headaches and GI disturbance. Some cardiologists discourage the use of cisapride in patients with underlying cardiac arrhythmias.

(Continued.)

Drug/How Supplied	Dose and Route	Remarks
CITRATE MIXTURES *Alkalinizing agent, electrolyte supplement* Each ml contains (mEq):	Dilute in water or juice **All mEq doses based on citrate** *Children:* 5–15 ml/dose Q6–8 hr PO or 2–3 mEq/kg/24 hr PO ÷ Q6–8 hr *Adult:* 15–30 ml/dose Q6–8 hr PO or 100–200 mEq/24 hr ÷ Q6–8 hr	Adjust dose to maintain desired pH. 1 mEq of citrate is equivalent to 1 mEq HCO_3. Use with **caution** in patients already receiving potassium supplements. May have laxative effect.

	Na	K	Citrate
Polycitra	1	1	2
Polycitra-K	0	2	2
Bicitra	1	0	1
Oracit	1	0	1

Drug/How Supplied	Dose and Route	Remarks
CLARITHROMYCIN (Biaxin) *Antibiotic, macrolide* Film tabs: 250, 500 mg Granules for suspension: 125, 250 mg/5 ml (50, 100 ml)	*Children:* 15 mg/kg/24 hr PO ÷ Q12 hr; **max dose:** 1 g/24 hr *Adult:* 250–500 mg/dose Q12 hr PO	Side effects: diarrhea, nausea, abnormal taste, dyspepsia, abdominal discomfort, headache. May increase carbamazepine, theophylline levels. **Contraindicated** in patients sensitive to erythromycin. May cause cardiac arrhythmias in patients also receiving terfenadine and cisapride.
CLINDAMYCIN (Cleocin-T, Cleocin, and others) *Antibiotic* Caps: 75, 150, 300 mg Oral liquid: 75 mg/5 ml (100 ml) Injection: 150 mg/ml (contains 9.45 mg/ml benzyl alcohol)	*Neonates:* IV, IM: 5 mg/kg/dose *≤7 days:* *≤2 kg:* Q12 hr *>2 kg:* Q8 hr *>7 days:* *<1.2 kg:* Q12 hr *1.2–2 kg:* Q8 hr *>2 kg:* Q6 hr	Not indicated in meningitis. Pseudomembraneous colitis may occur up to several weeks after cessation of therapy. May cause diarrhea, rash, Stevens-Johnson syndrome, granulocytopenia, thrombocytopenia, or sterile abscess at injection site.

Solution, topical: 1% (30, 60, 480 ml)
Gel: 1% (7.5, 30 g)

Children: 20–30 mg/kg/24 hr ÷ Q6 hr PO;
25–40 mg/kg/24 hr ÷ Q6–8 hr IM/IV
Adults: 150–450 mg/dose Q6–8 hr PO;
600–2700 mg/24 hr IM/IV ÷ Q6–12 hr;
Max dose: IV/IM: 4.8 g/24 hr
PO: 1.8 g/24 hr
Topical: apply to affected area BID

CLONAZEPAM
(Klonopin)
Benzodiazepine
Tabs: 0.5, 1, 2 mg
Suspension*: 100 mcg/ml

Children: ≤10 yr or <30 kg:
Initial: 0.01–0.03 mg/kg/24 hr ÷ Q8 hr
PO
Increment: 0.25–0.5 mg/24 hr Q3 days,
up to **max maintenance dose** of
0.1–0.2 mg/kg/24 hr ÷ Q8 hr
Adult:
Initial: 1.5 mg/24 hr PO ÷ TID
Increment: 0.5–1 mg/24 hr Q3 days;
max dose: 20 mg/24 hr

Drowsiness, behavior changes, increased
bronchial secretions, GI, CV, GU, and
hematopoietic toxicity
(thrombocytopenia, leukopenia) may
occur. Use with **caution** in patients
with renal impairment. **Therapeutic
levels:** 20–80 ng/ml. Do not
discontinue abruptly. $T_{1/2}$ = 24–36 hr.

CLONIDINE
(Catapres, Catapres TTS)
Central alpha-adrenergic agonist,
antihypertensive
Tabs: 0.1, 0.2, 0.3 mg
Transdermal patch: 0.1, 0.2, 0.3 mg/24 hr
(7 day)

Children, PO: 5–7 mcg/kg/24 hr ÷ Q6–12
hr; if needed, increase at 5–7 day
intervals to 5–25 mcg/kg/24 hr ÷ Q6
hr
Max dose: 0.9 mg/24 hr
Adult, PO: 0.1 mg BID initially; increase in
0.1 mg/24 hr increments until desired
response is achieved, **max dose:** 2.4
mg/24 hr

$T_{1/2}$: 6–20 hr. Applying >2 of the 0.3
mg/24 hr patches does not provide
additional benefit. Side effects: dry
mouth, dizziness, drowsiness, fatigue,
constipation, anorexia, arrhythmias,
local skin reactions with patch. **Do not**
abruptly discontinue; signs of

*Indicates suspensions not commercially available; need to be extemporaneously compounded by a pharmacist. See references 1
and 2 for specific formulations.

(Continued.)

Drug/How Supplied	Dose and Route	Remarks
	Transdermal patch, adults: Initial 0.1 mg/24 hr patch for first week. May increase dose of patch to 0.3 mg/24 hr PRN. Patches last for 7 days.	sympathetic overactivity may occur; taper gradually over >1 wk. May need dosage adjustment in renal impairment.
CLOTRIMAZOLE (Lotrimin, Mycelex, Mycelex G) *Antifungal* Cream: 1% (15, 30, 45, 90 g) Solution: 1% (10, 30 ml) Vaginal tabs: 100, 500 mg Vaginal cream: 1% (45, 90 g) Oral troche: 10 mg Lotion: 1% (30 ml) Twin Pack: Tab 500 mg (1) and vaginal cream 1% (7 g)	*Topical:* apply to skin BID × 4–8 wks *Vaginal Candidiasis:* (vaginal tabs) 100 mg/dose QHS × 7 days, or 200 mg/dose QHS × 3 days, or 500 mg/dose QHS × 1, or 1 applicator dose (5 g) of 1% vaginal cream QHS × 7–14 days *Thrush:* Dissolve slowly one troche in the mouth 5 times/24 hr × 14 days	May cause erythema, blistering, or urticaria where applied. Nausea and vomiting may occur with troches.
CLOXACILLIN (Tegopen, Cloxapen) *Antibiotic, penicillin (penicillinase resistant)* Caps: 250, 500 mg Oral solution: 125 mg/5 ml (100, 200 ml) Sodium content: 250 mg tab = 0.6 mEq 125 mg suspension = 0.48 mEq	*Infant/child:* 50–100 mg/kg/24 hr PO ÷ Q6 hr *Adults:* 250–500 mg/dose PO Q6 hr **Max dose:** 4 g/24 hr	Same side effects as other penicillins. Give on an empty stomach.

CODEINE

(Various brands)

Narcotic, analgesic, antitussive

Tabs: 15, 30, 60 mg

Injection: 30, 60 mg/ml

Syrup: 10, 60 mg/5 ml

Oral solution: 15 mg/5 ml

In combination with acetaminophen

Elixir (7% alcohol), Suspension, Solution:
Acetaminophen 120 mg and codeine
12 mg/5 ml

Caps: Acetaminophen 325 + 15 mg
codeine

Acetaminophen 325 + 30 mg codeine

Acetaminophen 325 + 60 mg codeine

Tabs: (all contain 300 mg acetaminophen
per tab)

Tylenol #1: 7.5 mg codeine

Tylenol #2: 15 mg codeine

Tylenol #3: 30 mg codeine

Tylenol #4: 60 mg codeine

Tabs:

Acetaminophen 650 mg + codeine 30
mg

Acetaminophen 500 mg + codeine 30
mg

Analgesic:

Children: 0.5–1 mg/kg/dose Q4–6 hr
IM, SC, or PO; **max dose:** 60
mg/dose

Adults: 15–60 mg/dose Q4–6 hr IM,
SC, or PO

Antitussive (all doses PRN): 1–1.5
mg/kg/24 hr ÷ Q4–6 hr; alternatively
dose by age

Children (2–6 yr): 2.5–5 mg/dose Q4–6
hr; **max** 30 mg/24 hr

Children (6–12 yr): 5–10 mg/dose Q4–6
hr; **max** 60 mg/24 hr

Adults: 10–20 mg/dose Q4–6 hr; **max**
120 mg/24 hr

Side effects: CNS and respiratory
depression, constipation, cramping.
May be habit forming. For analgesia,
use with acetaminophen orally. **Do not
use in children <2 yr old as
antitussive.** Not intended for IV use,
due to large histamine release and
cardiovascular effects. See Chapter 27
for equianalgesic dosing.

(Continued.)

Drug/How Supplied	Dose and Route	Remarks
COLFOSCERIL PALMITATE	See Surfactant, pulmonary	
CORTISONE ACETATE (Cortone acetate) *Corticosteroid* Tabs: 5, 10, 25 mg Injection: 25, 50 mg/ml (IM only)	*Anti-inflammatory/immunosuppressive:* PO: 2.5–10 mg/kg/24 hr ÷ Q6–8 hr IM: 1–5 mg/kg/24 hr ÷ Q12–24 hr *Physiologic replacement:* PO: 0.5–0.75 mg/kg/24 hr ÷ Q8 hr IM: 0.25–0.35 mg/kg/dose QD	See Chapter 28 for doses based on body surface area and other uses. IM form slowly absorbed over several days. May produce glucose intolerance, Cushing's syndrome, edema, hypertension, adrenal suppression, cataracts, hypokalemia, and skin atrophy.
CO-TRIMOXAZOLE (Trimethoprim-Sulfamethoxazole) (Bactrim, Septra, TMP-SMX, Sulfatrim, others) *Antibiotic, sulfonamide derivative* Tabs (reg strength): 80 mg TMP/400 mg SMX Tabs (double strength): 160 mg TMP/800 mg SMX Suspension: 40 mg TMP/200 mg SMX per 5 ml (20, 100, 150, 200, 480 ml) Injection: 16 mg TMP/ml and 80 mg SMX/ml	**Doses based on TMP component.** *Minor infections (PO or IV):* *Child:* 8–10 mg/kg/24 hr ÷ Q12 hr *Adult (>40 kg):* 160 mg/dose Q12 hr *UTI prophylaxis:* 2–4 mg/kg/24 hr PO QD *Severe infections and Pneumocystis carinii pneumonitis (PO or IV):* 20 mg/kg/24 hr ÷ Q6–8 hr *Pneumocystis prophylaxis (PO or IV):* 5–10 mg/kg/24 hr ÷ Q12 hr or 150 mg/m² 24 hr ÷ Q12 hr for 3 consecutive days/wk; **max dose:** 320 mg/24 hr	Not recommended for use with infants <2 mo. May cause kernicterus in newborns; may cause blood dyscrasias, crystalluria, glossitis, renal or hepatic injury, GI irritation, allergy, hemolysis in patients with G6PD deficiency. Reduce dose in renal impairment. See Chapter 18 for PCP prophylaxis guidelines.

CROMOLYN
(Intal, Nasalcrom, Crolom, Gastrocrom)

Anti-allergic agent

Caps: 20 mg (for inhalation via "spinhaler")

Nebulized solution: 10 mg/ml (2 ml)

Aerosol inhaler: 800 mcg/spray (8.1, 14.2 g)

Capsule: 100 mg

Ophthalmic: 4% (2.5, 10 ml)

Nasal spray: 4% (5.2 mg/spray) (13, 26 ml)

Spin Inhalant: 20 mg Q6–8 hr

Nebulization: 20 mg Q6–8 hr

Nasal: 1 spray each nostril TID-QID

Aerosol inhaler: 2 puffs TID-QID

Ophthalmic: 1–2 gtts 4–6 ×/24 hr

Food Allergy/Inflammatory Bowel disease

Children: 100 mg PO QID; give 15–20 min AC and QHS; **max dose:** 40 mg/kg/24 hr

Adults: 200–400 mg PO QID; give 15–20 min AC and QHS

Systemic mastocytosis:

<2 yr: 20 mg/kg/24 hr ÷ QID PO; **max dose:** 30 mg/kg/24 hr

2–12 yr: 100 mg PO QID; **max dose:** 40 mg/kg/24 hr

Adults: 200 mg PO QID

Allow 2–4 weeks of use for adequate trial. May cause rash, cough, bronchospasm, nasal congestion. May cause headache, diarrhea with oral use. Use with caution in patients with renal or hepatic dysfunction. Bronchospasm and pharyngeal irritation may occur when using spinhaler product. For exercise induced asthma, give no longer than 1 hour before activity.

CYCLOPENTOLATE
(Cyclogyl, and others)

Anticholinergic, mydriatic agent

Solution: 0.5%, 1%, 2% (2, 5, 15 ml)

Infant: 1 drop of 0.5% OU 5–10 min before exam

Children: 1 drop of 0.5–1% OU, followed by repeat drop if necessary

Adult: 1 drop of 1% OU followed by another drop OU in 5 min; use 2% solution for heavily pigmented iris

Do not use in narrow-angle glaucoma. May cause a burning sensation, behavioral disturbance, loss of visual accommodation. To minimize absorption, apply pressure over nasolacrimal sac for at least 2 min. Observe patient closely for at least 30 min after dose.

(Continued.)

Drug/How Supplied	Dose and Route	Remarks
CYCLOPENTOLATE/ PHENYLEPHRINE (Cyclomydril) *Anticholinergic/sympathomimetic, mydriatic agent* Solution: 0.2% cyclopentolate/1% phenylephrine (2, 5 ml)	1 drop OU Q5–10 min; **max dose: 3 drops per eye**	Used to induce mydriasis. See cyclopentolate for comments.
CYCLOSPORINE (Sandimmune) **CYCLOSPORINE MICROEMULSION** (Neoral) *Immunosuppressant* Injection: 50 mg/ml Oral solution: 100 mg/ml (50 ml) Cap: 25, 100 mg Neoral Cap: 25, 100 mg Neoral Solution: 100 mg/ml (50 ml) *Oral solution contains 12.5% alcohol Injection contains 32.9% alcohol Neoral products contain 9.5% alcohol*	Neoral manufacturer recommends a 1:1 conversion ratio with Sandimmune. Due to its better absorption, however, lower doses of Neoral may be required. *Oral:* 15 mg/kg as a single dose given 4–12 hr pre-transplant; give same daily dose for 1–2 wk post-transplant, then reduce by 5% per wk to 5–10 mg/kg/24 hr ÷ Q12–24 hr *IV:* 5–6 mg/kg as a single dose given 4–12 hr pretransplant; administer over 2–6 hr; give same daily dose post-transplant until patient able to tolerate oral form	Plasma concentrations increased with the use of ketoconazole, erythromycin, and corticosteroids. Plasma concentrations decreased with the use of rifampin, phenobarbital, and phenytoin. Plasma half-life 5–40 hrs. May cause nephrotoxicity, hepatotoxicity, hypomagnesemia, hypertension, hirsutism, acne, GI symptoms, tremor, leukopenia, sinusitis. **Monitor trough levels. Interpretation will vary based on treatment protocol and assay methodology (RIA monoclonal vs. RIA polyclonal vs. HPLC) as well as whole blood vs. serum sample.**

CYPROHEPTADINE
(Periactin)
Antihistamine
Tabs: 4 mg
Syrup: 2 mg/5 ml (473 ml); 5% alcohol

Children: 0.25–0.5 mg/kg/24 hr PO ÷ Q8–12 hr PO
Adult: 12–32 mg/24 hr ÷ TID PO
Max dose:
2–6 yr: 12 mg/24 hr
7–14 yr: 16 mg/24 hr
Adults: 32 mg/24 hr

Contraindicated in neonates, patients currently on MAO inhibitors, and patients suffering from asthma, glaucoma, or GI/GU obstruction. May produce anti-cholinergic side effects including appetite stimulation.

DANTROLENE
(Dantrium)
Skeletal muscle relaxant
Cap: 25, 50, 100 mg
Injection: 20 mg
Suspension*: 5 mg/ml

Chronic spasticity:
Children: (<5 yr)
Initial: 0.5 mg/kg/dose PO BID
Increment: Increase frequency to TID-QID at 4–7 day intervals, then increase doses by 0.5 mg/kg/dose
Max dose: 3 mg/kg/dose PO BID-QID, up to 400 mg/24 hr
Malignant Hyperthermia:
Prevention:
PO: 4–8 mg/kg/24 hr ÷ Q6 hr × 1–3 days before surgery
IV: 2.5 mg/kg over 1 hr beginning 1.25 hr before anesthesia, additional doses PRN
Treatment: 1 mg/kg IV, repeat PRN to **max** cumulative dose of 10 mg/kg, then continue 4–8 mg/kg/24 hr PO ÷ Q6 hr for 3 days

Contraindicated in active hepatic disease. Monitor transaminases for hepatotoxicity. May cause change in sensorium, weakness, diarrhea, and enuresis. Avoid unnecessary exposure to sunlight. Avoid extravasation into tissues. A decrease in spasticity sufficient to allow daily function should be therapeutic goal. Discontinue if benefits are not evident in 45 days. Use with **caution** in children with cardiac or pulmonary impairment.

(Continued.)

*Indicates suspensions not commercially available, need to be extemporaneously compounded by a pharmacist. See references 1 and 2 specific formulations.

Drug/How Supplied	Dose and Route	Remarks
DEFEROXAMINE MESYLATE (Desferal Mesylate) *Chelating agent* Injection: 500 mg	*Acute iron poisoning:* *Children:* IV: 15 mg/kg/hr or IM: 90 mg/kg/dose Q8 hr **Max dose:** 6 g/24 hr *Adult:* IV: 15 mg/kg/hr IM: 1 g × 1, then 0.5 g Q4 hr × 2; may repeat 0.5 g Q4–12 hr **Max dose:** 6 g/24 hr *Chronic iron overload:* *Children:* IV: 15 mg/kg/hr SC: 20–40 mg/kg/dose QD as infusion over 8–12 hr *Adult:* IM: 0.5–1 g/dose QD SC: 1–2 g/dose QD as infusion over 8–24 hr	**Contraindicated** in anuria, hemochromatosis. May cause flushing, erythema, urticaria, hypotension, tachycardia, diarrhea, leg cramps, fever, cataracts, hearing loss. Iron mobilization may be poor in children <3 yr.
DESMOPRESSIN ACETATE (DDAVP, Stimate) *Vasopressin analog, synthetic; hemostatic agent* Nasal Solution: DDAVP, 100 mcg/ml (2.5 ml); Stimate, 1500 mcg/ml (2.5 ml) Injection: 4 mcg/ml (1 ml)	*Diabetes insipidus:* 3 mo–12 yr: 5–30 mcg/24 hr ÷ QD- BID intranasally Adults: Intranasal, 10–40 mcg/24 hr ÷ QD-TID; titrate dose to achieve control of excessive thirst and urination; **max** intranasal dose: 40 mcg/24 hr IV/SC: 2–4 mcg/24 hr ÷ BID	Injection may be used SC or IV at approximately 10% of intranasal dose. Adjust fluid intake to decrease risk of water intoxication. Use with caution in hypertension and coronary artery disease. Peak effect is 1–5 hr. May cause headache, nausea, hyponatremia, nasal congestion, abdominal cramps, and hypertension.

Spray: 100 mcg/ml (5 ml)
Conversion: 100 mcg = 400 IU arginine
vasopressin

Hemophilia A and von Willebrand's
disease: 2–4 mcg/kg/dose intranasally
or 0.2–0.4 mcg/kg/dose IV over 15–30
min

Nocturnal enuresis (>6 yr): 20 mcg at
bedtime intranasally, range 10–40 mcg

For hemophilia A and von Willebrand's
disease administer dose intranasally, 2
hours before procedure; IV, 30 minutes
before procedure.

DEXAMETHASONE

(Decadron and other brand names)
Corticosteroid
Tabs: 0.25, 0.5, 1, 1.5, 2, 4, 6 mg
Injection: 4, 10, 20, 24 mg/ml (Sodium
phosphate)
IM Injection: 8, 16 mg/ml (acetate)
Elixir: 0.5 mg/5 ml (some preparations
contain 5% alcohol)
Oral Solution: 0.1, 1 mg/ml (some
preparations contain 30% alcohol)
Inhalation: 84 mcg/metered dose (12.6 g)

Cerebral Edema:
Loading dose: 1–2 mg/kg/dose PO, IV,
IM × 1
Maintenance: 1–1.5 mg/kg/24 hr ÷
Q4–6 hr
Airway Edema: 0.5–2 mg/kg/24 hr PO, IV,
IM ÷ Q6 hr (begin 24 hr before
extubation and continue for 4–6 doses
after extubation)
Croup: 0.6 mg/kg/dose IM × 1
Antiemetic:
Initial: 10 mg/m²/dose IV; **max:** 20 mg
Subsequent: 5 mg/m²/dose Q6 hr IV
Anti-inflammatory:
Children: 0.08–0.3 mg/kg/24 hr PO, IV,
IM ÷ Q6–12 hr
Adults: 0.75–9 mg/24 hr PO, IV, IM ÷
Q6–12 hr
Meningitis: 0.6 mg/kg/24 hr IV ÷ Q6 hr ×
4 days

Toxicity: same as for prednisone. Oral
peak serum levels occur 1–2 hr and
within 8 hr following IM administration.
Use in meningitis remains
controversial. Consult ID specialist or
latest edition of Red Book. For other
uses and doses based on body
surface area, see Chapter 28.

(Continued.)

Drug/How Supplied	Dose and Route	Remarks
DEXTROAMPHETAMINE (Dexedrine and many other brand names) *CNS stimulant* Tabs: 5, 10 mg Elixir: 5 mg/5 ml (10% alcohol) Sustained-release caps: 5, 10, 15 mg	*Attention Deficit Hyperactivity Disorder:* *3–5 yr:* 2.5 mg/24 hr QAM; increase by 2.5 mg/24 hr at weekly intervals to a **max dose** of 40 mg/24 hr *≥6 yr:* 5 mg/24 hr QAM; increase by 5 mg/24 hr at weekly intervals to a **max dose** of 40 mg/24 hr *Narcolepsy:* *6–12 yr:* 5 mg/24 hr ÷ QD-TID: increase by 5 mg/24 hr at weekly intervals to a **max dose** of 60 mg/24 hr *>12 yr:* 10 mg/24 hr ÷ QD-TID: increase by 10 mg/24 hr at weekly intervals to a **max dose** of 60 mg/24 hr	Use with caution in presence of hypertension or cardiovascular disease. **Not recommended for <3 yr olds.** Interrupt administration occasionally to determine need for continued therapy. Many side effects, including insomnia, restlessness, anorexia, psychosis, headache, vomiting, abdominal cramps, dry mouth, growth failure. Tolerance develops. (Same guidelines as for methylphenidate apply.) **Do not** give with MAO inhibitors, general anesthetics.
DIAZEPAM (Valium and others) *Benzodiazepine; anxiolytic, anticonvulsant* Tabs: 2, 5, 10 mg Oral solution: 1, 5 mg/ml Injection: 5 mg/ml Sustained-release cap: 15 mg	*Sedative/muscle relaxant:* *Children:* IM or IV: 0.04–0.2 mg/kg/dose Q2–4 hr **max dose:** 0.6 mg/kg within an 8-hr period PO: 0.12–0.8 mg/kg/24 hr ÷ Q6–8 hr *Adults:* IM or IV: 2–10 mg/dose Q3–4 hr PRN PO: 2–10 mg/dose Q6–12 hr PRN	Hypotension and respiratory depression may occur. Use with **caution** in glaucoma, shock, and depression. Give undiluted no faster than 2 mg/min. **Do not** mix with IV fluids. In status epilepticus, diazepam must be followed by long-acting anticonvulsants. For management of status epilepticus, see Chapter 1. For management of neonatal seizures, see Chapter 22.

Status epilepticus:
Neonate: 0.3–0.75 mg/kg/dose IV Q15–30 min × 2–3 doses
>1 mo: 0.2–0.5 mg/kg/dose IV Q15–30 min
Max total dose: <5 yr: 5 mg; ≥5 yr:10 mg
Adults: 5–10 mg/dose IV Q10–15 min
Max total dose: 30 mg
Rectal dose: 0.5 mg/kg/dose

DIAZOXIDE

(Hyperstat, Proglycem)
Antihypertensive agent, antihypoglycemic agent

Injection: 15 mg/ml
Caps: 50 mg
Suspension: 50 mg/ml (30 ml)

Hypertensive crisis: 1–3 mg/kg IV up to 150 mg; repeat Q5–15 min PRN, then Q4–24 hr
Hyperinsulinemic hypoglycemia (due to insulin-producing tumors):
Newborns and infants: 8–15 mg/kg/24 hr ÷ Q8–12 hr PO
Children and adults: 3–8 mg/kg/24 hr ÷ Q8–12 hr PO (start at lowest dose)

May cause hyponatremia, salt and water retention, GI disturbances, ketoacidosis, rash, hyperuricemia, weakness, hypertrichosis, and arrhythmias. Monitor BP closely for hypotension. Hyperglycemia occurs in majority of patients. Hypoglycemia should be treated initially with IV glucose; diazoxide should be introduced only if refractory to glucose infusion.

DICLOXACILLIN SODIUM

(Dynapen, and others)
Antibiotic, penicillin (penicillinase-resistant)

Caps: 125, 250, 500 mg
Oral suspension: 62.5 mg/5 ml (80, 100, 200 ml)

Children (<40 kg):
Mild/moderate infections: 12.5–25 mg/kg/24 hr PO ÷ Q6 hr
Severe infections: 50–100 mg/kg/24 hr PO ÷ Q6 hr
Adults (≥40 kg): 125–500 mg/dose PO Q6 hr; **max dose:** 4 g/24 hr

Toxicity and side effects similar to cloxacillin. Give 1–2 hr before meals or 2 hr after meals. Limited experience in neonates and very young infants. Higher doses (50–100 mg/kg/24 hr) are indicated following IV therapy for osteomyelitis.

(Continued.)

Drug/How Supplied	Dose and Route	Remarks
DIDANOSINE (DDI) (Dideoxyinosine, Videx) *Anti-viral agent* Tabs (buffered, chewable/dispersable): 25, 50, 100, 150 mg Oral powder, buffered (single-dose packets for solution): 100, 167, 250, 375 mg Oral pediatric powder (for solution): 2, 4 g	*Children:* 100–300 mg/m^2/24 hr ÷ Q12 hr Based on 200 mg/m^2/24 hr, the following are the doses: BSA / Tablets / Peds Powder Dose <0.4 — 25 mg Q12 hr — 31 mg Q12 hr 0.5–0.7 — 50 mg Q12 hr — 62 mg Q12 hr 0.8–1 — 75 mg Q12 hr — 94 mg Q12 hr 1.1–1.4 — 100 mg Q12 hr — 125 mg Q12 hr Patients >35 kg and adults: Weight (kg) / Tablets / Buffered Powder 35–49 — 125 mg Q12 hr — 167 mg Q12 hr 50–74 — 200 mg Q12 hr — 250 mg Q12 hr ≥75 — 300 mg Q12 hr — 375 mg Q12 hr	**Administer all doses on empty stomach.** Reported side effects in adults (in decreasing incidence): headaches (36%), diarrhea, peripheral neuropathy, nausea, vomiting, rash/pruritis, abdominal pain (21%), CNS depression, constipation, stomatitis, myalgia, arthritis (11%), pancreatitis (9%), alopecia (8%), dizziness, leukopenia, and anemia. Use with **caution** in patients on sodium restriction (264.5 mg Na/buffered tablet, 1380 mg Na/single dose packet). Impairs absorption of drugs requiring an acidic environment (i.e., ketoconazole, dapsone) and quinolones. **Consult package insert for additional details.**

DIGOXIN

(Lanoxin)
Antiarrhythmic agent, inotrope
Caps: 50, 100, 200 mcg
Tabs: 125, 250, 500 mcg
Elixir: 50 mcg/ml (60 ml)
Injection: 100, 250 mcg/ml

Digitalizing: Total digitalizing dose (TDD) and maintenance doses in mcg/kg/24 hr:

Age	TDD			Maintenance	
	PO	IV/IM	PO	IV/IM	
Premature	20	15	5	3–4	
Full term	30	20	8–10	6–8	
<2 yr	40–50	30–40	10–12	7.5–9	
2–10 yr	30–40	20–30	8–10	6–8	
>10 yr and <100 kg	10–15	8–12	2.5–5	2–3	

Initial: 1/2 TDD, then 1/4 TDD Q8–18 hr × 2 doses; obtain ECG 6 hr after dose to assess for toxicity.

Maintenance:
<10 yr: Give maintenance dose ÷ BID
≥10 yr: Give maintenance dose QD

Excreted via the kidney. Use with **caution** in renal failure. **Contraindicated** in patients with ventricular dysrhythmias. May cause AV block or dysrhythmias. In the patient treated with digoxin, cardioversion or calcium infusion may lead to ventricular fibrillation (pretreatment with lidocaine may prevent this). For signs and symptoms of toxicity, see Chapter 2. **Therapeutic concentration:** 0.8–2 ng/ml. Higher doses may be required for supraventricular tachycardia. Neonates may have falsely elevated digoxin levels, due to maternal digoxin-like substances.

DIGOXIN IMMUNE FAB (OVINE)

(Digibind)
Antidigoxin antibody
Injection: 40 mg

First, *determine total body digoxin load (TBL):* TBL(mg) = serum digoxin level (ng/ml) × 5.6 × wt (kg) ÷ 1000, or TBL (mg) = mg digoxin ingested × 0.8
Then, *calculate dose of digoxin immune Fab (mg):* Fab = TBL × 66.7;
Infuse IV over 15–30 min (through 0.22 micron filter).

May cause rapidly developing severe hypokalemia or decreased cardiac output. Digoxin therapy may be reinstituted in 3–7 days, when toxicity has been corrected. **Contraindicated** if hypersensitivity to sheep products, or if renal or cardiac failure.

(Continued.)

Drug/How Supplied	Dose and Route	Remarks
DIHYDROTACHYSTEROL (DHT, Hytakerol, DHT Intensol) *Fat-soluble vitamin D analog* Solution: 0.2 mg/ml (20% alcohol) Solution (in oil): 0.25 mg/ml (15 ml) Caps: 0.125 mg Tabs: 0.125, 0.2, 0.4 mg 1 mg = 120,000 IU vitamin D₂	*Hypoparathyroidism:* *Neonates:* 0.05–0.1 mg/24 hr PO *Infants/young children:* Initial, 1–5 mg/24 hr PO × 4 days, then 0.5–1.5 mg/24 hr PO *Older children/adults:* Initial, 0.75–2.5 mg/24 hr PO × 4 days, then 0.2–1.5 mg/24 hr PO *Nutritional Rickets:* 0.5 mg × 1 PO, or 13–50 mcg/24 hr PO QD until healing *Renal Osteodystrophy:* *Children/Adolescents:* 0.1–0.5 mg/24 hr PO *Adults:* 0.1–0.6 mg/24 hr PO	Monitor serum Ca⁺⁺ and PO₄. Toxicities include hypercalcemia or hypervitaminosis D. More potent than vitamin D₂ but more rapidly inactivated (half-life is hours vs. weeks). Titrate dose with patient response. Oral Ca⁺⁺ supplementation may be required. Activated by 25-hydroxylation in liver; does not require 1-hydroxylation in kidney.
DIMENHYDRINATE (Dramamine and other brand names) *Antiemetic, antihistamine* Tabs/Caps: 50 mg Tabs (chewable): 50 mg Injection: 50 mg/ml Solution: 12.5 mg/4 ml, 15.62 mg/5 ml	*Children (<12 yr):* 5 mg/kg/24 hr ÷ Q6 hr PO/IM/IV *Adult:* 50–100 mg/dose Q4–6 hr PRN PO/IM/IV **Max PO doses:** *2–6 yr:* 75 mg/24 hr *6–12 yr:* 150 mg/24 hr *Adults:* 400 mg/24 hr **Max IM dose:** 300 mg/24 hr	May mask vestibular symptoms. **Caution** when taken with ototoxic agents. Causes drowsiness. Use should be limited to management of prolonged vomiting of *known* etiology. **Not recommended in children <2 yr.** Toxicity resembles anti-cholinergic poisoning.

DIMERCAPROL

(BAL, British anti-Lewisite)
Heavy metal chelator *(arsenic, gold, mercury, lead)*
Injection (in oil): 100 mg/ml (3 ml)

Give all injections deep IM.
Lead poisoning: Administer BAL with Ca-EDTA. See Chapter 2 for details.
Arsenic or gold poisoning:
Days 1 and 2: 2.5–3 mg/kg/dose Q6 hr
Day 3: 2.5–3 mg/kg/dose Q12 hr
Days 4–14: 2.5–3 mg/kg/dose Q24 hr
Mercury poisoning: 5 mg/kg × 1, then 2.5 mg/kg/dose QD-BID × 10 days

May cause hypertension, tachycardia, GI disturbance, headache, fever (30% of children); transient neutropenia. Symptoms are usually relieved by antihistamines. **Contraindicated** in hepatic or renal insufficiency. Urine should be kept alkaline. May result in renal toxicity. Use **cautiously** in patients with G6PD deficiency. **Do not** use concomitantly with iron.

DIPHENHYDRAMINE

(Benadryl and other brand names)
Antihistamine
Elixir (14% alcohol): 12.5 mg/5 ml
Syrup (some contain 5% alcohol): 12.5 mg/5 ml
Caps/Tabs: 25, 50 mg
Injection: 10, 50 mg/ml
Cream: 2% (30, 60 g)
Lotion: 1% (75 ml)

Children: 5 mg/kg/24 hr ÷ Q6 hr PO/IM/IV;
max dose: 300 mg/24 hr
Adult: 10–50 mg/dose Q6–8 hr PO/IM/IV;
max dose: 400 mg/24 hr
For anaphylaxis or phenothiazine overdose: 1–2 mg/kg IV slowly

Side effects common to antihistamines. CNS side effects more common than GI disturbances. May cause paradoxical excitement.
Contraindicated with concurrent MAO inhibitor use or acute attacks of asthma.

DISOPYRAMIDE PHOSPHATE

(Norpace and others)
Antiarrhythmic agent, class Ia
Caps: 100, 150 mg
Extended-release caps (CR): 100, 150 mg

<1 yr: 10–30 mg/kg/24 hr ÷ Q6 hr PO
1–4 yr: 10–20 mg/kg/24 hr ÷ Q6 hr PO
4–12 yr: 10–15 mg/kg/24 hr ÷ Q6 hr PO
12–18 yr: 6–15 mg/kg/24 hr ÷ Q6 hr PO
Adult: 300–400 mg × 1 PO, then 400–800 mg/24 hr ÷ Q6 hr PO; **max dose:** 1.6 g/24 hr
With extended-release caps, give same daily dose ÷ Q12 hr

Modify dose in renal or hepatic failure. May cause decreased cardiac output. Anticholinergic effects may occur. Causes dose-related AV block, wide QRS, increased QTc, ventricular dysrhythmias. Erythromycin may increase serum levels. **Therapeutic levels: 3–7 mg/L.**

(Continued.)

Drug/How Supplied	Dose and Route	Remarks
DIVALPROEX SODIUM (Depakote) *Anticonvulsant* Enteric coated tabs: 125, 250, 500 mg Sprinkle caps: 125 mg	Dose: see Valproic Acid	Remarks: see Valproic Acid. Preferred over valproic acid for patients on ketogenic diet
DOBUTAMINE (Dobutrex) *Sympathomimetic agent* Injection: 12.5 mg/ml (contains sulfites)	*Continuous IV infusion:* 2.5–15 mcg/kg/min; **Max recommended dose:** 40 mcg/kg/min *To prepare infusion:* see inside front cover	Monitor BP and vital signs. $T_{1/2}$: 2 min. Peak effects in 10–20 min. **Contraindicated** in IHSS. Tachycardia, arrhythmias (PVCs), and hypertension may occasionally occur (especially at higher infusion rates). Correct hypovolemic states before use. Increases AV conduction, may precipitate ventricular ectopic activity.
DOCUSATE SODIUM (Colace and others) *Stool softener, laxative* Caps: 50, 100, 240, 250 mg Tabs: 100 mg Syrup: 16.7 mg/5 ml, 20 mg/5 ml Solution: 10 mg/ml, 50 mg/ml	*PO: (take with liquids)* <3 yr: 10–40 mg/24 hr ÷ QD-QID 3–6 yr: 20–60 mg/24 hr ÷ QD-QID 6–12 yr: 40–150 mg/24 hr ÷ QD-QID >12 yr: 50–500 mg/24 hr ÷ QD-QID *Rectal: Older children and adults:* add 50–100 mg of oral solution to enema fluid.	Oral dosage effective only after 1–3 days of therapy. Incidence of side effects is exceedingly low. Oral solution is bitter; give with milk, fruit juice, or formula to mask taste. A few drops of the 10 mg/ml solution may be used in the ear as a cerumenolytic. Effect is usually seen within 15 min.

DOPAMINE

(Intropin, Dopastat, and others)
Sympathomimetic agent
Injection: 40, 80, 160 mg/ml
Prediluted in D$_5$W: 0.8, 1.6, 3.2 mg/ml

Low dose: 2–5 mcg/kg/min IV; increases renal blood flow; minimal effect on heart rate and cardiac output
Intermediate dose: 5–15 mcg/kg/min IV; increases renal blood flow, heart rate, cardiac contractility, and cardiac output
High dose: >20 mcg/kg/min IV; alpha adrenergic effects are prominent; **decreases renal perfusion**
Max dose recommended: 20–50 mcg/kg/min IV
To prepare infusion: see inside front cover

Monitor vital signs and blood pressure continuously. Correct hypovolemic states. Tachyarrhythmias, ectopic beats, hypertension, vasoconstriction, vomiting may occur. Extravasation may cause tissue necrosis; treat with phentolamine. Use **cautiously** with phenytoin since hypotension and bradycardia may be exacerbated. **Do not use** in pheochromocytoma, tachyarrhythmias, or hypovolemia. Administration into an umbilical arterial catheter is **NOT recommended.**

DORNASE ALFA/DNASE

(Pulmozyme)
Inhaled mucolytic
Sol: 1 mg/ml (2.5 ml)

Patients > 5 yr: 2.5 mg via nebulizer QD. Some patients may benefit from 2.5 mg BID

Voice alteration, pharyngitis, laryngitis may result. These are generally reversible without dose adjustment. **Should not mix with other nebulized drugs.** A beta-agonist may be useful before administration to enhance drug distribution. Chest physiotherapy should be incorporated into treatment regimen

DOXAPRAM HCL

(Dopram)
CNS stimulant
Injection: 20 mg/ml (20 ml)
Contains 0.9% benzyl alcohol

Methylxanthine refractory neonatal apnea:
Load with 2.5–3 mg/kg over 15 min, followed by a continuous infusion of 1 mg/kg/hr titrated to the lowest responsive dose; **Max dose:** 2.5 mg/kg/hr

Hypertension occurs with higher doses (greater than 1.5 mg/kg/hr). May also cause tachycardia, arrhythmias, seizure, hyperreflexia, hyperpyrexia, and sweating. Avoid extravasation into tissues.

(Continued.)

Drug/How Supplied	Dose and Route	Remarks
DOXYCYCLINE (Vibramycin and others) *Antibiotic, tetracycline derivative* Caps: 50, 100 mg Tabs: 50, 100 mg Syrup: 50 mg/5 ml (30 ml) Suspension: 25 mg/5 ml (60 ml) Injection: 100, 200 mg	*Initial:* ≤45 kg: 5 mg/kg/24 hr ÷ BID PO/IV × 1 day to **max dose:** of 200 mg/24 hr >45 kg: 200 mg/24 hr ÷ BID PO/IV × 1 day *Maintenance:* ≤45 kg: 2.5–5 mg/kg/24 hr ÷ QD-BID PO/IV >45 kg: 100–200 mg/24 hr ÷ QD-BID PO/IV **Max adult dose:** 300 mg/24 hr *PID:* see Chapter 18.	Use with **caution** in hepatic and renal disease. May cause increased intracranial pressure. Do not use in children <9 yr: may result in tooth enamel hypoplasia and discoloration. May cause GI symptoms, photosensitivity, hemolytic anemia, hypersensitivity reactions. Infuse IV over 1–4 hr. Avoid direct sunlight. See Tetracycline.
DROPERIDOL (Inapsine) *Sedative, antiemetic* Injection: 2.5 mg/ml	*Antiemetic/Sedation:* 0.03–0.07 mg/kg/dose IV over 2 min; if needed, may give 0.1–0.15 mg/kg/dose; **max initial dose:** 2.5 mg/dose Administer PRN Q4–6 hr when used as an antiemetic	Onset in 3–10 minutes. Peak effects within 10–30 minutes. Duration of 2–4 hr. Often given as adjunct to other agents. Side effects include hypotension, dystonia, tachycardia, feeling of motor restlessness.

EDROPHONIUM CHLORIDE

(Tensilon)

Anti-cholinesterase agent, antidote for neuromuscular blockade

Injection: 10 mg/ml (1, 10, 15 ml)

Test for Myasthenia Gravis (IV):
Neonates; 0.1 mg single dose
Infants and Children:
Initial: 0.04 mg/kg/dose × 1
Max: 1 mg for <34 kg, 2 mg for ≥34 kg
If no response after 1 min, may give 0.16 mg/kg/dose for a total of 0.2 mg/kg
Total max dose: 5 mg for <34 kg, 10 mg for ≥34 kg
Adult: 2 mg test dose IV; if no reaction, give 8 mg after 45 sec

Keep atropine available in syringe and have resuscitation equipment ready. May precipitate cholinergic crisis, arrhythmias, bronchospasm. Hypersensitivity to test dose (fasciculations or intestinal cramping) is indication to stop giving drug. **Contraindicated** in GI or GU obstruction, or arrhythmias. Short duration of action (minutes). **Antidote:** Atropine 0.01–0.04 mg/kg/dose.

EDTA CALCIUM DISODIUM

(Calcium disodium versenate)

Chelating agent, antidote for lead toxicity

Injection: 200 mg/ml (5 ml)

Lead Poisoning: see Chapter 15 for classification, and Chapter 2 for treatment and dosing

May cause renal tubular necrosis. **Do not** use if anuric. Follow urinalysis and renal function. Monitor ECG continuously for arrhythmia when giving IV. Rapid IV infusion may cause sudden increase in intracranial pressure in patients with cerebral edema. May cause zinc and copper deficiency. Monitor Ca^{++} and PO$_4$. IM route preferred. Give IM with 0.5% procaine.

(Continued.)

Drug/How Supplied	Dose and Route	Remarks
EMLA *Eutectic mixture of local anesthetics* 5 g kit (with dressings), 30 g tube (lidocaine 2.5%, prilocaine 2.5%)	See Chapter 27 for maximum application area in cm².	Must apply 60–90 minutes in advance under an occlusive dressing. Wipe cream off before procedure. Use with caution in patients with G6PD deficiency and in patients with renal and hepatic impairment. Prilocaine has been associated with methemoglobinemia.
ENALAPRIL MALEATE (Vasotec) **ENALAPRIAT** (Vasotec IV) *Angiotensin converting enzyme inhibitor, antihypertensive* Tabs: 2.5, 5, 10, 20 mg (Enalapril) Injection: 1.25 mg/ml (Enalapriat)	*Children:* PO: 0.1 mg/kg/24 hr; increase PRN over 2 wk **Max dose: 0.5 mg/kg/24 hr** IV: 0.005–0.01 mg/kg/dose Q8–24 hr *Adult:* PO: 2.5–5 mg/24 hr QD initially to **max dose of 40 mg/24 hr ÷ QD-BID** IV: 0.625–1.25 mg/dose IV Q6 hr	Reduce dose in renal impairment. Administer IV over 5 min. Enalapril is converted to its active form (Enalapriat) by the liver. Side effects: nausea, diarrhea, headache, dizziness, hypotension, and hypersensitivity may occur. Cough is a reported side effect of ACE inhibitors.
EPINEPHRINE HCL (Adrenalin and others) *Sympathomimetic agent* 1:1000 (Aqueous): Injection: 1 mg/ml (1, 30 ml vials; 2 ml pre-filled syringe) 1:200 (Sus-phrine suspension): Injection: 5 mg/ml (0.3, 5 ml)	*Cardiac Uses:* *Neonate:* Asystole and bradycardia: 0.01–0.03 mg/kg of 1:10,000 solution (0.1–0.3 ml/kg) IV/ET Q3–5 min *Infants and Children:* Bradycardia/Asystole and Pulseless arrest: see inside front cover and decision trees	May produce arrhythmias, tachycardia, hypertension, headaches, nervousness, nausea, vomiting. Necrosis may occur at site of repeated local injection. ETT doses should be diluted with NS to a volume of 3–5 ml before administration. Follow with several positive pressure ventilations.

1:10,000 (Aqueous):
Injection: 0.1 mg/ml (3, 10 ml prefilled
  syringe)
1:100,000 (Aqueous):
Injection: 0.01 mg/ml (5 ml)
Epi-pen: 0.3 mg autoinjection (2 ml of
  1:1000 solution)
Epi-pen Jr: 0.15 mg autoinjection (2 ml of
  1:2000 solution)
Aerosol: 0.16, 0.2, 0.25 mg epinephrine
  base/spray (15, 22.5 ml)

*Bradycardia and asystole and
  pulseless arrest (first dose):* 0.01
  mg/kg of 1:10,000 solution (0.1
  ml/kg) IO/IV
*Asystole and pulseless arrest
  (subsequent doses) and all ET
  doses:* 0.1 mg/kg of 1:1000
  solution (0.1 ml/kg) IO/IV/ET Q3–5
  min

Adults:

Asystole: 1–5 mg IV/ET Q3–5 min
IV drip (all ages): 0.1–1 mcg/kg/min;
  titrate to effect; to prepare infusion,
  see inside front cover
Respiratory uses:
Bronchodilator:
1:1000 (Aqueous)
  Infants and Children: 0.01 ml/kg/dose
    SC (**max single dose** 0.3 ml);
    repeat Q15 min × 3–4 doses or
    Q4 hr PRN
  Adults: 0.3–0.5 ml/dose
1:200 (Susphrine suspension)
  Infants and Children: 0.005
    ml/kg/dose SC (**max single dose**
    0.15 ml); repeat Q8–12 hr PRN

(Continued.)

Drug/How Supplied	Dose and Route	Remarks
EPINEPHRINE HCL—(cont.)	*Adults:* 0.1–0.3 ml/dose *Inhalation:* 1–2 puffs Q4 hr PRN *Nebulization:* (alternative to racemic epinephrine): 0.5 ml/kg of 1:1000 solution diluted in 3 ml NS; **max doses:** ≤4 yr: 2.5 ml/dose; >4 yr: 5 ml/dose	Tachyarrhythmias, headache, nausea, palpitations reported. Rebound airway edema may occur. Monitoring should be considered if administered more frequently than Q1–2 hr.
EPINEPHRINE, RACEMIC (Vaponefrin, Micronefrin, Asthmanefrin) *Sympathomimetic agent* Solution: 2.25% (7.5, 15, 30 ml), 2% (15, 30 ml)	*Croup:* 0.05 ml/kg/dose diluted to 3 ml with NS. Given via nebulizer over 15 min PRN, but **not** more frequently than Q1–2 hr. **Max dose:** 0.5 ml	
EPOEITIN ALFA (Epogen, Procrit) *Recombinant human erythropoietin* Inj: 2000, 3000, 4000, 10,000 U/ml	*Renal failure: SC/IV* *Initial:* 50–100 U/kg 3×/wk; may increase dose if hematocrit does not rise by 5–6 points after 8 wk; maintenance doses are individualized *AZT treated HIV patients: SC/IV* 100 U/kg/dose 3×/wk × 8 wk; the dose may be increased by 50–100 U/kg/dose given 3×/wk; **max dose** 300 U/kg/dose given 3×/wk *Anemia of prematurity:* 25–100 U/kg/dose SC 3×/wk; alternatively, 200 U/kg/dose IV/SC QD to QOD for 2–6 wk may be used	Evaluate serum iron, ferritin, TIBC before therapy. Monitor Hct, BP, clotting times, platelets, BUN, serum creatinine. Peak effect in 2–3 wk. Reduce dose when target Hct is reached, or when Hct increases >4 points in any 2-wk period. May cause hypertension, seizure, hypersensitivity reactions, headache, edema, dizziness. SC route provides sustained serum levels compared to IV route.

ERGOCALCIFEROL
(Drisdol, Calciferol)
Vitamin D2
Caps/Tabs: 50,000 IU (1.25 mg)
Injection: 500,000 IU/ml
Drops: 8000 IU/ml (200 mcg/ml) (60 ml)
1 mg = 40,000 IU

Dietary supplementation:
Preterm: 400–800 IU/24 hr PO
Infants/Children: 400 IU/24 hr PO;
please refer to Chapter 23 for details
Renal Failure:
Children: 4000–40,000 IU/24 hr PO
Adult: 20,000 IU/24 hr PO
Rickets: Vitamin D dependent:
Children: 3000–5000 IU/24 hr PO;
some may require 60,000 IU/24 hr
Adults: 10,000–60,000 IU/24 hr PO;
some may require 500,000 IU/24 hr
Nutritional Rickets:
*Adults and Children with Normal GI
absorption:* 2000–5000 IU/24 hr PO
× 6–12 wk
Malabsorption:
Children: 10,000–25,000 IU/24 hr PO
Adults: 10,000–300,000 IU/24 hr PO
Vitamin D resistant rickets:
Children: Initial dose 400,000–800,000
IU/24 hr PO; increase dose by
10,000–20,000 IU/24 hr PO Q3–4
mo if needed
Adults: 10,000–60,000 IU/24 hr PO

Monitor serum Ca^{++}, PO_4, and alkaline
phosphate. Serum Ca^{++}, PO_4 product
should be <70 mg/dl. Titrate dosage
to patient response. Watch for
symptoms of hypercalcemia:
weakness, diarrhea, polyuria,
metastatic calcification,
nephrocalcinosis. Vitamin D_2 is
activated by 25-hydroxylation in liver
and 1-hydroxylation in kidney. May use
IM route in cases of fat malabsorption.
Injectable for IM administration only.

ERGOTAMINE
(Cafergot and others)
Ergot alkaloid

Older children and adolescents: 1 mg at
onset of attack, then 1 mg Q30 min
PRN up to **max** 3 mg

Caution in renal or hepatic disease. May
cause paresthesias, GI disturbance, or
muscle cramps.

(Continued.)

Drug/How Supplied	Dose and Route	Remarks
Tabs: 1 mg and 100 mg caffeine Sublingual tabs: 2 mg Suppository: 2 mg and 100 mg caffeine	*Adults:* 2 mg at onset of attack, then 1–2 mg Q30 min up to 6 mg per attack. *Suppository:* 2 mg at first sign of attack; follow with second dose (2 mg) after 1 hr, **max dose** 4 mg per attack, not to exceed 10 mg/week	
ERYTHROMYCIN PREPARATIONS (Erythrocin, Pediamycin, E-Mycin, Ery-Ped, and others) *Antibiotic, macrolide* *Erythromycin base:* Tabs: 250, 333, 500 mg Delayed release tabs: 333 mg Delayed release caps: 250 mg Topical Ointment: 2% (25 g) Topical Gel: 2% (30, 60 g) Topical Solution: 1.5%, 2% (60 ml) Ophthalmic ointment: 0.5% (3.5, 3.75 g) *Erythromycin Ethyl Succinate (EES):* Suspension: 200, 400 mg/5 ml (60, 100, 200 ml) Drops: 100 mg/2.5 ml (50 ml) Chewable Tabs: 200 mg Tabs: 400 mg *Erythromycin Estolate:* Suspension: 125, 250 mg/5 ml	*Oral:* *Neonates:* *<1.2 kg:* 20 mg/kg/24 hr ÷ Q12 hr *≥1.2 kg:* *0–7 days:* 20 mg/kg/24 hr ÷ Q12 hr *>7 days:* 30 mg/kg/24 hr ÷ Q8 hr *Children:* 30–50 mg/kg/24 hr ÷ Q6–8 hr; **Max dose:** 2 g/24 hr *Adults:* 1–4 g/24 hr ÷ Q6 hr; **max dose:** 4 g/24 hr *Parenteral:* *Children:* 20–50 mg/kg/24 hr ÷ Q6 hr IV *Adults:* 15–20 mg/kg/24 hr ÷ Q6 hr IV Max dose: 4 g/24 hr *Rheumatic fever prophylaxis:* 500 mg/24 hr ÷ Q12 hr PO *Endocarditis prophylaxis:* See Chapter 7 *Ophthalmic:* Apply 0.5 inch ribbon to affected eye BID-QID *Pertussis:* Estolate salt: 50 mg/kg/24 hr ÷ Q6 hr PO × 14 days	Avoid IM route (pain, necrosis). GI side effects common (nausea, vomiting, abdominal cramps). Give doses after meals. Use with **caution** in liver disease. Estolate may cause cholestatic jaundice, although hepatotoxicity is uncommon (2% of reported cases). May produce elevated digoxin, theophylline, carbamazepine, cyclosporine, methylprednisolone levels. Oral therapy should replace IV as soon as possible. Because of different absorption characteristics, higher oral doses of EES are needed to achieve therapeutic effects. May produce false positive urinary catecholamines. Formulations of IV lactobionate dosage form may contain benzyl alcohol.

Tabs: 500 mg
Caps: 250 mg
Erythromycin Stearate:
Tabs: 250, 500 mg
Erythromycin gluceptate:
Injection: 1000 mg
Erythromycin lactobionate:
Injection: 500, 1000 mg

ERYTHROMYCIN ETHYLSUCCINATE AND ACETYL SULFISOXAZOLE
(Pediazole)
Antibiotic, macrolide + sulfonamide derivative
Suspension: 200 mg erythromycin and 600 mg sulfa/5 ml (100, 150, 200 ml)

ESMOLOL HCL
(Brevibloc)
Beta-1-selective adrenergic blocking agent
Injection: 10, 250 mg/ml

Preoperative bowel prep: 20 mg/kg/dose PO erythromycin base × 3 doses, with neomycin, 1 day before surgery

Otitis media: 50 mg/kg/24 hr (as erythromycin) and 150 mg/kg/24 hr (as sulfa) ÷ Q6 hr PO, or give 1.25 ml/kg/24 hr ÷ Q6 hr PO
Max dose: 2 g erythromycin, 6 g sulfisoxasole/24 hr

Titrate to individual response.
IV: Loading dose: 100–500 mcg/kg over 1 min
Maintenance dose: 25–100 mcg/kg/min as infusion
If inadequate response, may re-administer loading dose above, and/or increase maintenance dose by 25–50 mcg/kg/min in increments of Q5–10 min
Usual maintenance dose range: 50–500 mcg/kg/min

See adverse effects of erythromycin and sulfisoxazole. **Not recommended** in infants <2 mo old.

$T_{1/2}$ = 9 minutes. May cause bronchospasm, congestive heart failure, nausea, vomiting. May increase digoxin level by 10%–20%. Morphine may increase esmolol level by 46%. Administer only in monitored setting.

(Continued.)

Drug/How Supplied	Dose and Route	Remarks
ETHAMBUTOL HCL (Myambutol) *Antituberculosis drug* Tabs: 100, 400 mg	*Children:* 15 mg/kg/24 hr PO QD *Adolescents and adults:* 15–25 mg/kg/24 hr as single PO dose or 50 mg/kg/dose twice weekly up to **max dose of 2.5 g/24 hr**	May cause reversible optic neuritis, especially with larger doses. Obtain baseline ophthalmologic studies before beginning therapy and then monthly. Follow visual acuity, visual fields, and (red-green) color vision. **Assessment of visual acuity may be difficult in young children.** Discontinue if any visual deterioration occurs. Monitor uric acid, liver function, heme status, and renal function. May cause GI disturbances. Give with food. Adjust dose with renal failure.
ETHOSUXIMIDE (Zarontin) *Anticonvulsant* Caps: 250 mg Syrup: 250 mg/5 ml	*Children:* *Oral:* ≤6 yr: Initial: 15 mg/kg/24 hr ÷ BID; **max:** 500 mg/24 hr; increase as needed Q4–7 days; usual maintenance dose: 15–40 mg/kg/24 hr ÷ BID >6 yr and Adults: 250 mg BID; increase by 250 mg/24 hr as needed Q4–7 days; usual maintenance dose: 20–40 mg/kg/24 hr ÷ BID **Max dose:** 1500 mg/24 hr	Monitor levels. Use with **caution** in hepatic and renal disease. Ataxia, anorexia, drowsiness, sleep disturbances, rashes, and blood dyscrasias are rare idiosyncratic reactions. May cause lupus-like syndrome; may increase frequency of grand mal seizures in patients with mixed type seizures. To minimize GI distress, may administer with food or milk. **Therapeutic levels:** 40–100 mg/L. $T_{1/2}$ = 24–42 hr.

FAMOTIDINE

(Pepcid, Pepcid AC [OTC])

Histamine-2-receptor antagonist

Injection: 10 mg/ml (multidose vials contain 0.9% benzyl alcohol)

Liquid: 40 mg/5 ml (contains parabens)

Tabs: 10 (OTC), 20, 40 mg

Children:

IV: Initial: 0.6–0.8 mg/kg/24 hr ÷ Q8–12 hr up to a **max** of 40 mg/24 hr

PO: Initial: 1–1.2 mg/kg/24 hr ÷ Q8–12 hr up to a **max** of 40 mg/24 hr

Adult:

PO: 20 mg BID or 40 mg QHS

IV: 20 mg BID

A Q12 hr dosage interval is generally recommended; however, infants and young children may require a Q8 hr interval because of enhanced elimination. Headaches, dizziness, constipation, diarrhea, and drowsiness have occurred. Dosage adjustment is required in severe renal failure.

FENTANYL

(Sublimaze, Duragesic, Fentanyl Oralet)

Narcotic; analgesic, sedative

Injection: 50 mcg/ml

SR patch: 25, 50, 75, 100 mcg/hr

Oralet lozenge: 200, 300, 400 mcg

Titrate dose to effect.

IV/IM: 1–2 mcg/kg/dose Q30–60 min PRN

Continuous IV infusion: 1 mcg/kg/hr; titrate to effect; usual infusion range 1–3 mcg/kg/hr

PO (Oralet): Sedation: 10–15 mcg/kg/dose up to **max** of 400 mcg/dose

Transdermal: Safety and efficacy have not been established in pediatrics

See Chapter 27 for equianalgesic dosing

Highly lipophilic and may deposit into fat tissue. Onset of action 1–2 minutes with peak effects in 10 minutes. Give IV dose over 3–5 minutes. Rapid infusion may cause respiratory depression and chest wall rigidity. Respiratory depression may persist beyond the period of analgesia.

(Continued.)

FERROUS SULFATE

See Iron Preparations

Drug/How Supplied	Dose and Route	Remarks
FILGRASTIM (G-CSF, Neupogen) *Colony stimulating factor* Injection: 300 mcg/ml	*IV/SC:* 5–10 mcg/kg/dose QD × 14 days or until ANC of 10,000/mm³. Dosage may be increased by 5 mcg/kg/24 hr if desired effect is not achieved within 7 days. Discontinue therapy when ANC > 10,000/mm³	Individual protocols may direct dosing. May cause bone pain, fever, rash. Monitor CBC, uric acid, and LFTs. Use with **caution** in patients with myeloid malignancies with myeloid characteristics. **Contraindicated** for patients sensitive to *E. coli*–derived proteins. SC routes of administration are preferred because of prolonged serum levels over IV route.

FLECAINIDE ACETATE
(Tambocor)
Antiarrhythmic, class Ic
Tabs: 50, 100, 150 mg
	Children: 3–6 mg/kg/24 hr ÷ Q8 hr PO, monitor serum levels to adjust dose if needed
	Adults:
	  Sustained V tach: 100 mg PO Q12 hr; may increase by 50 mg Q12 hr every 4 days to **max** dose of 600 mg/24 hr
	  PSVT/PAF: 50 mg PO Q12 hr; may increase dose by 50 mg Q12 hr every 4 days to **max** dose of 300 mg/24 hr
		May aggravate LV failure, sinus bradycardia, preexisting ventricular arrhythmias. May cause AV block, dizziness, blurred vision, dyspnea, nausea, headache, increased PR or QRS intervals. Reserve for life-threatening cases. Reduce dosage in renal failure. **Therapeutic trough level:** 0.2–1 mg/L.

FLUCONAZOLE
(Diflucan)
Antifungal agent
Tabs: 50, 100, 150, 200 mg
Injection: 2 mg/ml
Suspension: 10 mg/ml, 40 mg/ml

Children (3–13 yr):
Loading dose: 10 mg/kg IV/PO, then
Maintenance: (begin 24 hr after loading dose) 3–6 mg/kg/24 hr IV/PO QD
Adults:
Oropharyngeal and esophageal candidiasis: Loading dose of 200 mg PO/IV followed by 100 mg QD 24 hr after; doses up to **max** dose of 400 mg/24 hr may be used for esophageal candidiasis
Systemic candidiasis: Loading dose of 400 mg PO/IV, followed by 200 mg QD 24 hr later
Cryptococcal meningitis: Loading dose of 400 mg PO/IV, followed by 200–400 mg QD 24 hr later
Vaginal candidiasis: 150 mg PO × 1

PO and IV doses are equivalent. May cause nausea, headache, rash, vomiting, abdominal pain, and diarrhea. Reduce maintenance dose in renal dysfunction (see Chapter 29). May increase effects or levels of cyclosporin, phenytoin, theophylline, warfarin, oral hypoglycemics, and AZT. Rifampin increases fluconazole metabolism. Cardiac arrhythmias may occur when used with cisapride, terfenadine, astemizole. Concomitant administration of fluconazole with any of these drugs is **contraindicated.**

FLUCYTOSINE
(Ancobon, 5-FC, 5-Fluorocytosine)
Antifungal agent
Caps: 250, 500 mg
Oral liquid*: 10 mg/ml

Neonates: 80–160 mg/kg/24 hr ÷ Q6 hr PO
Children and Adults: 50–150 mg/kg/24 hr ÷ Q6 hr PO

Common side effects: nausea, vomiting, diarrhea, rash, CNS disturbance, anemia, leukopenia, thrombocytopenia. Monitor CBC, BUN, serum creatinine, alkaline phos, AST, ALT (see Chapter 29). **Therapeutic levels:** 25–100 mg/L. See references 1

(Continued.)

*Indicates suspensions not commercially available; need to be extemporaneously compounded by a pharmacist. See references 1 and 2 for specific formulations.

Drug/How Supplied	Dose and Route	Remarks
FLUDROCORTISONE ACETATE (Florinef acetate, 9-Fluorohydrocortisone) *Corticosteroid* Tabs: 0.1 mg	*Infants:* 0.05–0.1 mg/24 hr QD PO *Children and Adults:* 0.05–0.2 mg/24 hr QD PO	**Contraindicated** in CHF and systemic fungal infections. Has primarily mineralocorticoid activity. Monitor BP and serum electrolytes. 0.1 mg of fludrocortisone has the same mineralocorticoid effect as 1 mg DOCA. See Chapter 28 for steroid potency comparison.
FLUMAZENIL (Romazicon) *Benzodiazepine antidote* Injection: 0.1 mg/ml (5, 10 ml)	*Children, IV; reversal of benzodiazepine sedation:* Start with 0.1 mg. If no response in 30–60 seconds, repeat dose of 0.1–0.2 mg. May repeat above doses to a **max** total cumulative dose of 1 mg **or** 3 mg in 1 hour.	Onset of benzodiazepine reversal occurs in 1–3 minutes. Reversal effects of flumazenil ($T_{1/2}$ approx 1 hr) may wear off sooner than benzodiazepine effects. **Does not reverse narcotics.** May precipitate seizures, especially in patients taking benzodiazepines for seizure control or in patients with tricyclic antidepressant overdose. If patient does not respond after cumulative 1–3 mg dose, suspect agent other than benzodiazepines. See Chapter 2 for complete management of suspected ingestions.

Drug Doses   **541**

FLUNISOLIDE

(Nasalide, Aerobid, Aerobid-M)
Corticosteroid

Nasal solution: 25 mcg/spray (200 sprays/bottle) (25 ml)

Aerosol inhaler: 250 mcg/dose (50 doses/inhaler) (7 g)

For all dosage forms, reduce to lowest effective maintenance dose to control symptoms

Nasal Solution:

Children (6–14 yr):

Initial: 1 spray per nostril TID or 2 sprays per nostril BID; **max dose:** 4 sprays per nostril/24 hr

Adults:

Initial: 2 sprays per nostril BID; **max dose:** 8 sprays per nostril/24 hr

Inhaler:

Children >4 yr: 1 puff BID up to **max 4** puffs/24 hr

Adults: 2 puffs BID up to **max 8** puffs/24 hr

Stop gradually after 3 wk if no clinical improvement is seen. Shake inhaler well before use. In children, spacer devices may enhance drug delivery of inhaled form. Rinse mouth after administering drug by inhaler to prevent thrush. Patients using nasal solution should clear nasal passages before use.

FLUORIDE

(Luride, Fluoritab, and others)
Mineral

Concentrations based on fluoride ion:

Oral Solution: 0.5, 2, 2.25, 5.5, 5.9 mg/ml

Chewable Tabs: 0.25, 0.5, 1 mg

Tabs: 1 mg

All dose/24 hr:

Concentration of fluoride in drinking water (ppm):

Age	<0.3	0.3–0.7	>0.7
2 wk–2 yr	0.25 mg	0	0
2–3 yr	0.5 mg	0.25 mg	0
3–16 yr	1 mg	0.5 mg	0

Statement from Pediatrics, 5/95

Concentration of fluoride in drinking water (ppm):

Acute overdose: GI distress, salivation, CNS irritability, tetany, seizures, hypocalcemia, hypoglycemia, cardiorespiratory failure. Chronic excess use may result in mottled teeth or bone changes. Take with food, but not milk, to minimize GI upset. The statement from *Pediatrics*, 5/95 is an interim policy recommendation from the AAP. The doses have been decreased due to concerns over dental fluorosis.

(Continued.)

Drug/How Supplied	Dose and Route				Remarks

FLUORIDE —(cont.)

Age	<0.3	0.3–0.6	>0.6
Birth–6 mo	0	0	0
6 mo–3 yr	0.25 mg	0	0
3–6 yr	0.5 mg	0.25 mg	0
6–16 yr	1 mg	0.5 mg	0

FLUOXETINE HYDROCHLORIDE
(Prozac)
Antidepressant, selective serotonin reuptake inhibitor
Liquid: 20 mg/5 ml
Caps: 10, 20 mg

Depression:
Children >5 yr:
5–10 mg QD PO.
Max dose: 20 mg/24 hr
Adults: Start at 20 mg QD PO. May increase after several weeks by 20 mg/24 hr increments to **max** of 80 mg/24 hr. Doses > 20 mg/24 hr should be divided BID.

May cause headache, insomnia, nervousness, drowsiness, GI disturbance, and weight loss. **Contraindicated** in patients taking MAO inhibitors due to possibility of seizures, hyperpyrexia, and coma. May increase the effects of tricyclic antidepressants. May displace other highly protein bound drugs.

FLUTICASONE PROPIONATE
(Flonase, Cutivate)
Corticosteroid
Nasal Spray: 50 mcg/actuation (9, 16 g)
Topical Cream: 0.05% (15, 30, 60 g)
Topical Ointment: 0.005% (15, 60 g)

Children >12 yr: 1 spray per nostril QD
Max dose: 2 sprays per nostril/24 hr ÷ QD-BID; reduce to lowest effective maintenance dose

Patients should clear nasal passages prior to use. Effective for treatment of allergic rhinitis.

FOLIC ACID
(Folvite and others)
Water-soluble vitamin
Tabs: 0.1, 0.4, 0.8, 1 mg
Oral solution*: 1 mg/ml
Injection: 5, 10 mg/ml

For RDA, see Chapter 23
Folic acid deficiency PO, IM, IV, SC

	Infants	Children	Adults (>11 yr)
INITIAL DOSE	15 mcg/kg/ dose; **max dose 50** mcg/24 hr	1 mg/dose	1–3 mg/dose ÷ QD-TID
MAINTENANCE	30–45 mcg/ 24 hr QD	0.1–0.4 mg/24 hr QD	0.5 mg/24 hr QD; Pregnant/ lactating women: 0.8 mg/24 hr QD

Normal levels: serum >3 ng/ml, RBC 153–605 ng/ml. May mask hematologic effects of vitamin B$_{12}$ deficiency, but will not prevent progression of neurologic abnormalities. Women of child-bearing age considering pregnancy should take at least 0.4 mg QD before and during pregnancy to reduce risk of neural tube defects in the fetus.

FOSCARNET
(Foscavir)
Antiviral agent
Injection: 24 mg/ml (250, 500 ml)

Adolescents and Adults, IV:
CMV Retinitis:
  Induction: 180 mg/kg/24 hr ÷ Q8 hr × 14–21 days
  Maintenance: 90–120 mg/kg/24 hr QD
Acyclovir-resistant herpes simplex: virus infection: 40 mg/kg/dose Q8 hr or 40–60 mg/kg/dose Q12 hr for up to 3 weeks or until lesions heal

May cause peripheral neuropathy, seizures, hallucinations, GI disturbance, increased LFTs, and renal failure. Use with **caution** in patients with renal insufficiency. Discontinue use if Cr≥2.9 mg/dl. May cause hypocalcemia; this is augmented if given with pentamidine.

(Continued.)

*Indicates suspensions not commercially available; need to be extemporaneously compounded by a pharmacist. See references 1 and 2 for specific formulations.

Drug/How Supplied	Dose and Route	Remarks
FUROSEMIDE (Furomide, Lasix, and others) *Loop diuretic* Tabs: 20, 40, 80 mg Injection: 10 mg/ml Oral liquid: 10 mg/ml (60 ml), 40 mg/5 ml	*IM, IV, PO* *Neonates:* 0.5–1 mg/kg/dose Q8–24 hr; **max dose:** 6 mg/kg/dose PO, 2 mg/kg/dose IV *Infants and Children:* 0.5–2 mg/kg/dose Q6–12 hr; **max dose:** 6 mg/kg/dose *Adults:* 20–80 mg/24 hr ÷ Q6–12 hr; **max dose:** 600 mg/24 hr *Continuous infusion; IV:* *Children and Adults:* 0.05 mg/kg/hr, titrate to effect.	Ototoxicity may occur in presence of renal disease, especially when used with aminoglycosides. Use with **caution** in hepatic disease. May cause hypokalemia, alkalosis, dehydration, hyperuricemia, and increased calcium excretion. Prolonged use in premature infants may result in nephrocalcinosis. **Max rate of infusion:** 0.5 mg/kg/min.
GABAPENTIN (Neurontin) *Anticonvulsant* Caps: 100, 300, 400 mg	*>12 yr and Adults (PO):* Day 1: 300 mg at bedtime Day 2: 300 mg BID Day 3: 300 mg TID Usual effective doses: 900–1800 mg/24 hr ÷ TID Doses as high as 3.6 g/24 hr have been tolerated	May be taken with or without food. Side effects include somnolence, dizziness, ataxia, fatigue, and nystagmus. Do not withdraw medication abruptly. Adjust dosage in renal impairment. In TID dosing schedule, interval between doses should not exceed 12 hrs.

GANCICLOVIR

(Cytovene)
Antiviral agent
Injection: 500 mg
Caps: 250 mg

Cytomegalovirus infections:
Children >3 mo and adults:
Induction therapy (duration 14–21 days): 10 mg/kg/24 hr ÷ Q12 hr IV
Maintenance therapy: 5 mg/kg/dose QD IV or 6 mg/kg/dose QD IV for 5 days/wk
Oral maintenance therapy (adults): 1000 mg PO TID with food

Limited experience with use in children <12 yr old. **Use with extreme caution.** Reduce dose in renal failure (see Chapter 29). Common side effects: neutropenia, thrombocytopenia, retinal detachment, confusion. Drug reactions alleviated with dose reduction or temporary interruption. Minimum dilution is 10 mg/ml and should be infused IV over ≥1 hr. IM and SC administration are **contraindicated** because of high pH (pH = 11).

GENTAMICIN

(Garamycin and others)
Antibiotic, aminoglycoside
Injection: 10, 40 mg/ml
Ophthalmic ointment: 0.3% (3.5 g)
Ophthalmic drops: 0.3% (5 ml)
Topical ointment: 0.1%
Intrathecal injection: 2 mg/ml

Parenteral (IM or IV):

Post-conceptional Age (wk)	Postnatal Age (days)	Dose (mg/kg/dose)	Interval (hr)
≤29*	0–28	2.5	24
	>28	3	24
30 to 36	0–14	3	24
	>14	2.5	12
≥37	0–7	2.5	12
	>7	2.5	8

*Or significant asphyxia

Children: 6–7.5 mg/kg/24 hr ÷ Q8 hr
Adults: 3–5 mg/kg/24 hr ÷ Q8 hr
Cystic Fibrosis: 7.5–10.5 mg/kg/24 hr ÷ Q8 hr

Monitor peak and trough levels. May cause nephrotoxicity and ototoxicity. Ototoxicity may be potentiated with the use of loop diuretics. Eliminated more quickly in patients with cystic fibrosis, neutropenia, and burns. Adjust dose in renal failure (see Chapter 29).
Therapeutic peak levels:
6–10 mg/L general
8–10 mg/L in pulmonary infections, neutropenia, and severe sepsis
Therapeutic trough levels: <2 mg/L

(Continued.)

Drug/How Supplied	Dose and Route	Remarks
GENTAMICIN—(cont.)	*Intrathecal/intraventricular:* *>3 mo:* 1–2 mg QD *Adult:* 4–8 mg QD *Ophthalmic ointment:* apply Q6–8 hr *Ophthalmic drops:* 1–2 drops Q4 hr	
GLUCAGON HCl (Glucagon) *Antihypoglycemic agent* Injection: 1, 10 mg/vial (1 unit = 1 mg)	*Hypoglycemia, IM, IV, SC:* *Neonates/Infants:* 0.025–0.3 mg/kg/dose Q30 min PRN; **max dose:** 1 mg/dose *Children:* 0.03–0.1 mg/kg/dose Q20 min PRN; **max dose:** 1 mg/dose *Adults:* 0.5–1 mg/dose Q20 min PRN	High doses have cardiac stimulatory effect and have had some success in beta-blocker overdose. Do not delay glucose infusion, dose for hypoglycemia is 2–4 ml/kg of Dextrose 25%.
GLYCOPYRROLATE (Robinul) *Anticholinergic agent* Tabs: 1, 2 mg Injection: 0.2 mg/ml	*Respiratory antisecretory:* *IM/IV:* *Children:* 0.004–0.01 mg/kg/dose Q4–8 hr *Adults:* 0.1–0.2 mg/kg/dose Q4–8 hr **Max dose:** 0.2 mg/dose or 0.8 mg/24 hr *Oral:* *Children:* 0.04–0.1 mg/kg/dose Q4–8 hr *Adults:* 1–2 mg/dose BID-TID	Atropine-like side effects: tachycardia, nausea, constipation, confusion, bronchospasm, blurred vision, and dry mouth. These may be potentiated if given with other drugs with anticholinergic properties. Use with **caution** in hepatic and renal disease, ulcerative colitis, asthma, glaucoma, ileus, or urinary retention.

Reverse neuromuscular blockade: 0.2 mg for every 1 mg neostigmine or 5 mg pyridostigmine

GRISEOFULVIN MICROCRYSTALLINE
(Grifulvin V, Grisactin, Fulvicin)
Antifungal agent
Microsize:
Tabs: 250, 500 mg
Caps: 125, 250 mg
Suspension: 125 mg/5 ml (120 ml)
Ultramicrosize tabs: 125, 165, 250, 330 mg
250 mg ultra is approx 500 mg micro

Microsize:
Children >2 yr: 10–15 mg/kg/24 hr PO QD; give with milk, eggs, fatty foods
Adult: 500–1000 mg/24 hr QD PO
Max dose: 1 g/24 hr
Ultramicrosize:
Children >2 yr: 7 mg/kg/24 hr PO QD
Adults: 330–750 mg/24 hr PO ÷ QD-BID

Monitor hematologic, renal, and hepatic function. May cause leukopenia. Possible cross-reactivity in penicillin-allergic patients. **Contraindicated** in porphyria, hepatic disease. Usual treatment period is 4–6 wk (for tinea unguium, 4–6 mo). Photosensitivity reactions may occur. May reduce effectiveness or decrease level of oral contraceptives, warfarin, and cyclosporin. Phenobarbital may enhance clearance of griseofulvin.

HALOPERIDOL
(Haldol and others)
Antipsychotic agent
Injection (IM use only):
Lactate: 5 mg/ml
Decanoate: 50, 100 mg/ml
Tabs: 0.5, 1, 2, 5, 10, 20 mg
Solution: 2 mg/ml

Children 3–12 yr:
Agitation: 0.01–0.03 mg/kg/24 hr QD PO
IM use (as lactate) 6–12 yr: 1–3 mg/dose Q4–8 hr; **max dose:** 0.15 mg/kg/24 hr
Psychosis: 0.05–0.15 mg/kg/24 hr ÷ BID-TID PO
Tourette's syndrome: 0.05–0.075 mg/kg/24 hr ÷ BID-TID PO; may increase dose by 0.5 mg/24 hr

Use with **caution** in patients with cardiac disease because of the risk of hypotension and in patients with epilepsy since the drug lowers the seizure threshold. Acutely aggravated patients may require doses as often as Q60 min. Extrapyramidal symptoms can occur. Decanoate salt is given every 3–4 wk in doses that are 10–15 times the individual patient's stabilized oral dose.

(Continued.)

Drug/How Supplied	Dose and Route	Remarks
HALOPERIDOL—(cont.)	*>12 yr:* *Acute agitation:* 2–5 mg/dose IM as lactate or 1–15 mg/dose PO; repeat in 1 hr PRN *Psychosis:* 2–5 mg/dose Q4–8 hr IM PRN or 1–15 mg/24 hr ÷ BID-TID PO *Tourette's:* 0.5–2 mg/dose BID-TID PO	
HEPARIN SODIUM (Various trade names) *Anticoagulant* Injection: 10, 100, 1000, 2500, 5000, 7500, 10,000, 20,000, 40,000 U/ml 120 U = approx 1 mg	*Anticoagulation:* *Infants and Children:* *Initial:* 50 U/kg IV bolus *Maintenance:* 10–25 U/kg/hr as IV infusion or 50–100 U/kg/dose Q4 hr IV *Adults:* *Initial:* 50–100 U/kg IV bolus *Maintenance:* 15–25 U/kg/hr as IV infusion or 75–125 U/kg/dose Q4 hr IV *DVT prophylaxis:* 5000 U/dose SC Q8–12 hr until ambulatory *Heparin flush:* *Peripheral IV:* 1–2 ml of 10 U/ml solution Q4 hr *Central lines:* 2–3 ml of 100 U/ml solution Q24 hr	Adjust dose to give PTT 1.5–2.5 times control value. PTT is best measured 6–8 hr after initiation or changes in infusion rate. For intermittent injection, PTT is measured 3.5–4 hrs after injection. Toxicities: bleeding, allergy, alopecia, thrombocytopenia. Use preservative-free heparin in neonates. **Note:** heparin flush doses may alter PTT in small patients; consider using more dilute heparin in these cases. **Antidote:** Protamine sulfate (1 mg per 100 U heparin in previous 4 hr).

TPN (central line) and arterial line: add heparin to make final concentration of 0.5–1 U/ml;

Flush dose should be less than heparinizing dose!

HYALURONIDASE
(Wydase)
Antidote, extravasation
Injection: 150 U/ml
Powder for injection: 150, 1500 U

Infants and Children: Dilute to 15 U/ml; give 1 ml (15U) by injecting 5 separate injections of 0.2 ml (3U) at borders of extravasation site SC or ID using a 25- or 26-gauge needle

Contraindicated in dopamine and alpha-agonist extravasation. May cause urticaria. Administer as early as possible (minutes to 1 hour) after IV extravasation.

HYDRALAZINE HYDROCHLORIDE
(Apresoline)
Antihypertensive, vasodilator
Tabs: 10, 25, 50, 100 mg
Injection: 20 mg/ml
Oral liquid*: 2 mg/ml

Hypertensive crisis:
Children: 0.1–0.2 mg/kg/dose IM or IV Q4–6 hr PRN (not to exceed 20 mg/dose)
Adults: 10–40 mg IM or IV Q3–6 hr PRN
Chronic hypertension:
Children: 0.75–3 mg/kg/24 hr ÷ Q6–12 hr PO; **max dose:** 200 mg/24 hr or 7.5 mg/kg/24 hr
Adults: 10–50 mg/dose PO QID; **max dose:** 300 mg/24 hr

Use with **caution** in severe renal and cardiac disease. Slow acetylators, patients receiving high dose chronic therapy and those with renal insufficiency are at highest risk of lupus-like syndrome (generally reversible). May cause reflex tachycardia. Maximum effect is seen in 3–4 days.

*Indicates suspensions not commercially available; need to be extemporaneously compounded by a pharmacist. See references 1 and 2 for specific formulations.

(Continued.)

Drug/How Supplied	Dose and Route	Remarks
HYDROCHLOROTHIAZIDE (Esidrix, Hydro-T, Thiuretic, Hydrodiuril, and others) *Diuretic, thiazide* Tabs: 25, 50, 100 mg Solution: 10, 100 mg/ml	*Infants and Children:* 2–3 mg/kg/24 hr ÷ BID PO *Adults:* 25–100 mg/24 hr ÷ QD-BID PO; **Max dose:** 200 mg/24 hr	See chlorothiazide. May cause fluid and electrolyte imbalances, hyperuricemia.
HYDROCORTISONE (Solu-cortef, Hydrocortone, Cortef, and others) *Corticosteroid* Cortef Tabs: 5, 10, 20 mg Suspension: 10 mg/5 ml (120 ml) *Na Phosphate* Injection: 50 mg/ml *Na Succinate (Solu-Cortef)* Injection: 100, 250, 500, 1000 mg/vial *Acetate (Hydrocortone)* Injection: 25, 50 mg/ml	*Status asthmaticus:* *Children:* Load (optional): 4–8 mg/kg/dose IV, **max dose:** 250 mg Maintenance: 8 mg/kg/24 hr ÷ Q6 hr IV *Adults:* 100–500 mg/dose Q6 hr IV *Physiologic Replacement:* PO: 0.5–0.75 mg/kg/24 hr ÷ Q8 hr IM: 0.25–0.35/kg/dose QD *Anti-inflammatory/immunosuppressive:* PO: 2.5–10 mg/kg/24 hr ÷ Q6–8 hr IM/IV: 1–5 mg/kg/24 hr ÷ Q6 hr	For doses based on body surface area and topical preparations, see Chapter 28. Na succinate used for IV, IM dosing. Na phosphate may be give IM, SC, or IV. Acetate form recommended for intraarticular, intralesional, soft tissue use, but **not** for IV use.

HYDROMORPHONE HCl

(Dilaudid and others)

Narcotic, analgesic

Injection: 1, 2, 3, 4, 10 mg/ml (contains benzyl alcohol)

Suppository: 3 mg

Oral liquid: 1 mg/ml

Analgesia, titrate to effect:

Children:

IV: 0.015 mg/kg/dose Q4–6 hr PRN

PO: 0.03–0.08 mg/kg/dose Q4–6 hr PRN

Adolescents and Adults:

IM, IV, PO, SC: 1–4 mg/dose Q4–6 hr PRN

Refer to Chapter 27 for equianalgesic doses and patient-controlled analgesia dosing. Less pruritus than morphine. Similar profile of side effects to other narcotics.

HYDROXYZINE

(Atarax, Vistaril)

Antihistamine, anxiolytic

Tabs (HCl): 10, 25, 50, 100 mg

Caps (pamoate): 25, 50, 100 mg

Syrup (HCl): 10 mg/5 ml

Suspension (pamoate): 25 mg/5 ml (120 ml)

Injection (HCl): 25, 50 mg/ml

Oral:

Children: 2 mg/kg/24 hr ÷ Q6 hr

Adult: 25–100 mg/dose TID-QID

IM:

Children: 0.5–1 mg/kg/dose Q4–6 hr PRN

Adult: 25–100 mg/dose Q4–6 hr PRN;

Max dose: 600 mg/24 hr

May potentiate barbiturates, meperidine, and other depressants. May cause dry mouth, drowsiness, tremor, convulsions, blurred vision, hypotension. May cause pain at injection site. IV administration is **not** recommended.

IBUPROFEN

(Motrin, Advil, Nuprin, Medipren, Children's Advil, Children's Motrin, and others)

Nonsteroidal anti-inflammatory agent

Suspension (Rx): 100 mg/5 ml (120, 480 ml)

Suspension (OTC): 100 mg/5 ml (60, 120 ml)

Oral Drops (OTC): 40 mg/ml (15 ml)

Chew Tabs (Rx): 50, 100 mg

Caplets (OTC): 100 mg

Tabs: 200 (OTC), 300, 400, 600, 800 mg

Children:

Analgesic/Antipyretic: 5–10 mg/kg/dose Q6–8 hr PO;

Max dose: 40 mg/kg/24 hr PO

JRA: 30–50 mg/kg/24 hr ÷ Q6 hr PO;

Max dose: 2400 mg/24 hr

Adults:

Inflammatory disease: 400–800 mg/dose Q6–8 hr PO

Pain/fever/dysmenorrhea: 200–400 mg/dose Q4–6 hr PO

Max dose: 3.2 g/24 hr

GI distress (lessened with milk), rashes, ocular problems, granulocytopenia, anemia may occur. Inhibits platelet aggregation. Use **caution** with aspirin hypersensitivity, or hepatic/renal insufficiency, dehydration. Use higher dose range for T>39.0° in children.

(Continued.)

Drug/How Supplied	Dose and Route	Remarks
IMIPENEM-CILASTATIN (Primaxin) *Antibiotic* Injection: 250, 500, 750 mg. Each gram contains 3.2 mEq Na.	*Children:* 50–100 mg/kg/24 hr ÷ Q6–8 hr IV **Max dose:** 4 g/24 hr *Adults:* 250–1000 mg/dose Q6–8 hr IV **Max dose:** 4 g/24 or 50 mg/kg/24 hr, whichever is less	For IV use, give slowly over 30–60 minutes. Adverse effects: pruritus, urticaria, GI symptoms, seizures, dizziness, hypotension, elevated LFTs, blood dyscrasias, and penicillin allergy. Dosage adjustment needed in renal insufficiency (see Chapter 29).
IMIPRAMINE (Tofranil, Janimine) *Antidepressant, tricyclic* Tabs: 10, 25, 50 mg Caps: 75, 100, 125, 150 mg Injection: 12.5 mg/ml	*Antidepressant:* *Children:* *Initial:* 1.5 mg/kg/24 hr ÷ TID PO; Increase 1–1.5 mg/kg/24 hr Q3–4 days to **max** of 5 mg/kg/24 hr *Adolescent:* *Initial:* 25–50 mg/24 hr ÷ QD-TID PO; advance to **max** of 100 mg/24 hr *Adult:* *Initial:* 75–100 mg/24 hr ÷ TID PO/IM *Maintenance:* 50–300 mg/24 hr QHS PO **Max PO dose:** 300 mg/24 hr **Max initial IM dose:** 100 mg/24 hr *Enuresis (≥6 yrs):* *Initial:* 10–25 mg QHS PO *Increment:* 10–25 mg/dose at 1–2 wk intervals until max dose for age or desired effect achieved. Continue × 2–3 mo, then taper slowly	Side effects include sedation, urinary retention, constipation, dry mouth, dizziness, drowsiness, and arrhythmia. QHS dosing during first weeks of therapy will reduce sedation. Monitor ECG, BP, CBC at start of therapy and with dose changes. Decrease dose if PR interval reaches 0.22 sec, QRS reaches 130% of baseline, HR rises above 140/min, or if BP is more than 140/90. Tricyclics may cause mania. Therapeutic reference range (sum of imipramine and desipramine) = 150–250 ng/ml. Janimine 10 and 25 mg tablets and Tofranil PM 100 and 125 mg capsules contain tartrazine, which may cause allergic reactions. PO route preferred. May be given IM.

Max dose:
6–12 yr: 50 mg/24 hr
12–14 yr: 75 mg/24 hr
Augment analgesia for chronic pain:
Initial: 0.2–0.4 mg/kg/dose QHS PO;
increase 50% every 2–3 days to **max**
of 1–3 mg/kg/dose QHS PO

Contraindicated in narrow-angle
glaucoma and patients who used MAO
inhibitors within 14 days. See Chapter
2 for management of toxic ingestion.

IMMUNE GLOBULIN
(IM: Gammar-IM, Gamastan)
IV: Sandoglobulin, Gammagard.
Gamimune-N, Gammar-IV, Iveegam,
Polygam, Venoglobulin)
Gammar-IM: 165 ± 15 mg/ml
Gamastan: 165 ± 5 mg/ml
IV preparations
Gamimune-N: 5%, 10%
Polygam S/D: 5%, 10%
Gammar-IV: 5%
Sandoglobulin: 6%, 12%
Venoglobulin I: 5%
Venoglobulin S: 5%
Gammagard S/D: 5%, 10%

See indications and doses in Chapter 16.
*General Guidelines for administration (see
package insert of specific products):*
Begin infusion at 0.01 ml/kg/min;
double rate every 15–30 min, up to
max of 0.08 ml/kg/min. If adverse
reactions occur, stop infusion until side
effects subside and may restart at rate
that was previously tolerated.

May cause flushing, chills, fever,
headache, hypotension.
Hypersensitivity reaction may occur
when IV form is administered rapidly.
Gamimune-N contains maltose and
may cause an osmotic diuresis. May
cause anaphylaxis in IgA-deficient
patients due to trace amounts of IgA.
Some products are IgA depleted.
Consult a pharmacist.

(Continued.)

Drug/How Supplied	Dose and Route	Remarks
INDOMETHACIN (Indocin) *Nonsteroidal antiinflammatory agent* Caps: 25, 50 mg Sustained-release caps: 75 mg Injection: 1 mg Suppositories: 50 mg Suspension: 25 mg/5 ml	*Anti-inflammatory:* >14 yr old: 1–3 mg/kg/24 hr ÷ TID-QID PO; **max dose:** 200 mg/24 hr Adults: 50–150 mg/24 hr ÷ BID-QID PO *Closure of ductus arteriosus:* Infuse intravenously over 20–30 minutes:	May cause (especially in neonates) decreased urine output, platelet dysfunction, decreased GI blood flow. Monitor renal and hepatic function before and during use. **Reduction in cerebral flow associated with rapid IV infusion. Contraindicated** in active bleeding, coagulation defects, necrotizing enterocolitis, and renal insufficiency. Fatal hepatitis reported in treatment of JRA.

	Dose (mg/kg/dose Q12–24 hr)		
Age	#1	#2	#3
<48 hr	0.2	0.1	0.1
2–7 days	0.2	0.2	0.2
>7 days	0.2	0.25	0.25

In <1500 g infants, 0.1–0.2 mg/kg/dose IV Q24 hr may be given for an additional 3–5 days

Drug/How Supplied	Dose and Route	Remarks
INSULIN *Pancreatic hormone* Many preparations, at concentrations of 40, 100 U/ml	*Insulin preparations:* See Chapter 28 *Hyperkalemia:* See Chapters 1 and 11 *DKA:* See Chapter 1	When using insulin drip, flush tubing with insulin infusion solution before beginning infusion. This will ensure proper drug delivery.

IPECAC
Emetic agent
Syrup: 70 mg/ml (15, 30, 473, 4000 ml)
(contains 1.5–2% alcohol)

See Chapter 2 for indications.
6–12 *mos:* 5–10 ml Ipecac followed by 10–20 ml/kg water
1–12 *yr:* 15 ml Ipecac followed by 10–20 ml/kg water
Adults: 30 ml followed by 200–300 ml of water

May cause GI irritation, cardiotoxicity, myopathy. Refer to Chapter 2 for indications. Do **not** use ipecac fluid extract as it is 14 times more potent. May repeat dose once if emesis does not occur within 20–30 minutes.

IPRATROPIUM BROMIDE
(Atrovent)
Anticholinergic agent
Aerosol: 18 mcg/dose (200 actuations per canister)
Nebulized Solution: 500 mcg/2.5 ml

Inhaler:
<12 *yr:* 1–2 puffs TID-QID
≥12 *yr:* 2–4 puffs QID up to 12 puffs/24 hr
Nebulized treatments:
<2 *yr:* 250 mcg/dose TID-QID
≥2 *yr:* 250–500 mcg/dose TID-QID

Some studies indicate that frequent dosing of ipratropium may have a role as an adjunct to beta-agonists in the treatment of acute bronchospasm (*J Pediatr* 126:639–645, 1995). If medication is administered frequently, consider cardiac monitoring. Shake inhaler well prior to use. Use with **caution** in narrow-angle glaucoma or bladder neck obstruction, though ipratropium has fewer anticholinergic systemic effects than atropine.

IRON DEXTRAN
(InfeD)
Parenteral iron
Injection: 50 mg/ml (contains 50 mg elemental Fe/ml)

Inject test dose (see comments)
Iron deficiency anemia: Total replacement dose of iron dextran (ml) = 0.0476 × wt(kg) × (desired Hgb [g/dl] – measured Hgb [g/dl]) + 1 ml/5 kg body weight (up to **max** of 14 ml).

Oral therapy with iron salts is preferred. Numerous adverse effects including anaphylaxis, fever, hypotension, rash, myalgias, arthralgias. Use "Z-track" technique for IM administration. Inject test dose: 25 mg (12.5 mg for infants).

(Continued.)

Drug/How Supplied	Dose and Route	Remarks

IRON DEXTRAN—(cont.)	*Acute blood loss:* Total replacement dose of iron dextran (ml) = 0.02 × blood loss (ml) × hematocrit expressed as fraction. Assumes 1 ml of RBC = 1 mg iron.
	
	If no reaction to test dose, give remainder of replacement dose ÷ over 2–3 daily doses.
	Max daily (IM) dose:
	  <5 kg: 0.5 ml (25 mg)
	  5–10 kg: 1 ml (50 mg)
	  >10 kg: 2 ml (100 mg)
		If well tolerated after 1 hour, begin therapy with maximum rate of IV infusion at 50 mg/min. For IV infusion, diluting in NS may lower the incidence of phlebitis.

IRON PREPARATIONS
(Fergon, Fer-In-Sol, Ferralet, Feosol, and others)
Oral iron supplements
Ferrous sulfate (20% elemental Fe):
Drops (Fer-In-Sol): 75 mg (15 mg Fe)/0.6 ml (50 ml)
Syrup (Fer-In-Sol): 90 mg (18 mg Fe)/5 ml
Elixir (Feosol): 220 mg (44 mg Fe)/5 ml (5% alcohol)
Capsules: 250 mg (50 mg Fe)
Tabs: 195 mg (39 mg Fe), 300 mg (60 mg Fe), 324 mg (65 mg Fe)
	Iron deficiency anemia:
	  Children: 3–6 mg elemental Fe/kg/24 hr ÷ QD-TID PO
	  Adult: 60 mg elemental iron BID-QID
	Prophylaxis:
	  Children: Give dose below PO ÷ QD-TID
	  Premature: 2 mg elemental Fe/kg/24 hr
	  Full-term: 1–2 mg elemental Fe/kg/24 hr
	  Max dose: 15 mg elemental Fe/24 hr
	  Adults: 60 mg elemental Fe/24 hr PO ÷ QD-BID
		Iron preparations are variably absorbed. Less GI irritation when given with or after meals. Vitamin C, 200 mg per 30 mg iron, may enhance absorption. Liquid iron preparations may stain teeth. Give with dropper or drink through straw. May produce constipation, dark stools, nausea, and epigastric pain. Iron and tetracycline inhibit each other's absorption. Antacids may decrease iron absorption.

Ferrous gluconate (12% elemental Fe):
Elixir: 300 mg (34 mg Fe)/5 ml (7% alcohol)
Tabs: 300 mg (34 mg Fe), 320 mg (37 mg Fe), 325 mg (38 mg Fe)
Sustained-release caps: 320 mg (37 mg Fe), 435 mg (50 mg Fe)
Caps: 86 mg (10 mg Fe), 325 mg (38 mg Fe), 435 mg (50 mg Fe)

ISONIAZID
(INH, Nydrazid, Laniazid)
Antituberculous agent
Tabs: 50, 100, 300 mg
Syrup: 50 mg/5 ml (473 ml)
Injection: 100 mg/ml

See Chapter 18 for details and length of therapy.
Prophylaxis:
Infants and Children: 10–15 mg/kg (up to 300 mg) per dose PO QD, or 20–40 mg/kg (up to 900 mg) per dose PO, given twice weekly (after 1 mo of daily therapy)
Adults: 300 mg PO QD
Treatment:
Infants and Children:
10–20 mg/kg (up to 300 mg) per dose PO QD or 20–40 mg/kg (up to 900 mg) per dose twice weekly with Rifampin
Adults:
5–10 mg/kg (up to 300 mg) per dose PO QD or 15 mg/kg (up to 900 mg) per dose twice weekly with Rifampin
For INH-resistant TB: Discuss with Health Dept., or consult ID specialist

Should **not** be used alone for treatment. Peripheral neuropathy, optic neuritis, seizures, encephalopathy, psychosis, hepatic side effects may occur with higher doses, especially in combination with Rifampin. Follow LFTs monthly. Supplemental pyridoxine (1–2 mg/kg/24 hr) is recommended. May cause false positive urine glucose test. Inhibits hepatic microsomal enzymes; decrease dose of carbamazepine, diazepam, phenytoin, and prednisone. May be given IM when oral therapy is not possible.

(Continued.)

Drug/How Supplied	Dose and Route	Remarks
ISOPROTERENOL (Isuprel) *Adrenergic agonist* *Isoproterenol HCl:* Tabs: 10, 15 mg (sublingual) Solutions for nebulization: 0.25% (2.5 mg/ml) (0.5 ml, 15 ml) 0.5% (5 mg/ml) (0.5, 10, 60 ml) 1% (10 mg/ml) (10 ml) Aerosol: 80, 131 mcg/dose; about 300 metered doses per container (15 ml) Injection: 0.2 mg/ml (1, 5 ml ampules)	*Aerosol:* 1–2 puffs up to 5×/24 hr *Nebulized solution:* *Children:* 0.05 mg/kg/dose = 0.01 ml/kg/dose of 0.5% Sol (min dose: 0.5 mg; **max dose:** 1.25 mg) diluted with NS to 2 ml Q4 hr PRN *Adults:* 2.5–5 mg/dose = 0.25–0.5 ml of 1% solution diluted with NS to 2 ml Q4 hr PRN *IV Infusion:* *Children:* 0.1–2 mcg/kg/min; start at minimum dose and increase every 5–10 min by 0.1 mcg/kg/min until desired effect or onset of toxicity; **max dose:** 2 mcg/kg/min *Adults:* 2–5 mcg/kg/min See inside front cover for preparation of infusion	Use with care in CHF, ischemia, or aortic stenosis. May cause flushing, ventricular arrhythmias, profound hypotension, anxiety, and myocardial ischemia. Patients with continuous IV infusion should have heart rate, respiratory rate, and blood pressure monitored. **Not** for treatment of asystole or for use in cardiac arrests, unless bradycardia is due to heartblock. Continuous infusion use for bronchodilatation must be gradually tapered over a 24–48 hr period.

ISOTRETINOIN
(Accutane)
Retinoic acid, vitamin A derivative
Caps: 10, 20, 40 mg

Cystic acne: 0.5–2 mg/kg/24 hr ÷ Q12 hr
PO × 15–20 wk
Dosages as low as 0.05 mg/kg/24 hr
have been reported to be beneficial

Caution in females during childbearing years. **Contraindicated** during pregnancy; known teratogen. May cause conjunctivitis, xerosis, pruritus, epistaxis, anemia, hyperlipidemia, pseudotumor cerebri, cheilitis, bone pain, muscle aches, skeletal changes, lethargy, nausea, vomiting, elevated ESR. To avoid additive toxic effects, do not take vitamin A concomitantly. Monitor CBC, ESR, triglycerides, and LFTs.

KANAMYCIN
(Kantrex)
Antibiotic, aminoglycoside
Caps: 500 mg
Injection: 37.5, 250, 333 mg/ml

Neonatal IV/IM administration:

	<7 days	≥7 days
BW <2 kg	15 mg/kg/ 24 hr ÷ Q12 hr	22.5 mg/kg/ 24 hr ÷ Q8 hr
BW ≥2 kg	20 mg/kg/ 24 hr ÷ Q12 hr	30 mg/kg/ 24 hr ÷ Q8 hr

Infants and Children: IM/IV: 15–30 mg/kg/24 hr ÷ Q8–12 hr
Adults: IV/IM: 15 mg/kg/24 hr ÷ Q8–12 hr
PO Administration: 150–250 mg/kg/24 hr ÷ Q6 hr; **max dose:** 4 g/24 hr

Renal toxicity and ototoxicity may occur. Give over 30 min if IV. Reduce dosage frequency with renal impairment. Poorly absorbed orally, PO used to treat GI bacterial overgrowth. **Therapeutic levels:** peak: 15–30 mg/L; trough: <5–10 mg/L.

(Continued.)

Drug/How Supplied	Dose and Route	Remarks
KETAMINE (Ketalar) *General anesthetic* Injection: 10, 50, 100 mg/ml	*Children:* *IV; sedation for procedures:* 0.25–1 mg/kg *IM:* 2–5 mg/kg *Adults:* *IV:* 1–4.5 mg/kg *IM:* 3–8 mg/kg	May cause hypertension, hypotension, and emergence reactions, tachycardia, laryngospasm, respiratory depression, and stimulation of salivary secretions. **Contraindicated** in elevated ICP, hypertension, aneurysms, thyrotoxicosis, CHF, angina, and psychotic disorders. Rate of infusion should **not** exceed 0.5 mg/kg/min or be administered in less than 60 seconds.
KETOCONAZOLE (Nizoral) *Antifungal agent* Tabs: 200 mg Suspension*: 100 mg/5 ml (120 ml) Cream: 2% (15, 30, 60 g) Shampoo: 2%	*Children ≥2 yr:* 5–10 mg/kg/24 hr ÷ QD-BID PO *Adult:* 200–400 mg/24 hr QD PO **Max dose:** 800 mg/24 hr *Topical:* 1–2 applications/24 hr *Shampoo:* Twice weekly for 4 weeks with at least 3 days between applications; intermittently as needed to maintain control	Monitor liver function tests in long-term use. Drugs that decrease gastric acidity will decrease absorption. May cause nausea, vomiting, rash, headache, pruritus, and fever. Cardiac arrhythmias may occur when used with cisapride, terfenadine, astemizole. **Concomitant administration of ketoconazole with any of these drugs is contraindicated.**

KETOROLAC

(Toradol, Accular (ophth))
Nonsteroidal anti-inflammatory agent

Injection: 15, 30 mg/ml
Tab: 10 mg
Ophthalmic: 0.5% (5 ml)

Children:

0.5 mg/kg/dose IM/IV Q6 hr. **Max dose:** 30 mg Q6 hr or 120 mg/24 hr
Adults: 30 mg IM/IV Q6 hr. **Max dose:** 30 mg Q6 hr or 120 mg/24 hr
PO: (Children >50 kg and adults): 10 mg PRN Q6 hr; **max dose:** 40 mg/24 hr

Ketorolac therapy is not to exceed 5 days. May cause GI bleeding, nausea, dyspepsia, drowsiness, decreased platelet function, and interstitial nephritis. Not recommended in patients at increased risk of bleeding. Do not use in hepatic or renal failure. The IV route of administration in children is not yet recommended by the manufacturer although it is well supported in the literature and in practice.

LABETALOL

(Normodyne, Trandate)
Adrenergic antagonist (alpha and beta), antihypertensive

Tabs: 100, 200, 300 mg
Injection: 5 mg/ml
Suspension*: 10 mg/ml

Children:

PO: Initial: 4 mg/kg/24 hr ÷ BID. May increase up to 40 mg/kg/24 hr
IV: Hypertensive emergency:
Intermittent dose: 0.3–1 mg/kg/dose Q10 min PRN; **max:** 20 mg/dose
Infusion: 0.4–1 mg/kg/hr, to **max** of 3 mg/kg/hr; may initiate with a 0.2–1 mg/kg bolus; **max bolus:** 20 mg

Adults:

PO: 100 mg BID, increase Q2–3 days PRN to **max** of 2.4 g/24 hr

May cause orthostatic hypotension, edema, CHF, bradycardia, AV conduction disturbances, bronchospasm, urinary retention, and skin tingling. **Contraindicated** in asthma, pulmonary edema, cardiogenic shock, and heart block. **Patient should remain supine during IV administration.**

(Continued.)

*Indicates suspensions not commercially available; need to be extemporaneously compounded by a pharmacist. See references 1 and 2 for specific formulations.

Drug/How Supplied	Dose and Route	Remarks
LABETALOL—(cont.)	*IV: Hypertensive emergency:* *Intermittent dose:* 20–80 mg/dose (begin with 20 mg) Q10 min PRN; **max:** 300 mg total dose *Infusion:* 2 mg/min, increase to titrate to response	
LACTULOSE (Cephulac, and others) *Ammonium detoxicant, laxative* Syrup: 10 g/15 ml	*Chronic constipation:* *Children:* 7.5 ml/24 hr PO after breakfast *Adults:* 15–30 ml/24 hr PO to **max** of 60 ml/24 hr *Portal systemic encephalopathy:* *Infants:* 2.5–10 ml/24 hr PO ÷ TID-QID *Children:* 40–90 ml/24 hr PO ÷ TID-QID *Adults:* 30–45 ml/dose PO TID-QID; acute episodes 30–45 ml Q1–2 hr until 2–3 soft stools/day *Rectal (adults):* 300 ml diluted in 700 ml water or NS in 30–60 min retention enema; may give Q4–6 hr	Use with **caution** in diabetes mellitus. GI discomfort and diarrhea may occur. Adjust dose to achieve 2–3 soft stools per day. **Contraindicated** in galactosemia. Do **not** use with antacids.

LAMOTRIGINE
(Lamictal)
Anticonvulsant
Tabs: 25, 100, 150, 200 mg

Children: Start with low dose and increase gradually
Without valproic acid: 2–15 mg/kg/24 hr ÷ BID PO
With valproic acid: 0.5–5 mg/kg/24 hr ÷ BID PO
>16 yr and Adults:
Without valproic acid: 50 mg QD PO × 2 weeks, then increase to 50 mg BID × 2 weeks; may increase to 300–500 mg/24 hr to maintain therapeutic levels
With valproic acid: 25 mg QOD PO × 2 weeks, then increase to 25 mg QD × 2 weeks; may increase to 75 mg BID; **max dose:** 200 mg/24 hr

Used in conjunction with other anticonvulsants. May cause fatigue, drowsiness, ataxia, rash, headache, nausea, vomiting, and abdominal pain. Diplopia, nystagmus, alopecia have also been reported. Reduce dose in renal failure. **Monitor levels carefully.** **Therapeutic monitoring:** plasma trough 1–5 mg/L. Withdrawal symptoms may occur if discontinued suddenly.

LEVOCARNITINE
(Carnitor, VitaCarn)
L-carnitine
Tabs: 330 mg
Caps: 250 mg
Solution: 100 mg/ml (10 ml)
Injection: 1 g/5 ml

Children: 50–100 mg/kg/24 hr PO ÷ Q8–12 hr; increase slowly to **max dose** of 3 g/24 hr
Adults: 330 mg to 1 g/dose BID-TID PO
IV; children and adults: 50 mg/kg/24 hr IV infusion; maintenance: 50 mg/kg/24 hr ÷ Q4–6 hr; increase to **maximum** of 300 mg/kg/24 hr if needed.

May cause nausea, vomiting, abdominal cramps, diarrhea, body odor. Give bolus IV infusion over 2–3 minutes.

(Continued.)

Drug/How Supplied	Dose and Route	Remarks
LEVOTHYROXINE (T₄) (Synthroid, Levothroid) *Thyroid product* Tabs: 12.5, 25, 50, 75, 88, 100, 112, 125, 137, 150, 175, 200, 300 mcg Injection: 200, 500 mcg	*Children PO dosing:* 0–6 mo: 8–10 mcg/kg/24 hr QD 6–12 mo: 6–8 mcg/kg/24 hr QD 1–5 yr: 5–6 mcg/kg/24 hr QD 6–12 yr: 4–5 mcg/kg/24 hr QD >12 yr: 2–3 mcg/kg/24 hr QD IM/IV dose: 50%–75% of oral dose QD *Adults:* PO: *Initial:* 12.5–50 mcg/24 hr QD *Increment:* Increase by 25–50 mcg/24 hr at intervals of Q2–4 wk *Average adult dose:* 100–200 mcg/24 hr IM/IV dose: 50% of oral dose QD *Myxedema coma or stupor:* 200–500 mcg × 1, then 100–300 mcg the next day if needed IV	Total replacement dose may be used in children unless there is evidence of cardiac disease; in that case, begin with 1/4 of maintenance and increase weekly. Titrate dosage with clinical status and serum T₄ and TSH. May cause hyperthyroidism, rash, growth disturbances. 100 mcg levothyroxine = 65 mg thyroid USP. **Contraindications** include acute MI, thyrotoxicosis uncomplicated by hypothyroidism, and uncorrected adrenal insufficiency. Interacts with warfarin.
LIDOCAINE (Xylocaine and others) *Antiarrhythmic class Ib, local anesthetic* Injection: 0.5%, 1%, 1.5%, 2%, 2.5%, 4%, 10%, 20% (1% sol = 10 mg/ml) Injection with 1:100,000 epi: 1%, 2% Injection with 1:200,000 epi: 0.5%, 1%, 1.5%, 2%, 4%	*Anesthetic:* Injection: *Without epi:* **max** dose of 4.5 mg/kg/dose (up to 300 mg) *With epi:* **max** dose of 7 mg/kg/dose (up to 500 mg); do **not** repeat within 2 hours	Side effects include hypotension, asystole, seizures, and respiratory arrest. Decrease dose in hepatic failure or decreased cardiac output. **Contraindicated** in Stokes-Adams attacks, SA, AV, or intraventricular heart block without a pacemaker. Do **not** use topically for teething.

Ointment: 2.5% (37.5 g), 5% (50 g)
Cream: 0.5% (120 g)
Jelly: 2% (30 ml)
Liquid (viscous): 2% (20, 100 ml)
Solution (topical): 2% (15, 240 ml), 4% (50 ml)
Oral Spray: 10% (26.8 ml aerosol)
Topical 2.5% (with 2.5% prilocaine): See EMLA and Chapter 29

Topical: 3 mg/kg/dose no more frequently than Q2 hr
Antiarrhythmic: Bolus with 1 mg/kg/dose slowly IO, IV; may repeat in 10–15 minutes × 2; **max** total dose 3–5 mg/kg within the first hour
ETT dose = 2–2.5× IV dose
Continuous Infusion: 20–50 mcg/kg/min IV; see inside cover for infusion preparation

Prolonged infusion may result in toxic accumulation of lidocaine. Do **not** use epinephrine-containing solutions for treatment of arrhythmias. **Therapeutic levels** 1.5–5 mg/L. Toxicity occurs at >7 mg/L. Toxicity in neonates may occur at >5 mg/L.

LINDANE
(Gamma benzene hexachloride)
(Kwell, Scabene)
Scabicidal agent
Shampoo: 1% (30, 60, 473, 3800 ml)
Lotion: 1% (30, 60, 473, 3800 ml)
Cream: 1% (60 g)

Scabies: Apply thin layer of cream or lotion to skin. Bathe and rinse off medication in adults after 8–12 hr; children 6–8 hr. May repeat × 1 in 7 days PRN.
Pediculosis capitis: Apply 15–30 ml of shampoo, lather for 4–5 minutes, rinse hair and comb with fine comb to remove nits. May repeat × 1 in 7 days PRN.
Pediculosis pubis: May use lotion or shampoo (applied locally) as above.

Systemically absorbed. Risk of toxic effects is greater in young children; use other agents (permethrin) in infants, young children, and during pregnancy. Avoid contact with face, urethral meatus, or mucous membranes. May cause a rash; rarely may cause seizures or aplastic anemia. For scabies, change clothing and bedsheets after starting treatment and treat family members. For pediculosis pubis, treat sexual contacts.

(Continued.)

Drug/How Supplied	Dose and Route	Remarks
LITHIUM (Eskalith, Lithane, Lithonate, Lithotabs, Lithobid, Cibalith-S) *Antimanic agent* *Carbonate:* 300 mg carbonate = 8.12 mEq lithium Caps: 150, 300, 600 mg Tabs: 300 mg Controlled-release tabs: 450 mg Slow-release tabs: 300 mg *Citrate:* Syrup: 8 mEq/5 ml (10, 480 ml); 5 ml is equivalent to 300 mg Li carbonate Cibalith-S is citrate; all other brands are carbonate.	*Children:* *Initial:* 15–60 mg/kg/24 hr ÷ TID-QID PO. Adjust as needed to achieve therapeutic levels. *Adults:* *Initial:* 300 mg TID PO. Adjust as needed to achieve therapeutic levels. Usual dose is about 300 mg TID-QID. **Max dose: 2.4 g/24 hr**	Increased sodium intake will depress lithium levels. Decreased sodium intake or increased sodium wasting will increase lithium levels. **Therapeutic levels: 0.6–1.5 mEq/L.** May cause goiter, nephrogenic diabetes insipidus, or sedation at therapeutic doses. In either acute or chronic toxicity, confusion and somnolence may be seen at levels of 2–2.5 mEq/L. Seizures or death may occur at levels >2.5 mEq/L.
LOPERAMIDE (Imodium, Imodium AD, and others) *Antidiarrheal* Caps: 2 mg Tabs: 2 mg Liquid: 1 mg/5 ml (60, 90, 120 ml)	*Active diarrhea:* *Children:* *2–6 yr (13–20 kg):* 1 mg PO TID *6–8 yr (20–30 kg):* 2 mg PO BID *8–12 yr (>30 kg):* 2 mg PO TID **Max single dose 2 mg** *Adults:* 4 mg/dose × 1, followed by 2 mg/dose after each stool up to **max dose** of 16 mg/24 hr *Chronic diarrhea:* *Children:* 0.08–0.24 mg/kg/24 hr ÷ BID-TID **Max dose: 2 mg/dose**	May cause nausea, vomiting, constipation, cramps, dry mouth, CNS depression. Avoid use in children <2 yr. Discontinue use if no clinical improvement is observed within 48 hr. Naloxone may be administered for CNS depression.

LORACARBEF
(Lorabid)
Antibiotic, cephalosporin (2nd generation)
Susp: 100 mg/5 ml, 200 mg/5 ml (50, 100 ml)
Caps: 200, 400 mg

Infants and Children: (6 mo–12 yr)
Acute Otitis Media: 30 mg/kg/24 hr ÷ Q12 hr PO
Pharyngitis, Skin/soft tissue infection:
15 mg/kg/24 hr ÷ Q12 hr PO
≥ 13 yr and adults:
Uncomplicated cystitis: 200 mg PO Q24 hr
Sinusitis/uncomplicated pyelonephritis:
400 mg PO Q12 hr
Pharyngitis, Skin/soft tissue infection:
200 mg PO Q12 hr
Lower respiratory infections: 200–400 mg PO Q12 hr

Use with **caution** in penicillin-allergic patients. Adjust dose in renal impairment. Use suspension for acute otitis media due to higher peak plasma levels. Adverse effects similar to other orally administered beta-lactam antibiotics. Administer on an empty stomach 1 hour before or 2 hours after meals.

LORATADINE
(Claritin)
Antihistamine, less sedating
Tabs: 10 mg
Syrup: 10 mg/10 ml

≥6 yr: 10 mg PO QD
Reduce dose to 10 mg PO QOD in hepatic failure.

May cause fatigue, dry mouth, and dizziness. At time of publication, has not been implicated in causing cardiac arrhythmias when used with other drugs that are metabolized by hepatic microsomal enzymes (e.g., ketoconazole, erythromycin)

(Continued.)

Drug/How Supplied	Dose and Route	Remarks
LORAZEPAM (Ativan) *Benzodiazepine anticonvulsant* Tabs: 0.5, 1, 2, mg Injection: 2, 4 mg/ml (each contains 2% benzyl alcohol) Oral Sol conc: 2 mg/ml	*Status Epilepticus:* *Neonates, Infants, Children, and Adolescents:* 0.05–0.1 mg/kg/dose IV over 2–5 min. May repeat 0.05 mg/kg × 1 in 10–15 min. *Adult:* 4 mg/dose given slowly over 2–5 minutes. May repeat in 5–15 minutes. Usual total **max** dose in 12 hour period = 8 mg. *Antiemetic adjunct therapy:* *Children:* 0.04–0.08 mg/kg/dose IV Q6 hr PRN. **Max** single dose: 4 mg *Anxiolytic/Sedation:* *Children:* 0.05 mg/kg/dose Q4–8 hr PO/IV. May also give IM for preprocedure sedation *Adults:* 1–10 mg/24 hr PO ÷ BID-TID	May cause respiratory depression, especially in combination with other sedatives. May also cause sedation, dizziness, mild ataxia, mood changes, rash, and GI symptoms. Injectable product may be given rectally. Benzyl alcohol may be toxic to newborns in high doses. Onset of action for sedation: PO, 1 hour; IM, 30–60 minutes; IV, 15–30 minutes.

LYPRESSIN
(8-lysine vasopressin)
(Diapid)
Posterior pituitary hormone
Nasal spray: 185 mcg/ml; each spray
delivers 7 mcg or 2 posterior pituitary
(pressor) units.

Diabetes insipidus:
1–2 sprays into each nostril QID and
HS. If patient requires more than 2–3
sprays per dose, increase frequency
of doses rather than amounts/dose.

Titrate dose to thirst, urinary frequency.
Coronary vasoconstriction may occur
with large doses. May cause nasal
congestion, headache, conjunctivitis,
and abdominal cramps. Allergic rhinitis
or nasal congestion may interfere with
absorption. Carbamazepine or
chlorpropamide may potentiate effect.

MAGNESIUM CITRATE
(16.17% Mg)
(Evac-Q-Mag)
Laxative/cathartic
Sol: (300 ml): 5 ml = 3.9–4.7 mEq Mg

Children:
<6 yr: 2–4 ml/kg/24 hr PO ÷ QD-BID
6–12 yr: 100–150 ml/24 hr PO ÷ QD-BID
>12 yr: 150–300 ml/24 hr PO ÷ QD-BID

Use with **caution** in renal insufficiency.
May cause hypermagnesemia,
hypotension, respiratory depression.
Up to about 30% of dose is absorbed.
May decrease absorption of H_2
antagonists, phenytoin, iron salts,
tetracycline, steroids, and ciprofloxacin.

MAGNESIUM HYDROXIDE
(Milk of magnesia)
(41.69% Mg)
Antacid, laxative
Liquid: 390 mg/5 ml, 400 mg/5 ml (Milk
of Magnesia), 800 mg/5 ml (Milk of
Magnesia concentrate)
Susp: 2.5 g/30 ml
Chewable Tabs: 311 mg

All doses based on 400 mg/5 ml
Magnesium hydroxide
Laxative:
Children:
  Dose/24 hr ÷ QD-QID PO
  <2 yr: 0.5 ml/kg
  2–5 yr: 5–15 ml
  6–12 yr: 15–30 ml
  ≥12 yr: 30–60 ml
Antacid:
  Children: 2.5–5 ml/dose QD-QID PO
  Adults: 5–15 ml/dose QD-QID PO
  Tabs: 622–1244 mg/dose QD-QID PO

See Magnesium citrate.

(Continued.)

Drug/How Supplied	Dose and Route	Remarks
MAGNESIUM OXIDE (60.32% Mg) (Maox) *Oral Magnesium salt* Tabs: 400, 420, 500 mg Caps: 140 mg (241.3 mg Mg/400 mg oxide)	Doses expressed in Mg oxide salt *Magnesium supplementation:* *Children:* 5–10 mg/kg/24 hr ÷ TID-QID PO *Adults:* 400–800 mg/24 hr ÷ BID-QID PO *Hypomagnesemia:* *Children:* 65–130 mg/kg/24 hr ÷ QID PO *Adults:* 2000 mg/24 hr ÷ QID PO	See Mg citrate. For RDA for Magnesium, see Chapter 23.
MAGNESIUM SULFATE (Epsom salts) (9.9% Mg) *Magnesium salt* Inj: 100 mg/ml (0.8 mEq/ml), 125 mg/ml (1 mEq/ml), 250 mg/ml (2 mEq/ml), 500 mg/ml (4 mEq/ml) Oral Sol: 50% Granules: approx 40 mEq Mg per 5 g (240 g)	All doses expressed in MgSO₄ salt *Cathartic:* *Child:* 0.25 g/kg/dose PO Q4–6 hr *Adult:* 10–30 g/dose PO Q4–6 hr *Hypomagnesemia or hypocalcemia:* *IV/IM:* 25–50 mg/kg/dose Q4–6 hr × 3–4 doses; repeat PRN. **Max single dose:** 2 g *PO:* 100–200 mg/kg/dose QID PO *Daily Maintenance:* 0.25–0.5 mEq/kg/24 hr or 30–60 mg/kg/24 hr IV **Max dose:** 1 g/24 hr	When given IV beware of hypotension, respiratory depression, complete heart block, hypermagnesemia. Calcium gluconate (IV) should be available as antidote. Use with **caution** in patients with renal insufficiency and with patients on digoxin.

MANNITOL
(Osmitrol, Resectisol)
Osmotic diuretic
Inj: 50, 100, 150, 200, 250 mg/ml (5%, 10%, 15%, 20%, 25%)

Anuria/Oliguria:
  Test Dose: to assess renal function: 0.2 g/kg/dose IV; **max:** 12.5 g over 3–5 min. If there is no diuresis within 2 hr, discontinue mannitol.
  Initial: 0.5–1 g/kg/dose
  Maintenance: 0.25–0.5 g/kg/dose Q4–6 hr IV
Cerebral Edema:
  0.25 g/kg/dose IV over 20–30 min. May increase gradually to 1 g/kg/dose if needed. (May give furosemide 1 mg/kg concurrently or 5 min before mannitol.)

May cause circulatory overload and electrolyte disturbances. For hyperosmolar therapy, keep serum osmolality at 310–320 mOsm/kg.
Caution: may crystallize with concentration ≥20%; use in-line filter. May cause hypovolemia, headache, and polydipsia. Reduction in ICP occurs in 15 minutes and lasts 3–6 hours.

MEBENDAZOLE
(Vermox)
Anthelmintic
Chewable tabs: 100 mg (May be swallowed whole or chewed)

Children and Adults:
Pinworms:
  100 mg PO × 1, repeat in 2 wk if not cured
Hookworms, roundworms (Ascaris), and whipworm (Trichuris):
  100 mg PO BID × 3 days. Repeat in 3–4 wk if not cured.
Capillariasis:
  200 mg PO BID × 20 days

May cause diarrhea and abdominal cramping in cases of massive infection. Use with **caution** in children <2 yr. Family may need to be treated as a group. Therapeutic effect may be decreased if administered to patients receiving carbamazepine or phenytoin. Administer with food.

(Continued.)

Drug/How Supplied	Dose and Route	Remarks
MEPERIDINE HCL (Demerol and others) *Narcotic, analgesic* Tabs: 50, 100 mg Syrup, elixir: 50 mg/5 ml Inj: 10, 25, 50, 75, and 100 mg/ml	*PO, IM, IV, and SC:* *Children:* 1–1.5 mg/kg/dose Q3–4 hr PRN **Max dose:** 100 mg *Adults:* 50–150 mg/dose Q3–4 hr PRN	See Chapter 27 for details of use and equianalgesic dosing. **Contraindicated** in cardiac arrhythmias, asthma, increased ICP. Potentiated by MAO inhibitors, tricyclic antidepressants, phenothiazines, other CNS-acting agents. Meperidine may increase the adverse effects of isoniazid. May cause nausea, vomiting, respiratory depression, smooth muscle spasm, pruritis, constipation, and lethargy. **Caution:** in renal failure, sickle cell disease, and seizure disorders, accumulation of normeperidine metabolite may precipitate seizures.
METAPROTERENOL (Metaprel, Alupent, and others) *Beta-2-adrenergic agonist* Syrup: 10 mg/5 ml Tabs: 10, 20 mg Inhaler: 650 mcg/actuation (5, 10 ml) Approx 100 actuations/5 ml Inhalant solution: 5% (50 mg/ml) (0.3, 10, 30 ml) Single-dose inhalant solution: 0.4% (4 mg/ml), 0.6% (6 mg/ml) (2.5 ml)	*Inhalation:* *Aerosol:* 2–3 puffs Q3–4 hr to **max dose** of 12 puffs/24 hr *Nebulized Solution:* Dilute 0.1–0.3 ml of 5% solution in 2.5 ml NS; administer Q4–6 hr PRN *Single-dose solutions:* *Infants:* 2.5 ml of 0.4% *Children:* 2.5 ml of 0.6% *Usual dose:* Q4–6 hr. May give more frequently for acute bronchospasm.	Adverse reactions as with other β-adrenergic agents. Excessive use may result in cardiac arrhythmias and death. Also causes tachycardia, increased myocardial O_2 consumption, hypertension, nausea, palpitations, and tremor. The use of tube spacers may enhance efficacy of administering doses via metered dose inhaler. Nebulizers may be given more frequently in the acute setting.

Oral:
Children: 0.3–0.5 mg/kg/dose Q6–8 hr
Adults: 20 mg/dose Q6–8 hr

METHADONE HCL
(Dolophine)
Narcotic, analgesic
Tabs: 5, 10 mg
Tabs (dispersible): 40 mg
Sol: 5, 10 mg/5 ml
Conc. Sol: 10 mg/ml
Inj: 10 mg/ml

Children: 0.7 mg/kg/24 hr ÷ Q4–6 hr PO, SC, IM, or IV PRN pain. **Max dose:** 10 mg/dose
Adults: 2.5–10 mg/dose Q3–4 hr PO, SC, IM, or IV PRN pain.
Detoxification or maintenance: See package insert

May cause respiratory depression, hypotension, and bradycardia. Average T$_{1/2}$: children 19 hr, adults 35 hr. Oral duration of action is 6–8 hours initially and 22–48 hours after repeated doses. Respiratory effects last longer than analgesia. Accumulation may occur with continuous use making it necessary to adjust dose. See Chapter 27 for equianalgesic dosing and onset of action.

METHICILLIN
(Staphcillin)
Antibiotic, penicillin (penicillinase-resistant)
Inj: 1, 4, 6, 10 g (2.6–3.1 mEq Na/g)

Neonates: IM/IV
≤7 days:
  <2 kg: 50–100 mg/kg/24 hr ÷ Q12 hr
  ≥2 kg: 75–150 mg/kg/24 hr ÷ Q8 hr
>7 days:
  <1.2 kg: 50–100 mg/kg/24 hr ÷ Q12 hr
  1.2–2 kg: 75–150 mg/kg/24 hr ÷ Q8 hr
  ≥2 kg: 100–200 mg/kg/24 hr ÷ Q6 hr
Infants >1 mo and children: 150–400 mg/kg/24 hr ÷ Q4–6 hr IV/IM
Adults: 4–12 g/24 hr ÷ Q4–6 hr IV/IM
Max dose: 12 g/24 hr

Allergic cross-reactivity with and same toxicity as penicillin. May cause agranulocytosis, positive Coomb's test, hairy tongue, eosinophilia, and phlebitis at infusion site. Adjust dose in patients with renal failure, see Chapter 29. Methicillin has been associated with interstitial nephritis and hemorrhagic cystitis. Alternative agents are Oxacillin and Nafcillin.

(Continued.)

Drug/How Supplied	Dose and Route	Remarks
METHIMAZOLE (Tapazole) *Antithyroid agent* Tabs: 5, 10 mg	*Children:* *Initial:* 0.4–0.7 mg/kg/24 hr or 15–20 mg/m²/24 hr PO ÷ Q8 hr *Maintenance:* 1/3–2/3 of initial dose PO ÷ Q8 hr **Max dose:** 30 mg/24 hr PO *Adults:* *Initial:* 15–60 mg/24 hr PO ÷ TID *Maintenance:* 5–15 mg/24 hr PO ÷ TID **Max dose:** 30 mg/24 hr	Readily crosses placental membranes. Blood dyscrasias, dermatitis, hepatitis, arthralgia, CNS reactions, pruritis, nephrotic syndrome, agranulocytosis, headache, fever, hypothyroidism may occur. Switch to maintenance dose when patient is euthyroid.
METHSUXIMIDE (Celontin Kapseals) *Anticonvulsant* Caps: 150, 300 mg	*Children PO:* 10–15 mg/kg/24 hr ÷ Q6–8 hr. Increase weekly up to **max 30 mg/kg/24 hr** *Adults PO:* *Initial:* 300 mg/24 hr ÷ BID-QID for 1 wk. May increase by 300 mg/24 hr each wk to **max dose** of 1.2 gm/24 hr ÷ BID-QID	GI symptoms, blood dyscrasias, mental status changes, periorbital edema, drowsiness, Stevens-Johnson syndrome may occur. Use with **caution** in the presence of renal or liver disease. Follow CBC, LFTs, and urinalysis. Avoid abrupt withdrawal. Measure therapeutic range for metabolite, N-desmethylmethsuximide. **Therapeutic reference range: 10–40 mg/L**

METHYLDOPA
(Aldomet)
*Central alpha-adrenergic blocker,
antihypertensive*
Tabs: 125, 250, 500 mg
Inj: 50 mg/ml
Susp: 250 mg/5 ml

Hypertension:
Children: 10 mg/kg/24 hr ÷ Q6–12 hr
PO; increase PRN Q2 days. **Max
dose:** 65 mg/kg or 3 g/24 hr,
whichever is less.
Adults: 250 mg/dose BID-TID PO.
Increase PRN Q2 days to **max:** 3
g/24 hr
Hypertensive Crisis:
Children: 2–4 mg/kg/dose IV to **max** of
5–10 mg/kg/dose IV Q4–6 hr. **Max
dose** (whichever is less): 65
mg/kg/24 hr or 3 g/24 hr.
Adults: 250–1000 mg IV Q6 hr. **Max:** 4
g/24 hr

Contraindicated in pheochromocytoma
and active liver disease. Positive
Coombs' test, fever, hemolytic anemia,
leukopenia, sedation, GI disturbances,
orthostatic hypotension, black tongue,
and gynecomastia may occur. Use with
caution if patient is receiving
haloperidol, propranolol, lithium,
sympathomimetics. May interfere with
lab tests for creatinine, urinary
catecholamines.

METHYLENE BLUE
(Urolene Blue)
*Antidote, drug-induced
methemoglobinemia, and cyanide
toxicity*
Tabs: 65 mg
Inj: 10 mg/ml (1%)

Methemoglobinemia:
Adults and Children:
1–2 mg/kg/dose IV over 5 min. May
repeat in 1 hr if needed.

At high doses, may cause
methemoglobinemia. Use with **caution**
in G6PD deficiency or renal
insufficiency. May cause nausea,
vomiting, headache, diaphoresis,
stained skin, and abdominal pain.
Causes blue-green discoloration of
urine and feces.

METHYLPHENIDATE HCL
(Ritalin, Ritalin SR, others)
CNS stimulant
Tabs: 5, 10, 20 mg
Slow-release tabs: 20 mg (8-hr duration)

Attention deficit hyperactivity disorder:
≥6 yr:
Initial: 0.3 mg/kg/dose (or 2.5–5
mg/dose) given before breakfast
and lunch. May increase by 0.1
mg/Kg/dose PO (or 5–10 mg/dose)
weekly until maintenance dose
achieved.

Insomnia, weight loss, anorexia, rash,
nausea, emesis, abdominal pain,
hyper- or hypotension, tachycardia,
arrhythmias, hallucination, fever,
tremor may occur. High dose may slow
growth by appetite suppression.

(Continued.)

Drug/How Supplied	Dose and Route	Remarks
METHYLPHENIDATE HCL—(cont.)	*Maintenance dose range:* 0.6–1 mg/kg/24 hr **Max dose:** 2 mg/kg/24 hr or 60 mg/24 hr. May give extra afternoon dose if needed.	**Contraindicated** in glaucoma, anxiety disorders, motor tics and Tourette's syndrome. Use with **caution** in patients with hypertension and epilepsy. May increase serum concentrations of tricyclic antidepressants, phenytoin, phenobarbital, and warfarin. Effect of methylphenidate may be potentiated by MAO inhibitors.
METHYLPREDNISOLONE (Medrol, Solu-Medrol, Depo-Medrol, and others) *Corticosteroid* Tabs: 2, 4, 8, 16, 24, 32 mg Inj: Na succinate (Solu-Medrol) 40, 125, 500, 1000, 2000 mg (IV/IM use) Inj: Acetate 20, 40, 80 mg/ml (IM repository) (Depo-Medrol)	*Antiinflammatory/immunosuppressive:* PO/IM/IV: 0.5–1.7 mg/kg/24 hr ÷ Q6–12 hr *Status Asthmaticus:* Children: IM/IV: Loading dose: 2 mg/kg/dose × 1 Maintenance: 2 mg/kg/24 hr ÷ Q6 hr Adults: 10–250 mg/dose Q4–6 hr IM/IV *Acute spinal cord injury:* 30 mg/kg IV over 15 minutes followed in 45 minutes by a continuous infusion of 5.4 mg/kg/hr × 23 hr	See Chapter 28 for relative, steroid potencies and doses based on body surface area. Not all practitioners use loading dose for status asthmaticus. Acetate form may be used for intra-articular and intralesional injection; it should *not* be given IV. Like all steroids, may cause hypertension, pseudotumor cerebri, acne, Cushing's syndrome, adrenal axis suppression, GI bleeding, and osteoporosis.

METOCLOPRAMIDE
(Clopra, Maxolon, Reglan, and others)
Antiemetic, prokinetic agent
Tabs: 5, 10 mg
Inj: 5 mg/ml
Syrup (sugar-free): 5 mg/5 ml
Conc sol: 10 mg/ml

Gastroesophageal reflux (GER) or GI dysmotility:
Infants and Children: 0.1 mg/kg/dose up to QID IV/IM/PO
Max dose: 0.8 mg/kg/24 hr
Adult: 10–15 mg/dose QAC and QHS IV/IM/PO
Antiemetic:
1–2 mg/kg/dose Q2–6 hr IV/IM/PO. Premedicate with diphenhydramine to reduce EPS.

For GER, give 30 min before meals and at bedtime. May cause extrapyramidal symptoms (EPS), especially at higher doses. **Contraindicated** in GI obstruction, seizure disorder, pheochromocytoma, or in patients receiving drugs likely to cause EPS.

METOLAZONE
(Zaroxolyn, Diulo, Mykrox)
Diuretic
Tabs: 0.5 (Mykrox), 2.5, 5, 10 mg
Susp*: 1 mg/ml

Dosage based on Zaroxolyn
Children: 0.2–0.4 mg/kg/24 hr ÷ QD-BID PO
Adults:
Hypertension: 2.5–5 mg QD PO
Edema: 5–20 mg QD PO

Mykrox and oral suspension have increased bioavailability; therefore lower doses may be necessary when using these dosage forms. Electrolyte imbalance, GI disturbance, hyperglycemia, marrow suppression, chills, hyperuricemia, and rash may occur.

(Continued.)

*Indicates suspensions not commercially available; need to be extemporaneously compounded by a pharmacist. See references 1 and 2 for specific formulations.

Drug/How Supplied	Dose and Route	Remarks
METRONIDAZOLE (Flagyl, Protostat, Metro, and others) *Antibiotic, antiprotozoal* Tabs: 250, 500 mg Susp*: 100 mg/5 ml, or 50 mg/ml Inj: 500 mg Ready to use inj: 5 mg/ml (28 mEq Na/g)	*Amebiasis:* *Children:* 35–50 mg/kg/24 hr PO ÷ TID × 10 days *Adults:* 750 mg/dose PO TID × 10 days *Anaerobic Infection:* *Neonates: PO/IV:* *<7 days: <1.2 kg:* 7.5 mg/kg Q48 hr *1.2–2 kg:* 7.5 mg/kg Q24 hr *≥2 kg:* 15 mg/kg/24 hr ÷ Q12 hr *≥7 days: <1.2 kg:* 7.5 mg/kg Q48 hr *1.2–2 kg:* 15 mg/kg/24 hr ÷ Q12 hr *≥2 kg:* 30 mg/kg/24 hr ÷ Q12 hr *Infants/Children/Adults:* *IV/PO:* 30 mg/kg/24 hr ÷ Q6 hr **Max dose:** 4 g/24 hr *Bacterial Vaginosis:* *Children:* 15–20 mg/kg/24 hr PO ÷ Q8 hr × 7 days *Adults:* 500 PO BID × 7 days *Giardiasis:* *Children:* 15 mg/kg/24 hr PO ÷ TID × 5 days *Adults:* 250 mg PO TID × 5 days *Trichomoniasis: Treat sexual contacts* *Children:* 15 mg/kg/24 hr PO ÷ TID × 7 days *Adolescents/Adults:* 2 g PO × 1 or 250 mg PO TID × 7 days	Nausea, diarrhea, urticaria, dry mouth, leukopenia, vertigo, metallic taste, peripheral neuropathy may occur. Candidiasis may worsen. May discolor urine. Patients should not ingest alcohol for 24 hr after dose (disulfuram-type reaction). IV infusion must be given slowly over 1 hr. Avoid use in first-trimester pregnancy. Use with **caution** in patients with liver or renal disease (GFR <10 ml/min), see Chapter 29. For intravenous use in all ages, some references recommend a 15 mg/kg loading dose. May increase levels or toxicity of phenytoin, lithium, and warfarin. Phenobarbital and rifampin may increase metronidazole metabolism.

C. difficile infection:

    Children: 20–35 mg/kg/24 hr ÷ Q6 hr
    PO × 10 days

    Adults: 250–500 mg TID-QID × 10 days

Helicobacter pylori infection:

    Use in combination amoxicillin and
    bismuth subsalicylate.

    Children: 15–20 mg/kg/24 hr ÷ BID PO
    × 4 weeks

    Adults: 250–500 mg TID PO × 14 days

Inflammatory bowel disease (as alternative
to sulfasalazine):

    Adults: 400 mg BID PO

Perianal Disease: 20 mg/kg/24 hr PO in
3–5 divided doses

MEZLOCILLIN
(Mezlin)
Antibiotic, penicillin (extended spectrum)
Inj: 1, 2, 3, 4, 20 g (contains 1.85 mEq
Na/g)

Neonates: IM/IV:

    <1.2 kg: 150 mg/kg/24 hr ÷ Q12 hr

    ≥1.2 kg:

        ≤7 days: 150 mg/kg/24 hr ÷ Q12 hr

        >7 days: 225 mg/kg/24 hr ÷ Q8 hr

Infants and Children, IM/IV: 200–300
mg/kg/24 hr ÷ Q4–6 hr

Cystic Fibrosis:

    300–450 mg/kg/24 hr ÷ Q4–6 hr

    Max dose: 24 g/24 hr

Adults, IM/IV: 1.5–4 g/dose Q4–6 hr

    Max dose: 24 g/24 hr

May cause seizures, nausea, vomiting,
bone marrow suppression, blood
dyscrasias, elevated BUN/Cr, and
elevated LFTs. Use with **caution** in
biliary obstruction and renal
impairment, see Chapter 29. Causes
false-positive direct Coombs' test and
urinary protein.

---

*Indicates suspensions not commercially available; need to be extemporaneously compounded by a pharmacist. See references 1
and 2 for specific formulations.

(Continued.)

Drug/How Supplied	Dose and Route	Remarks
MICONAZOLE (Monistat) *Antifungal agent* Cream: 2% (15, 30, 90 g) Vaginal cream: 2% (45 g) Vaginal suppository: 100 mg (7's), 200 mg (3's) Powder: 2% (45, 90 g) Spray: 2% (105 ml) Inj: 1% (10 mg/ml)	*Topical:* Apply BID × 2–4 wk *Vaginal:* 1 applicator full of cream or 100 mg suppository QHS × 7 days **or** 200 mg suppository QHS × 3 days *IV: Neonates:* 5–15 mg/kg/24 hr ÷ Q8–24 hr *Infants and Children:* 20–40 mg/kg/24 hr ÷ Q8 hr *Adult:* 1.2–3.6 g/24 hr ÷ Q8 hr	Side effects include phlebitis (IV route), pruritis, rash, nausea, vomiting, fever, drowsiness, diarrhea, anemia, lipemia, thrombocytopenia, anorexia, and flushing. CN XII nerve palsy and arachnoiditis have been reported.
MIDAZOLAM (Versed) *Benzodiazepine* Inj: 1, 5 mg/ml Oral Sol:* 2.5 mg/ml, 3 mg/ml	**Titrate to effect under controlled conditions.** See Chapter 27 for additional routes of administration. *Sedation for procedures:* *Children:* *IV:* 0.05–0.1 mg/kg over 2 min. May repeat 0.05 mg/kg PRN in 2–3 min intervals up to **max total dose** of 0.2 mg/kg.	Causes respiratory depression, hypotension and bradycardia. Cardiovascular monitoring is recommended. Use lower doses or reduce dose when given in combination with narcotics or in patients with respiratory compromise. **Contraindicated** in patients with narrow angle glaucoma and shock.

Adults:
IV: 0.5–2 mg/dose over 2 min. May
repeat PRN in 2–3 min intervals
until desired effect. Usual total
dose: 2.5–5 mg.

Sedation with mechanical ventilation:
Intermittent:
Infants and Children: 0.05–0.15
mg/kg/dose Q1–2 hr PRN
Continuous IV infusion:
Neonates: 0.2–1 mcg/kg/min
Infants and Children: 0.5–3
mcg/kg/min
See inside front cover for infusion
preparation.

Serum concentrations may be increased
by cimetidine and erythromycin.
Sedative effects may be antagonized
by theophylline. Effects may be
reversed by flumazenil.

MINERAL OIL
(various names)
Laxative, lubricant
Liquid: various sizes
Rectal preparation: 133 ml

Children 5–11 yr:
PO: 5–15 ml/24 hr ÷ QD-TID
Rectal: 30–60 ml as single dose
Children ≥12 yr and Adults:
PO: 15–45 ml/24 hr ÷ QD-TID
Rectal: 60–150 ml as single dose

May cause lipid pneumonitis via
aspiration, diarrhea, cramps. Onset of
action is approximately 6–8 hrs. Do
not give QHS dose and use with
caution in children <5 years to
minimize risk of aspiration.

MINOCYCLINE
(Minocin and others)
Antibiotic, tetracycline derivative
Tabs: 50, 100 mg
Caps: 50, 100 mg
Oral susp: 50 mg/5 ml (60 ml)
Inj: 100 mg

Children (8–12 yr): 4 mg/kg/dose × 1
PO/IV, then 2 mg/kg/dose Q12 hr
PO/IV
Max dose: 200 mg/24 hr
Adolescent and Adults: 200 mg/dose × 1
PO/IV, then 100 mg Q12 hr PO/IV

Nausea, vomiting, allergy, photophobia,
injury to developing teeth. High
incidence of vestibular dysfunction,
30%–90%. **Do not take** with milk or
dairy products.

*Indicates suspensions not commercially available; need to be extemporaneously compounded by a pharmacist. See references 1
and 2 for specific formulations.
(Continued.)

Drug/How Supplied	Dose and Route	Remarks
MITHRAMYCIN	See *Plicamycin*	
MORPHINE SULFATE (various brand names) *Narcotic, analgesic* Oral Sol: 10 mg/5 ml, 20 mg/5 ml Conc. Oral Sol: 100 mg/5 ml Tabs: 15, 30 mg Controlled release tabs: 15, 30, 60, 100 mg Sustained release tabs: 30, 60, 100 mg Soluble tabs: 10, 15, 30 mg Rectal suppository: 5, 10, 20, 30 mg Inj: 0.5, 1, 2, 3, 4, 5, 8, 10, 15, 25 mg/ml	**Titrate to effect** *Analgesia/tetralogy (cyanotic) spells:* *Neonates:* 0.05–0.2 mg/kg/dose IM, slow IV, SC Q4 hr *Neonatal opiate withdrawal:* 0.08–0.2 mg/dose Q3–4 hr PRN *Infants and Children:* PO: 0.2–0.5 mg/kg/dose Q4–6 hr PRN (immediate release) or 0.3–0.6 mg/kg/dose Q12 hr PRN (controlled release) IM/IV/SC: 0.1–0.2 mg/kg/dose Q2–4 hr PRN *Adults:* PO: 10–30 mg Q4 hr PRN (immediate release) or 15–30 mg Q8–12 hr PRN (controlled release) IM/IV/SC: 2–15 mg/dose Q2–6 hr PRN *Continuous IV infusion: (Dosing ranges, titrate to effect)* *Neonates:* 0.01–0.02 mg/kg/hr *Infants and Children:* 0.025–2.6 mg/kg/hr *Adults:* 0.8–10 mg/hr	Dependence, CNS and respiratory depression, nausea, vomiting, urinary retention, constipation, hypotension, bradycardia, increased ICP, miosis, biliary spasm, allergy may occur. Naloxone may be used to reverse effects, especially respiratory depression. Causes histamine release resulting in itching and possible bronchospasm. Neonates may require higher doses due to decreased amounts of active metabolites. See Chapter 27 for equianalgesic dosing.

MUPIROCIN
(Bactroban)
Topical antibiotic
Ointment: 2% (15 g)

Topical: apply small amount TID to affected area × 5–14 days

Intranasal use: apply small amount intranasally 2–4 times/24 hr for 5–14 days

If clinical response is not apparent in 3–5 days with topical use, reevaluate infection. Intranasal administration may be used to eliminate carriage of S. aureus. May cause minor local irritation.

NAFCILLIN
(Unipen, Nafcil, Nallpen, and others)
Antibiotic, penicillin (penicillinase resistant)
Tabs: 500 mg
Caps: 250 mg
Oral Sol: 250 mg/5 ml
Inj: 0.5, 1, 2, 4, 10 g
Contains 2.9 mEq Na/g

Neonates: IM/IV:
≤7 days:
  <2 kg: 50 mg/kg/24 hr ÷ Q12 hr
  ≥2 kg: 75 mg/kg/24 hr ÷ Q8 hr
>7 days:
  <1.2 kg: 50 mg/kg/24 hr ÷ Q12 hr
  1.2–2 kg: 75 mg/kg/24 hr ÷ Q8 hr
  ≥2 kg: 100 mg/kg/24 hr ÷ Q6 hr
Infants and Children:
PO: 50–100 mg/kg/24 hr ÷ Q6 hr
IM/IV: (mild to moderate infections):
  50–100 mg/kg/24 hr ÷ Q6 hr
  (severe infections): 100–200
  mg/kg/24 hr ÷ Q4–6 hr
Adults:
PO: 250–1000 mg Q4–6 hr
IV: 500–2000 mg Q4–6 hr
IM: 500 mg Q4–6 hr
Max dose: 12 g/24 hr

Allergic cross-sensitivity with penicillin. Oral route **not** recommended due to poor absorption. High incidence of phlebitis with IV dosing. Use with **caution** in patients with combined renal and hepatic impairment. Nafcillin may increase elimination of warfarin. Acute interstitial nephritis is rare. May cause rash and bone marrow suppression.

(Continued.)

Drug/How Supplied	Dose and Route	Remarks
NALOXONE (Narcan) *Narcotic antagonist* Inj: 0.4, 1 mg/ml Neonatal Inj: 0.02 mg/ml	*Opiate intoxication:* *Neonates, Infants, Children <20 kg:* IM/IV/SC/ETT: 0.1 mg/kg/dose. May repeat PRN Q2–3 min. *Children ≥20 kg or >5 yr:* 2 mg/dose. May repeat PRN Q2–3 min *Continuous Infusion:* 0.005 mg/kg loading dose followed by infusion of 0.0025 mg/kg/hr has been recommended. A range of 0.0025–0.16 mg/kg/hr has been reported in children.	Does not cause respiratory depression. Short duration of action may necessitate multiple doses. For severe intoxication, doses of 0.2 mg/kg may be required. In the nonarrest situation, use the lowest dose effective (may start at 0.001 mg/kg/dose). See Chapter 27. The neonatal concentration (0.02 mg/ml) is no longer recommended in most instances due to large volumes of administration, 2 mg=100 ml. Will produce narcotic withdrawal syndrome in patients with chronic dependence. Use with **caution** in patients with chronic cardiac disease. Abrupt reversal of narcotic depression may result in nausea, vomiting, diaphoresis, tachycardia, hypertension, and tremulousness.
NAPROXEN/NAPROXEN SODIUM (Naprosyn, Anaprox, Aleve [OTC]) *Nonsteroidal antiinflammatory agent* Tabs (Naproxen): 250, 375, 500 mg Tabs (Naproxen sodium): Anaprox: 275 mg (250 mg base), 550 mg (500 mg base) Aleve: 220 mg (200 mg base) Susp: Naproxen 125 mg/5 ml	**All doses based on Naproxen base** *Children >2 yr:* *Analgesia:* 5–7 mg/kg/dose Q8–12 hr PO *JRA:* 10–20 mg/kg/24 hr ÷ Q12 hr PO **Usual max dose range:** 1000–1250 mg/24 hr	May cause GI bleeding, thrombocytopenia, heartburn, headache, drowsiness, vertigo, tinnitus. Use with **caution** in patients with GI disease, cardiac disease, renal or hepatic impairment, and those receiving anticoagulants. See Ibuprofen for other side effects.

	Rheumatoid arthritis, ankylosing spondylitis: Adults: 250–500 mg BID PO. *Dysmenorrhea:* 500 mg × 1, then 250 mg Q6–8 hr PO; **Max dose:** 1250 mg/24 hr.	
NEDOCROMIL SODIUM (Tilade) *Antiallergic agent* Aerosol Inhaler: 1.75 mg/actuation (112 actuations/inhaler, 16.2 g)	*Children >12 yr and adults:* 2 puffs QID. May reduce dosage to BID-TID once clinical response is obtained.	May cause dry mouth/pharyngitis, unpleasant taste, cough, nausea, headache, and rhinitis.
NEOMYCIN SULFATE (Mycifradin) *Antibiotic, aminoglycoside; ammonium detoxicant* Tabs: 500 mg Sol: 125 mg/5 ml (contains parabens) Cream: 0.5% Ointment: 0.5%	*Preterm and newborns:* *Diarrhea:* 50 mg/kg/24 hr ÷ Q6 hr PO *Hepatic Encephalopathy:* *Infants and Children:* 50–100 mg/kg/24 hr ÷ Q6–8 hr PO × 5–6 days. **Max dose:** 12 g/24 hr *Adults:* 4–12 g/24 hr ÷ Q6 hr PO × 5–6 days *Bowel prep:* *Children:* 90 mg/kg/24 hr PO ÷ Q4 hr × 2–3 days *Adults:* 1 g Q1 hr PO × 4 doses, then 1 g Q4 hr PO × 5 doses. (Many other regimens exist)	Monitor for nephrotoxicity and ototoxicity. **Contraindicated** in ulcerative bowel disease or intestinal obstruction. Oral absorption is limited, but levels may accumulate. May cause itching, redness, edema, colitis, candidiasis, or failure to heal if applied topically.
NEOMYCIN/POLYMYXIN B/ ± BACITRACIN (Neosporin) *Topical antibiotic*	*Topical:* apply to minor wounds and burns TID *Ophthalmic:* apply small amount to conjunctiva QD-QID	Do not use for extended periods. May cause superinfection, delayed healing. See Neomycin. Ophthalmic preparation may cause stinging and sensitivity to bright light. *(Continued.)*

Drug/How Supplied	Dose and Route	Remarks
NEOMYCIN/POLYMYXIN B/ ± BACITRACIN—(cont.) Ointment: 3.5 mg neomycin, 400 U bacitracin, 5000 U polymyxin B/g Cream: 3.5 mg neomycin, 10,000 U polymyxin B/g Ointment (ophthalmic): 3.5 mg neomycin, 400 U bacitracin, 10,000 U polymyxin B/g		
NEOSTIGMINE (Prostigmin and others) *Anticholinesterase (cholinergic) agent* Tabs: 15 mg (bromide) Inj: 0.25, 0.5, 1 mg/ml (methylsulfate)	*Myasthenia gravis–Diagnosis:* Use with atropine (see comments). *Children:* 0.04 mg/kg IM × 1 *Adults:* 0.022 mg/kg IM × 1 *Treatment:* *Children:* IM, IV, SC: 0.01–0.04 mg/kg/dose Q2–3 hr PRN PO: 2 mg/kg/24 hr ÷ Q3–4 hr *Adults: IM, IV, SC:* 0.5–2.5 mg/dose Q1–3 hr PRN PO: 15 mg/dose TID. May increase every 1–2 days. Dosage requirements may vary from 15–375 mg/24 hr. *Reversal of nondepolarizing neuromuscular blocking agents:* Administer with atropine or glycopyrrolate.	Titrate for each patient, but avoid excessive cholinergic effects. **Caution** in asthmatics. For diagnosis of myasthenia gravis (MG), administer atropine 0.011 mg/kg/dose IV immediately before or IM (0.011 mg/kg/dose) 30 minutes before neostigmine. For treatment of MG, patients may need higher doses of neostigmine at times of greatest fatigue. **Contraindicated** in GI and urinary obstruction. May cause cholinergic crisis, bronchospasm, salivation, nausea, vomiting, diarrhea, miosis, diaphoresis, lacrimation, bradycardia, hypotension, fatigue, confusion, respiratory depression, seizures. **Antidote:** Atropine 0.01–0.04 mg/kg/dose.

NIFEDIPINE

(Adalat, Adalat CC, Procardia, Procardia XL, and others)

Calcium channel blocker, antihypertensive

Caps: (Adalat, Procardia): 10 mg (0.34 ml), 20 mg (0.45 ml)

Sustained Release Tabs: (Adalat CC, Procardia XL): 30, 60, 90 mg. Do not crush or chew.

Infants: 0.025–0.1 mg/kg/dose IV

Children: 0.025–0.08 mg/kg/dose IV

Adults: 0.5–2.5 mg/kg/dose IV. **Max dose:** 5 mg/dose

Children:

Hypertension: 0.25–0.5 mg/kg/dose Q4–6 hr PRN PO/SL. **Max dose:** 10 mg/dose or 3 mg/kg/dose

Hypertrophic Cardiomyopathy: 0.5–0.9 mg/kg/24 hr ÷ Q6–8 hr PO/SL

Adults:

Hypertension:

Caps: Start with 10 mg/dose PO TID. May increase to 10–30 mg/dose PO TID-QID.

Max dose: 180 mg/24 hr

Sustained Release: Start with 30–60 mg PO QD. May increase to **max dose:** 120 mg/24 hr

May cause severe hypotension, peripheral edema, flushing, tachycardia, headaches, dizziness, nausea, palpitations, syncope. For sublingual administration, capsule must be punctured and liquid expressed into mouth. A small amount is absorbed via the SL route. The majority of effects are due to swallowing and oral absorption. Use with caution in patients with CHF and aortic stenosis. Grapefruit juice may increase bioavailability. Nifedipine may increase phenytoin, cyclosporine, and digoxin levels.

NITROFURANTOIN

(Furadantin, Macrodantin, Macrobid, and others)

Antibiotic

Caps (Macrocrystals): 25, 50, 100 mg

Caps (Dual release, *Macrobid*): 100 mg (25 mg macrocrystal/75 mg monohydrate)

Susp: 25 mg/5 ml

Children >1 mo: 5–7 mg/kg/24 hr ÷ Q6 hr PO

UTI Prophylaxis: 1–2 mg/kg QHS PO

Max dose: 400 mg/24 hr

Adults:

(macrocrystals): 50–100 mg/dose Q6 hr PO

(dual-release): 100 mg/dose Q12 hr PO

UTI Prophylaxis (macrocrystals): 50–100 mg/dose PO QHS

May cause nausea, hypersensitivity reactions, vomiting, diarrhea, cholestatic jaundice, headache, polyneuropathy, and hemolytic anemia. Contraindicated in severe renal disease, G6PD deficiency, infants <1 mo of age, and pregnant women at term. Dosage reduction may be required with prolonged use (>2 wk). Give with food or milk.

(Continued.)

Drug/How Supplied	Dose and Route	Remarks
NITROGLYCERIN (Tridil, Nitro-bid, Nitrostat, and others) *Vasodilator, antihypertensive* Inj: 0.5, 0.8, 5, 10 mg/ml Sublingual tabs: 0.15, 0.3, 0.4, 0.6 mg	*Children:* *Continuous IV infusion:* Begin with 0.25–0.5 mcg/kg/min; may increase by 0.5–1 mcg/kg/min Q3–5 min PRN. **Max dose:** 5 mcg/kg/min *Adults:* 5 mcg/kg/min IV, then increase by 5 mcg/kg/min up to 20 mcg/kg/min; titrate to effect. *Sublingual:* 0.2–0.6 mg Q5 min. **Max of 3** doses in 15 min *To prepare infusion:* See inside front cover.	In small doses (1–2 mcg/kg/min) acts mainly on systemic veins and decreases preload. At 3–5 mcg/kg/min acts on systemic arterioles to decrease resistance. Must use polypropylene infusion sets to avoid plastic adsorbing drug. May cause headache, flushing, GI upset, blurred vision, methemoglobinemia. Use with **caution** in severe renal impairment, increased ICP, hepatic failure. **Contraindicated** in glaucoma and severe anemia.
NITROPRUSSIDE (Nipride and others) *Vasodilator, antihypertensive* Inj: 50 mg	Dilute with D5W and protect from light. *Children and Adults:* IV, *continuous infusion* *Dose:* Start at 0.3–0.5 mcg/kg/min, titrate to effect. Usual dose is 3–4 mcg/kg/min. **Max dose:** 10 mcg/kg/min. *To prepare infusion:* See inside front cover	Monitor for hypotension. **Contraindicated** in patients with decreased cerebral perfusion and in situations of compensatory hypertension. Nitroprusside is nonenzymatically converted to cyanide, which is converted to thiocyanate. Cyanide may produce metabolic acidosis and methemoglobinemia. Thiocyanate may produce psychosis and seizures. Monitor thiocyanate levels if used for >48 hrs. **Thiocyanate levels should be <50 mg/L.**

NOREPINEPHRINE BITARTRATE
(Levophed and others)
Adrenergic agonist
Inj: 1 mg/ml as norepinephrine base

Children: Continuous IV infusion
Doses as norepinephrine base. Start at 0.05–0.1 mcg/kg/min. Titrate to effect. **Max dose:** 2 mcg/kg/min.
To prepare infusion: See inside front cover.

May cause cardiac arrhythmias, hypertension, hypersensitivity, headaches, vomiting, uterine contractions, and organ ischemia. May cause decreased renal blood flow and urine output. Avoid extravasation into tissues. If this occurs, treat locally with phentolamine.

NORFLOXACIN
(Noroxin, Chibroxin)
Antibiotic, quinolone
Tabs: 400 mg
Ophthalmic drops: 3 mg/ml (5 ml)

Adults: 400 mg PO Q12 hr
N. gonorrheae: 800 mg once PO, followed by doxycycline.
Ophthalmic: 1–2 drops QID. May give up to Q2 hr for severe infections.

Like other quinolones, there is concern regarding arthropathy, which has been shown in immature animals. Use with **caution** in children <18 years. May increase serum theophylline levels. May prolong PT in patients on warfarin. See Ciprofoxacin for common side effects and drug interactions.

NORTRIPTYLINE HYDROCHLORIDE
(Pamelor, Aventyl, and others)
Antidepressant, tricyclic
Caps: 10, 25, 50, 75 mg
Sol: 10 mg/5 ml (4% alcohol)

Depression:
Children 6–12 years: 1–3 mg/kg/24 hr ÷ TID-QID PO **or** 10–20 mg/24 hr ÷ TID-QID PO
Adolescents: 1–3 mg/kg/24 hr ÷ TID-QID PO **or** 30–50 mg/24 hr ÷ TID-QID PO
Adults: 75–100 mg/24 hr ÷ TID-QID PO, up to 150 mg/24 hr
Nocturnal Enuresis:
6–7 years (20–25 kg): 10 mg PO QHS
8–11 years (25–35 kg): 10–20 mg PO QHS
>11 years (35–54 kg): 25–35 mg PO QHS

See Imipramine for common side effects. Less CNS and anticholinergic side effects than amitriptyline. Administer with food to decrease GI upset. Therapeutic antidepressant effects occur in 7–21 days. **Therapeutic nortriptyline levels for depression: 50–150 ng/ml.** Do not discontinue abruptly.

(Continued.)

Drug/How Supplied	Dose and Route	Remarks
NYSTATIN (Mycostatin, Nilstat, and others) *Antifungal agent* Tabs: 500,000 U Troches/pastilles: 200,000 U Susp: 100,000 U/ml (60,473 ml) Cream/Ointment: 100,000 U/g (15, 30 g) Topical powder: 100,000 U/g (15 g) Vaginal Tabs: 100,000 U (15s, 30s)	*Oral:* *Preterm infants:* 0.5 ml (50,000 U) to each side of mouth QID *Term infants:* 1 ml (100,000 U) to each side of mouth QID *Children/Adults:* Susp: 4–6 ml (400,000–600,000 U) swish and swallow QID Troche: 200,000–400,000 U 4–5 ×/24 hr *Vaginal:* 1 tab QHS × 14 days *Topical:* Apply BID-QID	May produce diarrhea and GI side effects. Treat until 48–72 hr after resolution of symptoms. Drug is poorly absorbed through the GI tract. Do not swallow troches whole.
OCTREOTIDE ACETATE (Sandostatin) *Somatostatin analog, antisecretory agent* Inj: 0.05, 0.1, 0.5 mg/ml	*Infants and Children, IV/SC:* 1–10 mcg/kg/24 hr ÷ Q12–24 hr. Dose may be increased within recommended range every 3 days. **Max dose:** 1500 mcg/24 hr	Cholelithiasis, hyperglycemia, hypoglycemia, nausea, diarrhea, abdominal discomfort, headache, paint at injection site may occur. Cyclosporine levels may be reduced in patients receiving this drug.

OMEPRAZOLE
(Prilosec)
Gastric acid pump inhibitor
Caps, sustained release: 20 mg

Children: 0.7–3.3 mg/kg/dose PO QD.
Administer before meals.

Capsules contain enteric-coated granules to ensure bioavailability. **Do not chew or crush capsule.** For doses unable to be divided by 20 mg, capsule may be opened and intact pellets may be administered in an acidic beverage (i.e., apple juice, cranberry juice). Increases $T_{1/2}$ of diazepam, phenytoin, and warfarin. May decrease absorption of itraconazole, ketoconazole, iron salts, and ampicillin esters. Common side effects: headache, diarrhea, nausea, and vomiting.

ONDANSETRON
(Zofran)
Antiemetic agent
Inj: 2 mg/ml
Premix Inj: 32 mg/50 ml
Tabs: 4, 8 mg

Oral:
Children:
<4 years: 2 mg Q4 hr PRN nausea
4–11 years: 4 mg Q4 hr PRN nausea
>12 years and adults: 8 mg Q4 hr PRN nausea
IV: Children >3 yr and Adults:
Moderately emetogenic drugs:
0.15 mg/kg/dose at 30 min before, 4 and 8 hrs after emetogenic drugs. Then same dose Q4 hr PRN nausea.
Highly emetogenic drugs:
0.45 mg/kg/dose (**max:** 32 mg/dose) 30 min before emetogenic drugs. Then 0.15 mg/kg/dose Q4 hr PRN.

Bronchospasm, tachycardia, hypokalemia, seizures, headaches, lightheadedness, constipation or diarrhea, and transient increases in AST, ALT, and bilirubin may occur.

(Continued.)

Drug/How Supplied	Dose and Route	Remarks
OPIUM TINCTURE (Deodorized tincture of opium) *Narcotic, analgesic* Liquid: 10% opium. Contains 17%–21% alcohol (1 ml equivalent to 10 mg morphine).	**Dilute 25-fold with water** to make a final concentration of 0.4 mg/ml morphine equivalent. Dose for the *dilution* is equivalent to paregoric doses (see *dilution*).	**Use 25-fold dilution** to treat neonatal abstinence syndrome (NAS). Doses for the *dilution* are equivalent to paregoric doses. Morphine may also be used to treat NAS.
OXACILLIN (Bactocil, Prostaphlin) *Antibiotic, penicillin (penicillinase resistant)* Caps: 250, 500 mg Oral Sol: 250 mg/5 ml Inj: 0.25, 0.5, 1, 2, 4, 10 g 1 g of drug contains 2.8–3.1 mEq Na	*Neonates, IM/IV:* doses are the same as for Nafcillin (see Nafcillin). *Infants and Children:* Oral: 50–100 mg/kg/24 hr ÷ Q6 hr IM/IV: 100–200 mg/kg/24 hr ÷ Q6 hr **Max dose:** 12 g/24 hr *Adults:* Oral: 500–1000 mg/dose Q4–6 hr IM/IV: 250–2000 mg/dose Q4–6 hr	Side effects include allergy, diarrhea, nausea, vomiting, leukopenia, and hepatotoxicity. Acute interstitial nephritis has been reported. Oral form should be administered on an empty stomach.
OXTRIPHYLLINE (Choledyl and others) *Bronchodilator, xanthine derivative* Many preparations (64% theophylline) Tabs: 100, 200 mg Extended release tabs: 400, 600 mg Elixir: 100 mg/5 ml (20% alcohol) Syrup: 50 mg/5 ml	See doses under Theophylline and convert: 16 mg theophylline = 25 mg oxytriphylline	Same as Theophylline

OXYBUTYNIN CHLORIDE

(Ditropan, Dridase)

Anticholinergic agent, antispasmodic

Tabs: 5 mg

Syrup: 5 mg/5 ml (473 ml)

Child ≤5 yr: 0.4–0.8 mg/kg/24 hr ÷ BID-QID PO

Child >5 yr: 10–15 mg/24 hr ÷ BID-TID PO

Adult: 10–20 mg/24 hr ÷ BID-QID PO

Anticholinergic side effects may occur. **Contraindicated** in glaucoma, GI obstruction, megacolon, myasthenia gravis, severe colitis, hypovolemia.

OXYCODONE

(Roxicodone)

Narcotic, analgesic

Sol: 1 mg/ml (8% alcohol), 20 mg/ml

Tabs: 5 mg

Dose based upon oxycodone salt:

Children: 0.05–0.15 mg/kg/dose Q4–6 hr PRN up to 10 mg/dose PO

Adults: 5–10 mg Q4–6 hr PRN PO

Abuse potential. CNS and respiratory depression, increased ICP, histamine release, constipation, GI distress may occur. **Naloxone is the antidote.** See Chapter 27 for equianalgesic dosing. Consider dosages of acetaminophen or aspirin when using combination products. Aspirin is not recommended in children due to concerns of Reye's syndrome.

OXYCODONE AND ACETAMINOPHEN

(Tylox, Roxilox, Percocet, and Roxicet 5/500)

Capsule/Caplet: acetaminophen 500 mg, oxycodone HCl 5 mg

Tabs: acetaminophen 325 mg, oxycodone HCl 5 mg

Sol: acetaminophen 325 mg, oxycodone HCl 5 mg/5 ml (0.4% alcohol)

Dose based on amount of oxycodone and acetaminophen.

See oxycodone and acetaminophen.

Drug/How Supplied	Dose and Route	Remarks
OXYCODONE AND ASPIRIN (Percodan, Percodan-Demi, Roxiprin, Codoxy) Tabs: aspirin 325 mg, oxycodone HCl 4.5 mg, and oxycodone tereph 0.38 mg; aspirin 325 mg, oxycodone HCl 2.25 mg, and oxycodone tereph 0.19 mg	*Dose based on amount of oxycodone and aspirin.*	See oxycodone and aspirin.
PANCREATIC ENZYMES See Chapter 28 for description and contents of lipase, protease, and amylase.	*Initial doses:* (actual requirements are patient specific) Enteric-coated *microspheres and microtabs:* *Infants:* 2000–4000 U lipase per 120 ml formula or per breast feeding *Children <4 yr:* 1000 U lipase/kg/meal *Children ≥4 yr:* 500 U lipase/kg/meal The total daily dose should include approximately three meals and two to three snacks per day. Snack doses are approximately 1/2-meal doses.	May cause occult GI bleeding, allergic reactions to porcine proteins, hyperuricemia, and hyperuricosuria with high doses. Dose should be titrated to eliminate diarrhea and to minimize steatorrhea. Do not chew microspheres or microtabs. Concurrent administration with H_2 antagonists may enhance enzyme efficacy. Doses higher than 6000 U lipase/kg/meal have been associated with colonic strictures in children <12 years of age. Powder dosage form is **not** preferred due to potential GI mucosal ulceration.

PANCURONIUM BROMIDE
(Pavulon)
Nondepolarizing neuromuscular blocking agent
Injection: 1, 2 mg/ml (contains 1% benzyl alcohol)

Neonate: Initial dose: 0.02 mg/kg/dose IV. Then 0.05–0.1 mg/kg/dose Q 0.5–4 hr PRN

1 mo–adult:
Initial: 0.04–0.1 mg/kg/dose IV
Maintenance: 0.015–0.1 mg/kg/dose IV Q30–60 min

Onset of action is 1–2 minutes. Drug effects may be accentuated by hypothermia, acidosis, neonatal age, decreased renal function, halothane, succinylcholine, hypokalemia, clindamycin, tetracycline, and aminoglycoside antibiotics. May cause tachycardia, salivation, and wheezing. **Antidote is neostigmine** (with atropine or glycopyrrolate).

PARALDEHYDE
(Paral)
Anticonvulsant, sedative-hypnotic
Oral or rectal liquid: 1 g/ml (30 ml)

Children:
Sedative: 0.15 ml (150 mg)/kg/dose PO (diluted in milk or fruit juice) or PR (diluted with equal volume of cottonseed or olive oil). **Max dose:** 5 ml

Anti-convulsant: 0.3 ml (300 mg)/kg/dose in 1:1 dilution with cottonseed or olive oil Q2–4 hr PR. **Max dose:** 5 ml

Do not use discolored or "vinegar scented" solutions. Avoid exposure to plastics, air, and light. **Contraindicated** in hepatic or pulmonary disease. Overdose may cause cardiorespiratory depression. Parenteral dosage form is no longer commercially available in the U.S. Less frequently used as an anti-convulsant.

(Continued.)

Drug/How Supplied	Dose and Route	Remarks
PAREGORIC (Camphorated opium tincture) *Narcotic, antidiarrheal* Camphorated tincture: 2 mg (morphine equivalent)/5 ml (some preparations contain up to 45% alcohol)	*Analgesia/Antidiarrheal:* *Children:* 0.25–0.5 ml/kg/dose PO QD-QID *Adults:* 5–10 ml/dose PO QD-QID *Neonatal opiate withdrawal:* *Initial:* 0.2–0.3 ml/dose Q3–4 hr *Increment:* 0.05 ml/dose until symptoms abate. Rare to exceed 0.7 ml/dose. **Max dose:** 1–2 ml/kg/24 hr.	Each 5 ml paregoric contains 2 mg morphine equivalent, 0.02 ml anise oil, 20 mg benzoic acid, 20 mg camphor, 0.2 ml glycerin, and alcohol. The final concentration of morphine equivalent is 0.4 mg/ml. **This is 25-fold less potent than undiluted deodorized tincture of opium (DTO: 10 mg morphine equivalent/ml). If using DTO to treat neonatal abstinence, must dilute 25-fold prior to use.** Similar side effects to morphine. After symptoms are controlled for several days, dose for opiate withdrawal should be decreased gradually over a 2- to 4-week period (e.g., by 10% Q2–3 days).
PAROMYCIN SULFATE (Humatin) *Amebicide, antibiotic (aminoglycoside)* Caps: 250 mg	*Intestinal Amebiasis:* *Children and Adults:* 25–35 mg/kg/24 hr PO ÷ Q8 hr × 5–10 days *Tapeworm* (see comments): *Children:* 11 mg/kg/dose Q15 min × 4 doses *Adults:* 1 g Q15 min × 4 doses *Tapeworm (Hymenolepis nana):* *Children and Adults:* 45 mg/kg/dose PO QD × 5–7 days	Tapeworms affected by short-duration therapy include *T. saginata, T. solium, D. latum,* and *D. caninum.* Drug is poorly absorbed and therefore not indicated for sole treatment of extraintestinal amebiasis. Side effects include GI disturbance, hematuria, rash, ototoxicity, and hypocholesterolemia.

Cryptosporidial diarrhea:
Adults: 1.5–3 g/24 hr PO ÷ 3–6 × daily. Duration varies from 10–14 days to 4–8 weeks. Maintenance therapy has also been used.

May cause insomnia, anorexia, depression, abdominal pain, movement disorders, drug dependence. Use with **caution in renal disease. Has been associated with life threatening hepatic failure.** Pemoline should not be considered as first line therapy for ADHD. **Contraindicated** in Tourette's syndrome. **Not recommended for children <6 years old.**

PEMOLINE
(Cylert)
CNS stimulant
Tabs: 18.75, 37.5, 75 mg
Chewable tabs: 37.5 mg

Children >6 yr:
Initial: 37.5 mg QAM PO
Increment: 18.75 mg/24 hr at weekly intervals
Maintenance: 0.5–3 mg/kg/24 hr (effective dose range: 56.25–75 mg/24 hr)
Max dose: 112.5 mg/24 hr
Effect may not be seen for 3–4 weeks. Do not abruptly discontinue drug.

PENICILLAMINE
(Cuprimine, Depen)
Heavy metal chelator
Tabs: 250 mg
Caps: 125, 250 mg
Susp*: 50 mg/ml

Lead chelation therapy (see also Chapter 2):
Children: 30–40 mg/kg/24 hr or 600–750 mg/m²/24 hr PO ÷ BID-TID. **Max dose:** 1.5 g/24 hr
Adults: 1–1.5 g/24 hr PO ÷ BID-TID Durations of treatment vary from 1–6 months.
Wilson's Disease:
Infants and Children: 20 mg/kg/24 hr PO ÷ BID-QID. **Max dose:** 1 g/24 hr
Adults: 250 mg/dose PO QID. **Max dose:** 2 g/24 hr

Dose should be given 1 hr before or 2 hr after meals. Must be in lead-free environment, since it can increase absorption of lead if present in GI tract. Follow CBC, LFTs, and urine. Can cause optic neuritis, fever, rash, nausea, altered taste, vomiting, lupuslike syndrome, peripheral neuropathy, leukopenia, eosinophilia, thrombocytopenia. May reduce serum digoxin levels. Avoid concomitant administration with iron, antacids, and food.

(Continued.)

*Indicates suspensions not commercially available; need to be extemporaneously compounded by a pharmacist. See references 1 and 2 for specific formulations.

Drug/How Supplied	Dose and Route	Remarks
	Arsenic poisoning: 100 mg/kg/24 hr PO ÷ Q6 hr × 5 days **Max dose:** 1 g/24 hr *Cystinuria:* *Infants and young children:* 30 mg/kg/24 hr ÷ QID PO *Older children and adults:* 1–4 g/24 hr ÷ QID PO *Primary biliary cirrhosis; Adults:* *Initial:* 250 mg/24 hr PO; increase by 250 mg Q2 wk to a total of 1 g/24 hr (given as 250 mg QID) *Juvenile Rheumatoid Arthritis:* 5 mg/kg/24 hr ÷ QD-BID PO × 2 mo, then 10 mg/kg/24 hr ÷ QD-BID PO × 4 mo	Patients treated for Wilson's disease, rheumatoid arthritis, or cystinuria should be treated with pyridoxine 25–50 mg/24 hr. Titrate urinary copper excretion to >1 mg/24 hr for patients with Wilson's disease. Patients with cystinuria should have doses titrated to maintain urinary cystine excretion at <100–200 mg/24 hr.

PENICILLIN G PREPARATIONS - POTASSIUM AND SODIUM

(Various trade names)

Antibiotic, aqueous penicillin

Inj (K⁺): 1, 5, 10, 20 million units (contains 1.7 mEq K and 0.3 mEq Na/1 million unit PenG)

Inj (Na⁺): 5 million units (contains 2 mEq Na/1 million unit PenG)

Tabs (K⁺): 200,000, 250,000, 400,000, 500,000, 800,000 U

Sol (K⁺): 200,000, 400,000 U/5 ml

Conversion: 250 mg = 400,000 U

Neonates: IM/IV

≤7 *days:*

≤2 *kg:* 50,000–100,000 U/kg/24 hr ÷ Q12 hr

>2 *kg:* 75,000–150,000 U/kg/24 hr ÷ Q8 hr

>7 *days:*

<1.2 *kg:* 50,000–100,000 U/kg/24 hr ÷ Q12 hr

1.2–2 *kg:* 75,000–225,000 U/kg/24 hr ÷ Q8 hr

≥2 *kg:* 100,000–200,000 U/kg/24 hr ÷ Q6 hr

Infants and Children:

PO: 40,000–80,000 U/kg/24 hr **or** 25–50 mg/kg/24 hr ÷ Q6–8 hr

IM/IV: 100,000–400,000 U/kg/24 hr ÷ Q4–6 hr

Max dose: 24 million U/24 hr

Adults:

PO: 200,000–800,000 U/dose **or** 125–500 mg/dose Q6–8 hr

IM/IV: 4–30 million U/24 hr ÷ Q4–6 hr

Congenital Syphilis, Neurosyphilis: See Chapter 18

Oral penicillin G should be taken 1–2 hr before or 2 hr after meals. Penicillin V Potassium is better orally absorbed. Side effects: anaphylaxis, urticaria, hemolytic anemia, interstitial nephritis, Jarisch-Herxheimer reaction. $T_{1/2} = 30$ min; may be prolonged by concurrent use of probenecid. For meningitis, use higher daily dose at shorter dosing intervals. Adjust dose in renal impairment; see Chapter 29 for details.

(Continued.)

Drug/How Supplied	Dose and Route	Remarks
PENICILLIN G PREPARATIONS - BENZATHINE (Permapen, Bicillin L-A) *Antibiotic, penicillin (very long-acting IM)* (may contain parabens and povidone). Injection should be IM only. Inj: 300,000, 600,000 U/ml	*Group A streptococci:* *Infants and Children:* 25,000–50,000 U/kg/dose IM × 1. **Max dose:** 1.2 million U/dose *Or* *>1 month and <27 kg:* 600,000 U/dose IM × 1 *≥27 kg:* 1.2 million U/dose IM × 1 *Adults:* 1.2 million U/dose IM × 1 *Rheumatic Fever prophylaxis:* *Infants and Children:* 25,000–50,000 U/kg/dose IM Q3–4 wk. **Max dose:** 1.2 million U/dose *Adults:* 1.2 million U/dose IM Q3–4 wk or 600,000 U/dose IM Q2 wk *Syphilis: early acquired and >1 year duration:* See Chapter 18.	Provides sustained levels for 2–4 weeks. Side effects same as for Penicillin G. **Do not administer intravenously;** cardiac arrest and death may occur. **Not recommended** for congenital syphilis.

PENICILLIN G PREPARATIONS - PROCAINE

(Wycillin, Cysticillin A.S., Pfizerpen-AS)
Antibiotic, penicillin (long-acting IM)
Inj: 300,000, 500,000, 600,000 U/ml (may contain parabens, phenol, providone, and formaldehyde). Contains 120 mg procaine per 300,000 U.

Newborns: 50,000 U/kg/24 hr IM QD; see comments
Infants and Children: 25,000–50,000 U/kg/24 hr ÷ Q12–24 hr IM. **Max dose:** 4.8 million U/24 hr
Adults: 0.6–4.8 million U/24 hr ÷ Q12–24 hr IM
Congenital syphilis, Syphilis, Neurosyphilis: See Chapter 18.

Provides sustained levels for 2–4 days. Use with **caution** in neonates due to higher incidence of sterile abscess at injection site and risk of procaine toxicity. Side effects similar to Penicillin G. In addition, may cause CNS stimulation and seizures. **Do not administer IV**; neurovascular damage may result. Large doses may be administered in two injection sites. No longer recommended for empiric treatment of gonorrhea due to resistant strains.

PENICILLIN G PREPARATIONS - PENICILLIN G BENZATHINE AND PENICILLIN G PROCAINE

(Bicillin C-R, Bicillin C-R 900/300)
Antibiotic, penicillin (very long acting)
Bicillin CR: 150,000 U PenG procaine + 150,000 U PenG benzathine/ml (10 ml vial) or
300,000 U PenG procaine + 300,000 U PenG benzathine/ml (1, 2 ml tubex, 4 ml syringe)
Bicillin CR (900/300): 150,000 U PenG procaine + 450,000 U PenG benzathine/ml (2 ml tubex)

Acute streptococcal infection: Dose such that PenG benzathine is given in recommended amount (Red Book, p. 435, 1994). See doses for PenG benzathine.

This preparation provides early peak levels in addition to prolonged levels of penicillin in the blood. **Do not administer IV.** The addition of procaine penicillin has not been shown to be more efficacious than benzathine alone. However, it may reduce injection discomfort.

(Continued.)

Drug/How Supplied	Dose and Route	Remarks
PENICILLIN V POTASSIUM (Pen Vee K, V-Cillin K, and others) *Antibiotic, penicillin* Tabs: 125, 250, 500 mg Oral Sol: 125 mg/5 ml, 250 mg/5 ml 250 mg = 400,000 U	*Children:* 25–50 mg/kg/24 hr ÷ Q6–8 hr PO. **Max dose:** 3 g/24 hr *Adults:* 250–500 mg/dose PO Q6–8 hr *Acute group A streptococcal pharyngitis:* Children: 250 mg PO BID-TID × 10 days *Secondary rheumatic fever/ pneumococcal prophylaxis:* ≤5 yr: 125 mg PO BID >5 yr: 250 mg PO BID	GI absorption is better than penicillin G. **Note:** Must be taken 1 hr before or 2 hr after meals. Penicillin will prevent rheumatic fever if started within 9 days of the acute illness. The BID regimen for streptococcal pharyngitis should be used only if good compliance is suspected.
PENTAMIDINE ISETHIONATE (Pentam 300, NebuPent) *Antibiotic, antiprotozoal* Inj: 300 mg (Pentam 300) Inhalation: 300 mg (NebuPent)	*Treatment:* *Pneumocystis carinii:* 4 mg/kg/24 hr IM/IV QD × 14–21 days *Trypanosomiasis (T. gambiense, T. rhodesiense):* 4 mg/kg/24 hr IM/IV QD × 10 days *Leishmaniasis (L. donovani):* 2–4 mg/kg/dose IM QD or QOD × 15 doses *Prophylaxis:* *Pneumocystis carinii:* 4 mg/kg/dose IM/IV Q2–4 wk OR ≥5 yr: 300 mg in 6 ml H₂O via inhalation Q month (Respigard II nebulizer). See also Chapter 18 for indications.	May cause hypoglycemia, hyperglycemia, hypotension (both IV and IM administration), nausea, vomiting, fever, mild hepatotoxicity, pancreatitis, megaloblastic anemia, nephrotoxicity, hypocalcemia, and granulocytopenia. Aerosol administration may also cause bronchospasm, oxygen desaturation, dyspnea, and loss of appetite. Infuse IV over 1 hour to reduce the risk of hypotension. **Sterile abscess** may occur at IM injection site.

Trypanosomiasis: (T. gambiense, T. rhodesiense) 4 mg/kg/24 hr IM q3–6mo.

Max single dose: 300 mg

PENTOBARBITAL
(Nembutal, others)
Barbiturate
Caps: 50, 100 mg
Suppository: 30, 60, 120, 200 mg
Inj: 50 mg/ml
Elixir: 18.2 mg/5 ml

Hypnotic
Children:
PO/PR.:
<4 years: 3–6 mg/kg/dose QHS
≥4 years: 1.5–3 mg/kg/dose QHS
IM: 2–6 mg/kg/dose. **Max dose:** 100 mg

Pre-procedure Sedation
Children:
PO/PR./IM: 2–6 mg/kg/dose. **Max dose:** 150 mg
IV: 1–3 mg/kg/dose. **Max dose:** 150 mg

Barbiturate coma
Children and Adults
IV: Load: 10–15 mg/kg given slowly over 1–2 hr
Maintenance: Begin at 1 mg/kg/hr. Dose range: 1–3 mg/kg/hr as needed.

No advantage over phenobarbital for control of seizures. Adjunct in treatment of ICP. May cause drug-related isoelectric EEG. Do not administer for >2 wk in treatment of insomnia. **Contraindicated** in liver failure. May cause hypotension, arrhythmias, hypothermia, respiratory depression, and dependence.
Onset of action: PO/PR: 15–60 min; IM: 10–15 min; IV: 1 min.
Administer IV at a rate of <50 mg/min.
Suppositories should not be divided.
Therapeutic serum levels:
Sedation: 1–5 mg/L
Hypnosis: 5–15 mg/L
Coma: 20–40 mg/L

(Continued.)

Drug/How Supplied	Dose and Route	Remarks
PERMETHRIN (Elimite, Nix) *Scabicidal agent* Cream: 5% (Elimite) Liquid cream rinse: 1% (Nix)	*Pediculus capitis, Pediculus humanis,* *Pthirus pubis:* *Head Lice:* Saturate hair and scalp with 1% cream rinse after shampooing, rinsing, and towel drying hair. Leave on 10 minutes, then rinse. May repeat in 7 days. May be used for lice in other areas of the body (i.e., pubic lice) in same fashion. *Scabies:* Apply 5% cream head to toe and wash off with water in 8–14 hours. May repeat in 7 days.	Avoid contact with eyes during application. Shake well before using. May cause pruritus, hypersensitivity, burning, stinging, erythema, and rash. For either lice or scabies, **instruct** **patient to launder bedding and** **clothing.**
PHENAZOPYRIDINE HCl (Pyridium) *Urinary analgesic* Tabs: 95, 100, 200 mg	*Children 6–12 yr:* 12 mg/kg/24 hr ÷ TID until symptoms of lower urinary tract irritation are controlled or 2 days. *Adults:* 200 mg TID until symptoms are controlled or 2 days.	May cause GI problems, or renal insufficiency. May cause methemoglobinemia, hemolytic, anemia. Colors urine orange; stains clothing. May also stain contact lenses. Give after meals.

PHENOBARBITAL

(Luminal, Solfoton, and others)

Barbiturate

Tabs: 15, 16, 30, 32, 60, 65, 100 mg

Caps: 16 mg

Elixir: 15, 20 mg/5 ml (contains alcohol)

Inj: 30, 60, 65, 130 mg/ml (some injectable products may contain benzyl alcohol and propylene glycol)

Status epilepticus:

Loading dose, IV:

Neonates, Infants, and Children: 15–20 mg/kg/dose in a single or divided dose. May give additional 5 mg/kg doses Q15–30 min to a **maximum** of 30 mg/kg.

Maintenance dose, PO./IV: **Monitor levels.**

Neonates: 3–5 mg/kg/24 hr ÷ QD-BID

Infants: 5–6 mg/kg/24 hr ÷ QD-BID

Children 1–5 yr: 6–8 mg/kg/24 hr ÷ QD-BID

Children 6–12 yr: 4–6 mg/kg/24 hr ÷ QD-BID

>12 yr: 1–3 mg/kg/24 hr ÷ QD-BID

Hyperbilirubinemia: <12 yr: 3–8 mg/kg/24 hr PO ÷ BID-TID. Doses up to 12 mg/kg/24 hr have been used.

Sedation, children: 6 mg/kg/24 hr PO ÷ TID

Pre-op sedation, children: 1–3 mg/kg/dose IM/IV/PO × 1. Give 60–90 minutes prior to procedure.

IV administration may cause respiratory arrest or hypotension. **Contraindicated** in hepatic or renal disease and porphyria. $T_{1/2}$ approximately 96 hr in children. Neonatal $T_{1/2}$ may be greater than 100 hours. Due to long half-life, consider other agents for sedation for procedures. Paradoxical reaction in children (not dose-related) may cause hyperactivity, irritability, insomnia. **Therapeutic levels: 15–40 mg/L.** Induces liver enzymes, thus decreases blood levels of many drugs (e.g., anticonvulsants). **IV push not to exceed 1 mg/kg/min.**

(Continued.)

Drug/How Supplied	Dose and Route	Remarks
PHENTOLAMINE MESYLATE (Regitine) *Adrenergic blocking agent (alpha); antidote, extravasation* Inj: 5 mg vial (contains 25 mg mannitol)	*Treatment of alpha adrenergic drug extravasation* (most effective within 12 hr of extravasation) *Neonates:* Make a solution of 0.25–0.5 mg/ml with normal saline. Inject 1 ml (in 5 divided doses of 0.2 ml) SC around site of extravasation; **max total dose:** 0.1 mg/kg or 2.5 mg total. *Infants, Children, and Adults:* Make a solution of 0.5–1 mg/ml with normal saline. Inject 1–5 ml (in 5 divided doses) SC around site of extravasation; **max total dose:** 0.1–0.2 mg/kg or 5 mg total. *Diagnosis of pheochromocytoma, IM/IV:* *Children:* 0.1 mg/kg/dose up to 5 mg *Adults:* 5 mg/dose	For diagnosis of pheochromocytoma, patient should be resting in a supine position. A blood pressure reduction of more than 35 mm Hg systolic and 24 mm Hg diastolic is considered a positive test for pheochromocytoma. For treatment of extravasation, use 27- to 30-gauge needle with multiple small injections.
PHENYLEPHRINE HCl (Neo-Synephrine and others) *Adrenergic agonist* Nasal drops: 0.125, 0.16, 0.25, 0.5% (15, 30 ml) Nasal spray: 0.25, 0.5, 1% (15, 30 ml) Ophthalmic drops: 0.12, 2.5, 10% Inj: 10 mg/ml (1%)	*Hypotension:* *Children:* *IM/SC:* 0.1 mg/kg/dose Q1–2 hr PRN; **max dose: 5 mg** *IV bolus:* 5–20 mcg/kg/dose Q10–15 min PRN *IV drip:* 0.1–0.5 mcg/kg/min; titrate to effect *Adults:* *IM/SC:* 2–5 mg/dose Q1–2 hr PRN; **max dose: 5 mg** *IV bolus:* 0.1–0.5 mg/dose Q10–15 min PRN	Use **cautiously** in presence of arrhythmias, hyperthyroidism, or hyperglycemia. May cause tremor, insomnia, palpitations. Metabolized by MAO. **Contraindicated** in pheochromocytoma and severe hypertension. Nasal decongestants may cause rebound congestion with excessive use (>3 days). Injectable product may contain sulfites. **Note:** Phenylephrine is found in a variety of combination cough and cold products.